365 WISE WAYS

TO HAPPINESS

With 365 Ways to Start A Happiness Support Group

By Janet Lindeman, Ph.D.

Introduction: Happiness is a one-day-at-a-time endeavor. It is also an inside-job. It helps to surround ourselves with others who practice happiness principles. It also helps to accept the fact that sometimes life just hands us disappointments and hardships, no matter what we do to avoid them. Therefore, having clear principles with which to handle hardships and relationships, plus a network of supportive others is essential.

This book is about practicing happiness principles 365 days out of the year. It is also about forming a circle of supportive relationships. 365 daily readings are introduced by gems of wisdom from ancient philosophers and teachers, as well as modern psychologists and teachers. Every reading includes a statement of a happiness principle, as well as a self-discovery question and an affirmation. Reading and meditating for five minutes every day with the help of this book, is sure to increase your happiness level. Reading Appendix One can also help you to understand the workings of the brain and heart and ways you can take care of them to promote your own happiness.

Forming a Happiness Support Group using this book could increase your happiness level even more than just personal study and meditation. Therefore, guidelines for forming and sustaining such a group are included in Appendix Two. Company IS stronger than will power. Getting together regularly with at least one other person to discuss these happiness principles can help immensely. Appendix Two explains ways that Happiness Group sharing can be productive and supportive. Such groups can meet in homes, schools, churches, synagogues, temples, mosques, libraries, senior centers, women's and men's resource centers, shelters, mental health centers and prisons and anywhere two people choose to meet to support each other in applying the principles outlined in this book. Appendix Three is a Happiness Skill Self Inventory. It summarizes the skills and attitudes most helpful in creating happiness. Appendix Four summarizes the 12 Steps and 12 Traditions mentioned in each successive month of the daily readings. The Subject Index in the back of this book and the daily self-discovery questions are all designed to suggest topics for sharing and discussion.

This book is designed to help create and sustain healthy individual, couple and family relationships in healthy democracies. They are respectful of diversity in cultural and religious backgrounds.

I wish you the best for your practice of happiness principles. You can reach me at the address below if you would like to give me feedback on your experiences with this book.

Acknowledgements and Permissions

While the 12 Steps and 12 Traditions in this book were inspired by the 12 Steps and Traditions of Alcoholics Anonymous, they are not an "adaptation" of the A.A. Steps and Traditions. They have been created specifically by this author for this book, The Alcoholics Anonymous World Services' office has requested this author to clarify that A.A. is a program concerned <u>only</u> with recovery from alcoholism, and is not affiliated with the publication of this book.

Brief quotes in this book are included under the "fair use" copyright provision. Authors of the quotes are acknowledged in the Authors and Sources Index. Some references to books and websites for further study are also included within the texts of the Daily Readings.

365 Wise Ways To Happiness

Table of Contents

365 WISE WAYS TO HAPPINESS

January 1   **Trust**

Principle: If we pay attention in every fearful situation, there is an opportunity for developing new awareness and strength.

Perennial Wisdom Quote: "Anything that has real and lasting value is always a gift from within." -- Franz Kafka

Discussion: Fear tends to prod us into "fight or flight" responses. Fear attempts to convince us that the danger comes from outside and can be either destroyed or escaped. But most often the danger actually comes from inside -- from the abandonment or avoidance of clear perception and/or effective following of personal principles.

When we take personal responsibility for our fears, we can face them, grow beyond them and become both stronger and more compassionate with ourselves and others. It is vital that we do not blame our fears on others. Our hearts know that real emotional security comes, not from outside defenses, but through loving connection to others and through the humble acceptance of our small, individual places in the natural universe. When we can trust ourselves to choose reliable, principled friends and to be such friends to others, our world becomes much safer. Building such trust in ourselves and others is what builds real security.

Self-exploration Question: How can I learn to better trust myself and my friends?

Affirmation: Today I trust my heart to teach me how to lovingly face my fears.

January 2   **Self-acceptance**

Principle: The soft pain of acceptance transforms the hard pain of struggling against suffering.

Perennial Wisdom Quote: "Our very defects are thus shadows of our virtues." -- Ralph Waldo Emerson

Discussion: When we try to avoid awareness of our shortcomings and mistakes, we just create more suffering. Everyone makes mistakes. Emotional pain is the normal flip-side of pleasure. It is as night is to day. When we accept unavoidable emotional pain, that pain which is out of our control, it softens and passes more quickly, making room for joy and the cultivation of new virtues. When we resist unavoidable pain, and blame and shame others or ourselves for it, the pain just hardens and lingers longer.

We live with ourselves longer than with anyone else, and befriending ourselves is a prerequisite for happiness. Befriending others also gives us important practice in learning how to better befriend ourselves. When we don't befriend others, we add to their and our own suffering. When we don't befriend ourselves, we add, not only to our own suffering, but tend to project negativity, which adds to the suffering of others. Accepting our shortcomings and gradually changing them into assets, is one important way to befriend ourselves. (See the Self-Inventory in Appendix 3.)

Self-exploration Question: How can I learn to more gracefully accept what is beyond my control, avoiding self-shame

Affirmation: Today I choose to accept unavoidable pain and learn from it.

Principle: When we value all others unconditionally, we can celebrate diversity, while also not condoning violence and prejudice.

Perennial Wisdom Quote: "If we really want to be genuinely pluralistic, we must support and encourage moral development as it moves from egocentric to ethnocentric to worldcentric. We must not sit back and say, 'Gee, all views are equally okay because we're celebrating rich diversity.'" -- Ken Wilber, Ph.D., *One Taste,* page 231

Discussion: Egocentric morality reasons that "What's good is what's good for me." Ethnocentric morality reasons that "What's good is what's good for my group, country or religious group." Worldcentric morality reasons that "What's good is what's good for all beings."

Modern convention usually involves ethnocentric morality, but, with the arrival of nuclear weapons, terrorism, the global economy, and global warming's threats to the global ecosystem, it becomes increasingly impossible to separate one group's fundamental interests from another's. Developing worldcentric morality may be necessary for the survival of our species on this planet. Our human fears divide neighbors and families, as well as nations. Therefore, individually learning how to manage our anxieties and take responsibility for our fears is fundamental to world peace and recovery from global warming. We can start with commitments to replace our violent and prejudicial "fight" defenses with efforts to understand and accept others, even when we disagree with them.

Self-exploration Question: How can I learn to more agreeably disagree with others?

Affirmation: Today I am valuing and accepting myself and others unconditionally.

Principle: Full awareness transforms denial, projection, distortion and ignorance.

Perennial Wisdom Quote: "Though we travel the world over to find the beautiful, we must carry it with us, or we will not find it." -- Ralph Waldo Emerson

Discussion: You've heard the old saying, "Beauty is in the eyes of the beholder." It follows, doesn't it, that ugliness is often also in the eyes of the beholder? There is a saying, "When we point at someone else, three fingers are pointing back at us."

When we project shame, blame or criticism onto others, we always do so in order to repudiate part or all of our own participation in interactions. We do this to reduce our own fear, anxiety or some other unpleasant emotion. This is why taking full responsibility for one's own fears and other unpleasant emotions is the foundation of mental health and effective, interpersonal relationships. It is vitally important for us to learn to recognize and check emotional projections because they are always used to justify emotional attacks or abandonment. When we project responsibility onto others for our own happiness, we set ourselves up to allow others to control us. When we do this, we are actually victimizing ourselves.

Self-exploration Question: How can I take more responsibility for all my own emotions and behaviors, especially my happiness?

Affirmation: Today I am practicing full awareness and self-responsibility, avoiding denial, projection and blame.

Principle: Paying attention to and taking responsibility for our nighttime dreams can also improve our wakeful hours.

Perennial Wisdom Quote: "Wisdom comes to us in dreams." -- Wovcoka, Paiute Native American

Discussion: Our night dreams are designed to show us our unconscious realities, our shadow selves. With a little practice, anyone can learn to remember and benefit from a night dream. All the characters, objects and drama of our dreams reflect parts of ourselves. The "I" in each dream is the most conscious part of one's self. Other people and animals and objects in our dreams reflect less conscious parts of ourselves. When there is a death in a dream, a part of one's self is being released. When there is a union in a dream, a part of one's self is connecting with another part of one's self. When there is a birth in a dream a new part of one's self is being born.

   We can change our night dreams by remembering them, writing them down, and responsibly sharing them with others. We can help ourselves by determining how we would like the endings of some of our dreams to be different. We can heal our inner anxieties by seeing how they show up in our dreams and determining how our dream dramas could end more productively. As we learn to do this, we can reduce the amount of drama we unconsciously create in our daytime lives. Those around us also benefit.

Self-exploration Question: How can I take my night dreams seriously, learn from them and share them? (See Appendix 5.)

Affirmation: Today I am benefiting from remembering, recording, contemplating and sharing my night dreams.

January 6   **Happiness Step One: Humility**

Principle: Happiness Step One is "We humbly give up our fearful escapes from awareness and our reactive attempts to control others."

Perennial Wisdom Quote: "Pride is the mask we make of our faults." -- Hebrew saying

Discussion: Having clear awareness, not distorting reality, and accepting what we see, are all fundamental to any happiness program. "Three A's" make up the core of any happiness program. Awareness is the essential first "A." This awareness includes awareness of self, awareness of others, and awareness of our interaction patterns.

Repressing and avoiding awareness usually are the results of the amygdala, the fear center of the low brain, becoming over stimulated so that blood in the brain does not flow sufficiently to the prefrontal cortex, the higher part of the brain which helps us to have good judgment (See Appendix 1).

In Step One of this book's Happiness Program we humbly witness our fearfulness when it appears, and we stay calm rather than acting out our fear or secondary anger. We witness our physiological reactivity. We witness our automatic thoughts. We take responsibility for our need to take no verbal or physical action unless it promotes our safety and is not harmful to others. We do not use our fear to try to angrily control others. We give our "low brains" time to connect to our "high brains." We humbly accept the limitations of our will and respect others' rights to make their own choices, as long as they are not aggressive. This principle is necessary in any functioning democracy.

Self-exploration Question: How have I escaped awareness and attempted to force solutions in the past?

Affirmation: Today I humbly give up my past attempts to force solutions on others.

January 7   Happiness Tradition One: Unity and respect for the common welfare

Principle: Tradition One of this Happiness Program is "Unity and respect for the common welfare of a support group promotes individual progress for the greatest number of members."

Perennial Wisdom Quote: "He who does me one favor I will recompense with two; he who respects me, I will respect him more." -- Lebanese saying

Discussion: Respect for the principle of unity is foundational for any fellowship. Occasionally situations arise in any group in which there is a conflict of interest between what appears to be helpful to an individual and what is helpful to the greatest number of participants in the group. When such a situation develops, Tradition One states the priority is always given to respect for the common welfare of the group.

        Sometimes one member will hurt another member and that hurt member will develop a resentment about it. The wisdom of Tradition One makes it clear that in such situations the alienated individuals either need to make amends and offer forgiveness to one another, or find some other ways to set aside their personal grievances so that they do not interfere with the health of the group. If necessary, one of the individuals involved can leave a former group and start a new group. New Happiness Support Groups can begin at any time (See Appendix 2).

Self-exploration Question: How do I practice putting principles above personalities for the welfare of all?

Affirmation: Today I am practicing putting principles above personality differences for the welfare of any group in which I participate.

Principle: Listening and attending transform self-absorption and inattention to others.

Perennial Wisdom Quote: "Study to be quiet." -- Saint Paul, *The Bible,* 1 Thess. 1:3

Discussion: We are only as powerful as our capacity to perceive, to receive information and insight from what is within us and around us. This takes a quiet mind, a mind not absorbed in fear or speech, a mind able to observe its own thoughts as well as the words and feelings of others. What we give attention to, we reinforce. If we are attending to what we like and appreciate in others, that's what we reinforce. If we are attending to what we dislike, criticize or fear in others, that's what we reinforce.

The same is true about what we attend to within ourselves. If we attend to our talents, our natural gifts and our virtues, that's what we reinforce. If we only attend to our shortcomings, we can fall into self-rejection and shame.

A quiet mind can observe not only the actions and words of others, but one's own thoughts, as well as one's body sensations and emotional feelings. When a mind is overly noisy, it is easy to identify with our thoughts and feelings and forget that we are not our thoughts and feelings. We are that which watches our thoughts and feelings, our Essence or our Soul. Our principled minds can control our brains and manage our moods. Developing a quiet, observing consciousness takes time and practice. It's very much worth the effort.

Self-exploration Question: How can I refine my listening and attention skills?

Affirmation: Today I am practicing "quiet mind," listening, observing and learning from all my experiences.

Principle: Looking for the wonder in life transforms boredom and despair.

Perennial Wisdom Quote: "Someone's boring me…I think it's me." -- Dylan Thomas

Discussion: As the 21st century Information Revolution swings into ever higher gear, it's easy to fall into a mindset which expects the world to entertain us. According to modern research, a passive response to multiple, electronic-stimulation sources actually promotes dissatisfaction and potentially boredom.

When we take responsibility ourselves for creating wonder and newness in our own experiences the results are much more satisfying. Brain research shows that the more we use our minds creatively and learn to observe and carefully choose our thoughts and behaviors the more our brains grow, even as adults. Finding a new hobby, meeting a new person, reading a new book, dancing, drawing, singing, running, swimming, walking -- all such activities stimulate the brain much more than does passive entertainment.

Wonder opens the doors to new knowledge, which keeps the brain stimulated and healthy. The Arapaho Indians put it this way, "If we wonder often, the gift of knowledge will come." When we wonder about nature's creations, we learn more about the life-sustaining principles exemplified in nature. When we learn about these principles and align our lives with them, life flows with heightened happiness and wonder.

Self-exploration Question: How can I make my life more wonder-full by exploring new feelings, new thoughts, new experiences and new observations?

Affirmation: Today I wonder about all that life brings me and about all that I bring to life.

Principle: Honesty is the foundation of all the other virtues and of happiness.

Perennial Wisdom Quote: "It is better to suffer from truth than to prosper by falsehood." -- Danish saying

Discussion: When we lie, we are hoping to prosper from our falsehoods. Yet in the process, we distance ourselves from real life. Lies are a way of trying to "play God," attempting to create reality consistent with our ego wills.

Dishonesty is most often rationalized on the basis of "The end justifies the means" theory. But life is about "the means," the "hows" of choices and events, more than any "ends." Life is not "an end" goal. Life is what happens moment by moment in a vast universe of interconnections. Dishonesty, lying, deception, and non-disclosure don't work because they are human attempts to deny these interconnections in order to escape self-created pain. If we avoid such pain, we never learn how to avoid the behaviors which create this pain. It's a Lose/Lose pattern.

Dishonesty generates fear, which generates hiding, which generates isolation, which generates separation from our true selves and others. All the founders of the world's major religions and the great philosophers have taught that honesty is a fundamental virtue. In order to maintain personal integrity, we have to be honest with ourselves. When we are honest with ourselves, it's much easier to be honest with others.

Self-exploratory Question: How can I improve my practice of honesty?

Affirmation: Today I choose to be completely honest with myself and everybody else.

Principle: Our bodies and minds require rest and relaxation to rejuvenate and strengthen themselves.

Perennial Wisdom Quote: "Every now and then go away, have a little relaxation, for when you come back to your work, your judgment will be surer, since to remain constantly at work will cause you to lose power of judgment." --Leonardo Da Vinci

Discussion: As the electronic, computer age brings data to us ever faster, creating ever more complex economic networks, fear can drive us to over-work and under-rest. This can both shorten our lives and emotionally empty them.

Perhaps the easiest way to relax one's mind and rejuvenate one's spirits is to breathe deeply, slowly and consciously. This means watching and actually thinking about our deep breaths. We can literally fill ourselves up with oxygen while letting go of muscular tension. This is a fascinating process to observe. The ancient yogis considered "the corpse pose" -- the pose of complete relaxation on one's back -- as the most fundamental of all their mind-enriching and body-strengthening yoga poses. We are only as strong as we can be relaxed. Body tension creates rigidity and rigidity creates fatigue and fatigue creates weakness. Deep relaxation creates fluidity and flexibility which creates rejuvenation, which creates strength. This is true of the mind as well as the body.

Often the most creative ideas come from one's night dreams or relaxed musings. Tension is necessary at times to protect ourselves and move objects, but it only promotes strength when we also know when to let go.

Self-exploration Question: How can I better balance effort with rest and relaxation?

Affirmation: Today I am finding a quiet half hour just for myself to rest and relax.

Principle: We are most empowered when we focus our energies on the present moment, not on the past or the future.

Perennial Wisdom Quote: "Every day is a little life; every awakening and rising a little birth; every fresh morning a little youth; every going to rest and sleep a little death. -- Aurther Schopenhauer, *Our Relation To Ourselves*

Discussion: The English word "present" originally meant "gift." Gifts come only in the present moment. But fear and distraction often get in the way of fully experiencing the moment. These happiness promoting slogans can help us to focus on the present moment: "One day at a time." "Keep life simple." "Stop expecting; start accepting."

Projecting into the past or future often just leads to the promotion of guilt, shame, resentment, and/or anxiety. Focusing on the present moment promotes an observing, pro-active mind. It also opens the heart. Our hearts resonate with our immediate environments. They feel and connect us to what is around us. When we spend time focusing on the past or the future, we become overly mental and less capable of connecting to present, life-supporting energies. Take time to connect to other human beings and nature every day, with an open heart.

Self-exploratory Question: How can I help myself to focus my attention more on present moments?

Affirmation: This very moment I am very aware of all sensations from within and without me.

Principle: Prayer is an attitude of patience, love and gratitude for life.

Perennial Wisdom Quote: "The greatest prayer is patience." -- Buddha

Discussion: A teacher once said, "We don't pray to change God; we pray to change ourselves." Having a deistic philosophy of life may be helpful for prayer, but it isn't completely necessary. A person can be agnostic and atheistic and still pray. Prayer is an attitude of the heart, more than a speaking of words with the mind. Prayer helps us to remember and appreciate our small place in a very large universe. It helps us to become less self-absorbed and more grateful for life itself and all that supports life.

A famous Christian theologian, Paul Tillich, actually defined God as "the ground of all being." Anyone can speak to this "ground" or energetic Source of life. Anyone can address this Source and feel blessed by it without having to define it. All the world's religious and spiritual teachers stress the importance of taking private time for silence, prayer and meditation.

Prayer can connect people of different religious affiliations or of no religious affiliation, rather than separate them. When we together honor a Source of life greater than ourselves, we are less likely to fight among ourselves. Our common respect for this Source can teach us to respect and love each other.

In schools "quiet time" can be established with the instruction to "rest, be quiet, and, if you wish, to respectfully consider a Source of power greater than yourself." This practice could help to teach self control, and a balanced commitment to both individuality and community, thus helping democracy to thrive.

Self-exploratory Question: How can I learn to pray, so as to deepen an attitude of patience, love, gratitude for life, and respect for the welfare of a diverse community?

Affirmation: Today I am opening my heart and mind to prayer. I do not have to believe in a deity to pray. (I can begin my words with, "May I/we/all beings be...." To affirm my hopes for myself and others.)

Principle: Meditation transforms distraction and teaches self-control.

Perennial wisdom quote: "In the solitude of your mind are the answers to all your questions about life. You must take the time to ask and listen." -- Bawa Mahaiyaddeen

Discussion: Some people say prayer is talking to God and meditation is listening to God, but a person doesn't have to believe in God to meditate. Meditation involves slowing down the restless mind and teaching it to relax and concentrate. Buddhists speak of meditation as "mindfulness" training. This involves practices which help the mind to stay alert and fully aware of the fullness of the present moment. Modern psychological research has shown how these kinds of practices are very effective in reducing fear and in rejuvenating and enriching the brain. Objects of fearful attention are simply pushed out of the mind with techniques such as concentrating on the breath, or on simple hand movements, on immediate sights and sounds, or on a repetitive phrase.

One creative American teacher, John Oliver in Danvers, Massachusetts, sets aside some "self-control time" regularly for his students. He uses simple breathing exercises, done while sitting quietly with eyes closed, to help his students become more focused and self-disciplined. Brain research shows how these practices help young minds to repair and grow. "Self-control time" is a form of meditation -- simply closing one's eyes and concentrating on the breath going in and out, so as to gradually slow it down and to be aware of one's feelings and behaviors and their impact on others.

Self-exploratory question: What form of daily meditation helps to sustain my life?

Affirmation: Today I am setting aside at least 15 minutes for quiet meditation.

Principle: Understanding transforms prejudice and intolerance.

Perennial wisdom quote: "Grant that we not so much seek to be understood as to understand." -- Saint Francis of Assisi

Discussion: When we "stand under" something we can usually see its shadow side; we also are standing in a lower position, a position of humility. When we seek to be understanding of others we are seeking to see and accept others' least admirable sides. We are humbly attempting to have empathy for others' losses and sufferings which might help to explain others' unkind behaviors. When we understand others, we are least apt to judge them harshly or be rejecting and violent towards them. Similarly, when we seek to understand ourselves, we can accept our damaged, shadowy parts and work on healing them. But we cannot understand ourselves if we have not learned how to observe our thoughts and feelings.

There is a modern saying, "What goes around comes around." It's an updated version of both what the Hindus call "karma" and the Biblical teaching that "as you sow, so shall you reap." When we can accept this principle, it is much easier to choose to be understanding, kind and compassionate towards others, because that behavior is what we all want to receive. Many scriptures teach us to attempt to understand even our enemies. We have to be patient, because when we offer another understanding, we may not receive it back from that specific person. It might take quite a while for the understanding to be returned, but eventually it will come from someone some time.

Self-exploratory question: When do I take time to understand others' thoughts, feelings, and behaviors, as well as my own?

Affirmation: Today I choose to focus on understanding – others, as well as myself.

Principle: When we are aware of grief and fear, and allow them to flow through us without acting them out toward others, they gradually pass, and we become resilient.

Perennial Wisdom Quote: "Between grief and nothing I will take grief." -- William Faulkner

Discussion: The alternative to painful feelings is numbness or emotional toughness. Both are the result of repressing feelings. Both reduce a person's capacity to fully experience life. Both tend to create personality disorders.

Feelings cannot stay repressed indefinitely. When forced down, they will pop back up just when we are feeling the weakest. Unfortunately, those are usually the times when we are least able to process our feelings effectively. Those are the times when we are most apt to get defensive, shaming and aggressive.

Pain and fear are designed to strengthen us and give us energy. When we avoid awareness of them through such escapes as addiction, intellectualization, self-pity, violence, self-shame and shaming others, we only weaken ourselves.

Fear and grief are best faced frontally, and lovingly shared with others. Otherwise they can make our lives too heavy to bear. First one needs to identify and accept a fear, dropping all shame, then determine a healthy source of safety and support. Finally, unless danger is very imminent, one needs to choose a response to the fear which allows for non-reactive flowing with feelings, rather than attempts at escape feelings and trying to control others.

Self-exploratory Questions: When was I last aware of grief and fear? What did I do about these feelings?

Affirmation: Today I am accepting and facing my grief and my fears.

Principle: Awareness of anger and using the "Anger Formula" and "Adult Time Out" transforms depression and rage.

Perennial Wisdom Quote: The powerful one is not the one who overthrows others, but the one who controls himself in anger. -- Muhammad, *The Hadith*

Discussion: The "Anger Formula" has three parts: 1) a responsible feeling statement such as "I feel angry", 2) a clear behavioral description of the other's stimulating behavior, such as "…when you keep interrupting me", and 3) a clear request for a positive substitute behavior, such as, "Please let me finish what I have to say."

If you are too angry or confused to make a respectful request for a corrective behavior, or if another person cannot respectfully accept your request, it is best to take an "Adult Time Out." This involves: 1) telling the other person that you need Time Out, 2) giving an estimate of about when you will be ready to call Time In, 3) temporarily detaching physically and emotionally from the interaction, and 4) later respectfully calling "Time In."

Adults who live together always benefit from having "Adult Time Out" agreements. This means they take responsibility for "Timing themselves Out" when necessary, and they also commit to respecting each other's Time Out calls. Many an intimate relationship can be saved by just using these two vital skills.

Self-exploratory Question: How can I more responsibly express my anger?

Affirmation: Today I am using the Anger Formula and, if necessary, Adult Time Out, whenever I become angry.

Principle: Using the Anger Formula teaches self-responsibility and respect for self and others.

Perennial Wisdom Quote: "Anyone can become angry -- that is easy. But to be angry with the right person, to the right degree, at the right time, for the right purpose, and in the right way -- that is not easy." -- Aristotle, *The Nichomachean Ethics*

Discussion: The first part of the Anger Formula involves taking responsibility for our own emotions and labeling them correctly, avoiding such irresponsible language as "You're making me angry."

The second part of the Anger Formula involves specifically and respectfully describing the other person's behavior to which we are responding, avoiding shaming, personality-assassination statements like, "Stop being a jerk (or other 4-letter words)!"

The third part of the Anger Formula involves responsibly requesting specific, corrective behavior from the person to whom you have responded with anger. (Sometimes the other person has no idea what behavior would be helpful to you.)

Following all three of these Anger Formula steps keeps ourselves healthy, even if the persons whom we confront do not themselves respond to the Anger Formula with respect. Statespersons and effective leaders know how to deal with anger in these ways.

Self-exploratory Question: How can I more effectively use the Anger Formula?

Affirmation: I am using the Anger Formula more effectively each time I use it.

January 19   **Taking "Adult Time Out" (ATO)**

Principle: When an adult can temporarily not use the Anger Formula effectively, it is always best to take an Adult Time Out (ATO) and call Time In later.

Perennial Wisdom Quote: "Anger and hatred are rooted in fear." -- Frances Vaughan

Discussion: Because anger is rooted in fear, sometimes we are too afraid to be able to responsibly share our feelings and make responsible, assertive requests for corrective behaviors. Sometimes the person to whom we are responding with anger is not acting responsibly and thinking clearly. Especially if the relationship with this person is one which we want to continue, taking an Adult Time Out can give everyone time to privately, more effectively, process the fear underneath the anger. This usually eventually reduces the anger. It also gives the brain time to properly do its work, rather than short-circuiting the brain's pre-frontal cortex which is designed to help out the brain's emotional, limbic systems. (See more brain information in Appendix 1.) It also gives the angry person time to get clear on what corrective behavior to request from the other person, or what apology to make for his or her own part of the problem.

If the person calling for Adult Time Out (ATO) can be relied upon for calling Time In at a later, appropriate time, usually the person who is left in the interaction feels respected rather than rejected. It is helpful when calling ATO to let the other person know where you are going and about when you might be ready to call Time In. This makes it easier for the one left behind to also detach from the negative interaction and not feel abandoned or rejected. The only reason to not do this would be if the other person is threatening violence, in which case just immediately take an Adult Time Out.

Using Adult Time Out creates interpersonal safety. Learning how to take ATO should be a part of all rehabilitation for anyone involved in domestic violence (both the victim and the perpetrator), and anyone involved in assault and felony violence. Correctional and probation officers also need to be familiar with the Anger Formula and Adult Time Out principles.

Self-exploratory Question: How well do I practice Adult Time Out?

Affirmation: I can count on myself to call Adult Time Out when it is needed.

Principle: Peacefulness involves a calm mind and an open heart.

Perennial Wisdom Quote: "Oppose not rage while rage is in its force, but give it way a while and let it waste." -- William Shakespeare

Discussion: Personality traits which are associated with peacefulness include patience, high frustration tolerance, an ability to tolerate criticism, a respect for others, an ability to have emotionally intimate relationships, and the ability to be introspective about one's own thoughts and feelings. Brain research shows how all these abilities stem from an "integrated," well-functioning brain. To develop such a brain takes patient observations of, and acceptance of, all of one's feelings and behaviors. It takes noticing and changing abrupt, emotional defenses which shut down awareness.

When another person has lost patience and is being critical and rejecting, the violated person can choose peace by taking an Adult Time Out and open-heartedly offering the other a later opportunity to work out the difficulty in a mutually respectful way. Non-violence is not acquiescence. It is assertiveness which promotes courage and self-esteem in all concerned.

Self-exploratory Question: How can I be more committed to patient observations of myself and others and the peaceful and respectful resolution of conflict?

Affirmation: Today I am patiently and peacefully responding to all conflict.

January 21   **Self-examination**

Principle: Self-examination can transform repression, avoidance and projection.

Perennial Wisdom Quote: "Nothing is easier than self-deceit. Not to alter one's faults is to be faulty indeed." -- Confucius

Discussion: Modern psychological research has confirmed that avoidance is one of the most common emotional defenses. Unfortunately, this defense reduces the effective functioning of the brain.

Honestly examining one's self and doing so without emotional self-rejection is very challenging. Many people just avoid it. Such avoidance, however, usually just leads to attempts by others to point out our faults.

Self-examination on a regular basis is like physical exercise and a healthy diet -- it prevents worse problems later. Most spiritual and ethical groups provide support for this kind of honest self-examination, as well as guidelines for promoting self-forgiveness. If you are not a member of a group, joining one in order to receive this kind of support is a good idea. Be sure that it is a group which does not reinforce shame and "black and white thinking." Choose a group which will offer suggestions, guidance, love, forgiveness, and respect while you are working through your shortcomings, not just tell you what you want to hear. If you cannot find such a group, consider forming a Happiness Support Group or Talking Circle (See Appendix 2) to learn safe sharing and support guidelines. Another option is to ask a counselor to start a Counseling Group using this book. Self-examination is the core of the Happiness Fourth Step. More will be said about this later.

Self-exploratory Question: How can I more regularly examine my own attitudes and behaviors? (See the Self-Evaluation Appendix.)

Affirmation: Today I am observing myself carefully and not avoiding honest self-examination.

Principle: Awareness of joy transforms anxiety.

Perennial Wisdom Quote: "Our need is not for pleasure but for joy -- a deep sense of fulfillment that not only never leaves us but actually increases with the passage of time. Fun is living for ourselves; joy comes from living for others, giving our time and love to a purpose greater than ourselves." -- Eknath Easwaran, *Thousand Names of Vishnu*

Discussion: Joy trusts life. Joy accepts life, even the unpleasant parts of it. Joy celebrates life, right now in the moment. Joy lives in the heart and needs to be unconditionally released from the heart, without allowing the mind to put conditions on its release. Joy thrives on concern for and service to others.

Anxiety lives in the mind and puts all kinds of conditions on the release of joy from the heart. Anxiety says, "I will only be joyful if…" Anxiety lives in the future and is conditioned by habits of the past. When we are aware of joy and its cultivation, we learn how to drop "If only." We don't dwell on regrets and disappointments. We accept our losses and sadness, and we move on to the next moment with an openness to whatever newness may come in it.

Appropriate medications can help to lift depression and anxiety, but to bring more joy into our lives we also need to learn how to generate it behaviorally.

Self-exploratory Question: How can I expand experiences of joy in my life?

Affirmation: Today I choose to open my heart to life and live it joyfully.

Principle: Personal autonomy and independence transforms dependence and co-dependence.

Perennial Wisdom Quote: "Learn to see, listen and think for yourself." -- Malcolm X

Discussion: Personal autonomy means the ability, not only to see, to listen and to think for ourselves, but also to feel for ourselves. When we become adults, we need to put away childish thoughts and dependencies. We need to accept that no one can make our most important life decisions for us. We need to realize that no one can protect us from pain and suffering and make all our hurts go away. We need to accept that we are responsible for learning from our own pain, for tolerating our own losses, for healing our own hurts. We need to responsibly develop our brains as well as our muscles.

Having trust in a Higher Power which can teach us how to do all this challenging adult work is, of course, very helpful but, ultimately, we have to learn these lessons for ourselves. We cannot ask another human being to do this work for us. We cannot blame another for our unhappiness. Loved ones can be supportive or hurtful, but they cannot ultimately determine our happiness. People who accept personal responsibility for their own feelings and who find joy in giving to others are ultimately the happiest.

All the major religions of the world in one way or another accept "free will" as a fundamental truth which each of us must responsibly accept. This means personal autonomy.

Self-exploratory Question: How can I accept more responsibility for my own happiness?

Affirmation: Today I accept full responsibility for my actions and happiness.

Principle: Emotional intelligence transforms immaturity and mis-education.

Perennial Wisdom Quote: Emotional intelligence includes "abilities such as being able to motivate oneself and persist in the face of frustrations; to control impulse and delay gratification; to regulate one's moods and keep distress from swamping the ability to think; to empathize and to hope." -- Daniel Goleman, Ph.D., *Emotional Intelligence*

Discussion: Daniel Goleman, Ph.D., an American psychologist, coined the term "emotional intelligence" because intelligence had for too many years in the United States been associated only with logical reasoning and perception. The emotional component of intelligence had been grossly overlooked by prior psychological and educational research and well as most school systems and educators. Attention to emotions, the ancient virtues, and perennial wisdom teachings had been neglected.

Recent psychological research as to what personality factors most determined adult career success clearly indicate that factors such as frustration tolerance, impulse control, the self-regulation of moods and the ability to delay gratification are of even more importance than advanced reading, writing and arithmetic skills. Yet, these skills are still underemphasized in school curriculums. Fortunately, Dr. Goleman's writings have been widely read, and attention is now being given by American educators to how to help children develop greater "emotional intelligence." Of course, one of the best ways that adults can improve children's emotional intelligence is to be good examples of such intelligence themselves. Scientists have recently discovered that the brain is continually capable of development. It is never too late to learn.

Self-exploratory Question: How can I improve my emotional intelligence?

Affirmation: I value emotional intelligence as much as academic intelligence.

January 25   **Sobriety and Abstinence from Mind Altering Substances**

Principle: Good judgment can't be exercised when a mind is altered by chemicals.

Perennial Wisdom Quote: "The desire to take drugs is finished when I see the real danger of them; I won't touch them. As long as I don't see the danger of it, I'll go on." -- J. Krishnamurti, *On Fear*

Discussion: One definition of addiction is a dependency on outside substances, objects or excitements to attempt to take care of inside needs and deficiencies. When we can see the danger and dead-end-street nature of these kinds of dependencies, we are much more able to find better ways to take care of our inside deficiencies. To use a chemical to change one's mood is always a dangerous choice, unless it is prescribed by a knowledgeable medical person. We all need to learn to alter negative moods without the use of alcohol or street drugs. If we are plagued with insomnia or dark moods, we need to see a medical person about an appropriate, safe, mood altering medication and we need to work with a counselor and/or support group to learn behavioral ways to improve our moods. We also need to learn to develop loving friendships to which we can turn for support when we are emotionally down.

Most inmates in U.S. prisons are people who have not yet learned this principle. They have not yet learned how to use appropriate counseling, medication and social support to take care of inside needs and deficiencies, and heal the impact on their brains of past losses and traumas. Somehow our culture needs to help such people learn to do this. By staying sober ourselves and helping those who haven't yet learned to do so, each of us can be part of the solutions to these problems. The modeling of statespersons and leaders who are able to do this is also important.

Self-exploratory Question: How can I avoid using alcohol or street drugs as mood medicines?

Affirmation: Today I choose not to use alcohol or street drugs for mood management.

Principle: Process addictions such as over-eating and gambling are also dangerous mood-altering dependencies.

Perennial Wisdom Quote: "The pleasure of doing good is the only one that will not wear out." -- Chinese proverb

Discussion: Dependency is always intertwined with fear, and using an outside "fix" to escape fear only strengthens it. Using an addictive process to escape awareness of our fears only furthers the deterioration of our brains. We have to face our emotional fears and losses and find healthy sources of pleasure. The Chinese thousands of years ago already discovered that the only pleasure that will not wear out is the pleasure of doing good.

Modern psychological research has shown that positive social connection is a much greater indicator of happiness than access to comfort foods, alcohol, drugs or money. To establish positive social connections, we have to learn to be good friends to others, in order to have good friends ourselves. We have to learn to give as much as we hope to receive, and value and respect others as much as we hope to be valued and respected ourselves. All this takes commitment, time and practice. We can start in small ways with just one or two persons and then gradually build our positive interpersonal attitudes and skills until our support circle is extended.

Self-exploratory Question: How can I abstain from using food, gambling or any process addiction to find happiness?

Affirmation: Today I am accepting my feelings and finding pleasure in doing good.

January 27
Questioning

Principle: A questioning mind transforms close-mindedness.

Perennial Wisdom Quote: "The important thing is not to stop questioning." -- Albert Einstein

Discussion: For human beings to learn to live together in peace and harmony, we need to be able to question ourselves as well as others. Sometimes our unconscious defenses sabotage us. Sometimes our intentions are kind, but our choices of behaviors are faulty. Sometimes our intentions themselves are hurtful and unkind. We always need to question both our own intentions and our own choice of behaviors. We also need to be able to question others, asking for their perceptions about our behaviors, and questioning them, so as to better understand their behaviors. Of course, we always need to be respectful when we question the intentions and behaviors of others.

Curiosity about the world around us can help us to make our places better in that world. This includes wanting to understand the whole planet and universe, as well as the people in it. When we question what we see, and when we respectfully ask others to share what they know, our minds are strengthened, and we have more opportunity to better our lives.

Self-exploratory Question: How can I more respectfully question myself and others?

Affirmation: Today I am respectfully questioning both myself and others.

Principle: Freedom cannot be sustained without self-education.

Perennial Wisdom Quote: "The one who asks questions doesn't lose his way. -- African (Akan) proverb

Discussion: Taking responsibility for educating our own minds is foundational to freedom and democracy. A nation cannot sustain liberty if its people cannot safely question its leaders. Members of any institution cannot ensure the quality of that institution if authority cannot be questioned. Secure, educated leaders welcome respectful questions. All the great spiritual teachers of the world have welcomed questions and have encouraged independence in their followers.

Nations and institutions are doomed to totalitarianism and stultifying, blind obedience if respectful questioning is not encouraged.

Different people have different capacities to learn in different areas, but everyone has some capacity to learn. Human brains are capable of growing throughout a lifetime, not just during childhood. The challenge is for each of us to learn to our greatest capacity so we can create satisfying, happy lives for ourselves. No one is a complete victim. As long as we are alive, we have the capacity to determine our own thoughts and attitudes. Even in prison we can find ways to educate ourselves. Self-education begins with self-knowledge and follows with knowledge about others, our interactions and the world.

Self-exploratory Question: How can I best avoid ignorance and practice assertive self-education?

Affirmation: Today I am liberating my mind with increasing self-education.

January 29   **Freedom from "Black and White**
Thinking"

Principle: Knowledge transforms "black and white thinking."

Perennial Wisdom Quote: "Knowledge of our own ignorance is the first step toward true knowledge." -- Socrates

Discussion: "Black and white thinking" is thinking which rigidly dwells on good/bad, right/wrong, beautiful/ugly, and for-me/against-me dualities. It is normal in childhood but needs to discontinue in adulthood because it is fear-based thinking, motivated by a belief that the only way to stay safe is to be "right" and separate from what is "wrong."

Adults with a lot of "black and white thinking" are usually very anxious people, often people who have been abused, neglected, abandoned, enmeshed or traumatized as children or people who have abused drugs as young adults. The limbic system in their brains tend to "highjack" their pre-frontal cortex functioning. (See Appendix 1.) Fear causes them to form quick pro/con attitudes and reject all that is feared or different from themselves. "Black and white thinking" breeds intolerance and prejudice. It thrives among people with damaged senses of self.

A person can be ethical, moral and clear on his or her own values and beliefs and still avoid "black and white thinking." "Black and white thinking" usually involves judging other people, without understanding them. Often labels are put on other people, without truly understanding their circumstances or motivation. Normal adults can unknowingly sometimes engage in "black and white thinking." This thinking is simply based on the ignorant belief that they understand another when in actuality their understanding is limited.

The first step out of "black and white thinking" is awareness of our own imperfect understanding. The second step is acceptance of our own damaged senses of self.

Self-exploratory Question: How can I best overcome "black and white thinking"?

Affirmation: Today I commit to avoiding "black and white thinking."

January 30
Wisdom

Principle: Wisdom transforms ignorance and fear.

Perennial Wisdom Quote: "Wisdom is knowledge plus; knowledge -- and the knowledge of one's own limits." -- Viktor E. Frankl, *The Unconscious God: Psychotherapy and Theology*

Discussion: To become wise a person both needs to have knowledge and experience. He or she needs to have developed the adult ability to experience himself or herself clearly and separately from others. Ignorance thrives in childlike, fearful avoidance and projection. Wisdom thrives in aware contact and good emotional boundaries.

Anthony de Mello in his book, *Awakenings,* outlines these "Four Steps to Wisdom": 1) identify all feelings as in yourself; 2) understand that they originate in you, not in the world of external reality; 3) dis-identify yourself from these feelings; 4) understand that, when you identify with your own true nature (love and freedom) you begin to feel happiness no matter what is going on "out there."

Wise people can look deeply into Nature and themselves and experience the love and freedom at Nature's very core. They find satisfaction and happiness in life through their own choices of loving and accepting attitudes and behaviors. They are not dependent on external situations for happiness. They lovingly relate to others because love is what they have in their hearts for life itself. They are committed to developing healthy brains and minds and resolving any past traumas which might be obstructions.

Self-exploratory Question: How would I describe the limits of my own knowledge?

Affirmation: Today I wisely remind myself of the limits of my own knowledge.

January 31
Identity

Principle: Self-identity creates the foundation for our experience.

Perennial Wisdom Quote: "A beautiful soul always dwells in a beautiful world." -- Ralph Waldo Emerson

Discussion: One's identity (or "sense of self") creates much of one's experience of reality. Many wise teachers have broken down a personal sense of self into several parts, because most of us perceive ourselves differently at different times. Often these parts are referred to as body, mind, and spirit (or soul).

All the major world religions stress the importance of taking good care of one's body and mind, and identifying primarily with one's spirit (or soul). Some teachers refer to the soul as "that which watches" or the "Higher Self", the part of one's self which can observe one's body and thoughts so, therefore, is in charge of one's body and brain. When we can identify ourselves as "that which watches," it is easier to develop a positive self of self, one worthy of respect and love.

Maybe, like Anthony de Mello, we can actually identify our own personal essence as "love and freedom." This means we can recognize that our minds may have fearful, manic or depressed thoughts, and our bodies might be sick, but still our souls are, in their very essence, simply love and freedom.

Why Smart People Can Be So Stupid, edited by Robert J. Sternberg discusses how, in order to be wise, we need to avoid four "fallacies: the "egocentrism fallacy," the "omniscience fallacy," the "omnipotence fallacy," and the "invulnerability fallacy." We need to accept that the world doesn't revolve around ourselves, that we don't know all there is to know, that our intelligence doesn't make us all-powerful, and that we are not invulnerable from hurt and exposure.

Self-exploratory Question: How would I describe my personal, core essence?

Affirmation: Today I am identifying myself as a beautiful, loving, free soul and similarly seeing the world around me as full of such souls.

February 1
Patience

Principle: Patience is one of the fundamental virtues.

Perennial Wisdom Quote: "Patience is the best remedy for any trouble." -- Plautus

Discussion: Fundamental to the development of patience is understanding the difference between the things we can change the things we can't. Many people become impatient with themselves and others because they mistakenly believe that they can or should have more control. In reality, generally as adults we cannot control other people, places and things. When we try to do so, our relationships become emotionally distant or at best tolerant. Attempting to control other adults minimizes intimacy and joyful spontaneity.

What we need to focus on controlling is ourselves. We need to learn how to observe our thoughts and behaviors and make them self-caring and respectful of ourselves and others. We need to learn how to regulate our moods, how to be patient with ourselves as we grow in maturity.

Nature teaches us that there is a natural order and flow to life which is subtle, quiet, and sometimes hidden. Yet this order it always bigger and wiser than any one person's individual will. When we are impatient with something, we need to step back, look for the bigger picture, and accept the life-sustaining flow of energy around us.

Self-exploratory Question: How can I learn to be more patient and accepting?

Affirmation: Today I am becoming more patient and accepting.

February 2
Perseverance

Principle: Hopeful perseverance transforms victim consciousness.

Perennial Wisdom Quote: "Perseverance opens up treasures which bring perennial joy." -- Mahatma Gandhi

Discussion: Patience, when complemented by perseverance, is very powerful, especially when it is focused on self-improvement. Together, perseverance and patience reinforce hope. When we learn what is in our control and what is not, and we don't persevere to try to manage what is unmanageable, our energies always flow in productive directions. Our brains are less stressed and function better.

In general, other adult people, places and things are unmanageable. Only our own thoughts, attitudes and behaviors are manageable. When we persevere in honoring our own highest values, our own integrity-filled behaviors, and our best intentions, usually we do not go wrong.

Many of us, unfortunately, persevere with trying to avoid pain and pursue pleasure. This intention is doomed to failure because nature gives us pain to attempt to correct our own misguided behavior. When we avoid awareness of this pain, we can persevere with misguided behavior and simply cause ourselves more pain at a future time. We need to be very clear to only persevere with behaviors which promote health and life, for ourselves as well as others.

Self-exploratory Question: How can I do more to persevere with behaviors which promote health and life, for myself and others?

Affirmation: Today I am persevering with behaviors which promote health and life.

Principle: Self-acceptance and self-esteem transform shame.

Perennial Wisdom Quote: "To accuse others for one's own misfortunes is a sign of want of education; to accuse oneself shows that one's education has begun; to accuse neither oneself nor others shows that one's education is complete." -- Epictetus

Discussion: Epictetus was a Greek philosopher and emancipated slave from 50-120 C.E. (Common Era). In the above quote he beautifully describes three levels of maturity. The lowest level is when we shame and blame another for our own troubles. This gets us nowhere. The next level is when we shame ourselves for our own mistakes. At this level of maturity at least we are taking responsibility for our own mistakes, but we haven't yet learned to positively learn from them while still maintaining self-esteem. At the highest level of maturity, we neither shame ourselves nor others. We notice our mistakes; we make amends for them; we learn from them, and we move on without damaging our self-esteem. When we notice others making mistakes, we only point them out, if we can do so respectfully and in ways which will help others to learn from their mistakes.

Incongruence between inner ideals and outer behaviors builds toxic shame and self-rejection. This is why it is so important to maintain behavior which is in line with our inner ideals. If we don't respect ourselves, we can't maintain respect of others.

Self-exploratory Question: How can I improve the alignment between my behavior and my inner ideals?

Affirmation: Today I am avoiding shame by aligning my behavior with my inner ideals.

February 4   **Self-appreciation**

Principle: It is just as important to appreciate ourselves as it is to appreciate others.

Perennial Wisdom Quote: "It is difficult to make a man miserable while he feels he is worthy of himself and claims kindred to the great God who made him." -- Abraham Lincoln

Discussion: Satisfaction in life is built by an upward spiral of first positive thought, then optimistic attitude, then effort to achieve positive goals, then self-appreciation, then improved self-confidence, then more effort toward achieving positive goals, etc.

Self-appreciation usually involves affirmative thoughts such as, "I did well," "I'm glad I did that," "I'm glad I said that," etc. It also involves awareness of our strengths and a commitment to build upon them.

Martin Seligman, Ph.D. has dedicated his life to researching what makes for increased life satisfaction. He has found that six types of strengths are most important: wisdom/knowledge, courage, love, justice, temperance, and transcendence/spirituality. A person can go to his website, www.authentichappiness.org, or read his book, *Authentic Happiness* to learn more about his research on creating life satisfaction.

When we appreciate ourselves, our behavior is in line with our inner highest ideals, and we celebrate this fact. In order to do this, we need to know what our highest ideals are so we can pursue them while using our primary strengths. Simple, positive self-appreciation can be shared with others who can join in our pleasure. This is different from bragging which involves being comparative and competitive, so that others don't share in our pleasure.

Self-exploratory Question: How can I recognize and appreciate my strengths? (See the Self-Inventory Appendix.)

Affirmation: I recognize and appreciate my strengths.

February 5
Remorse

Principle: Healthy remorse leads to making healthy amends for our wrongdoings.

Perennial Wisdom Quote: "Remorse begets reform." -- William Cowper

Discussion: Remorse is healthy, expiated guilt. It motivates a person to be aware of having done harm to another, to make amends, to compensate for the harm, and not to repeat the harm. This kind of guilt leads to improved self-esteem. Unhealthy guilt is un-expiated self-hatred (i.e. self-hatred which has not taken healing action.) It involves the defensive avoidance of responsibility for making amends. It avoids learning from mistakes. When a person carries around unresolved feelings of unhealthy guilt, he or she can become isolated, detached from reality, and more prone to repeating mistakes. This is why it is so important to learn to distinguish healthy remorse from unhealthy guilt.

Remorse opens up the way to self-forgiveness. Unhealthy guilt leaves a person feeling unworthy of forgiveness and consequently unable to work toward life's positive gifts. When we can feel healthy remorse, we can admit all our wrongs, suffer the natural consequences of them, make amends for them, and go on to rebuild our lives in more positive, creative ways. When we stay stuck in unhealthy guilt, we begin to identify ourselves as "bad" and begin to justify bad behavior as inherent to our "badness." Most people are capable of healthy remorse given a long enough time in a supportive enough environment.

Self-exploratory question: What amend could I now most benefit from making, in order to let go of guilt and forgive myself?

Affirmation: Today I choose to promptly make amends for any mistake I make.

February 6
Tolerance

Principle: Tolerance transforms fear, resentment and forced solutions.

Perennial Wisdom Quote: "Selfishness is not living as one wishes to live; it is asking others to live as one wishes to live." -- Oscar Wilde

Discussion: Intolerance is a form of selfishness. It is fear twisting and distorting reality. Nature herself is very tolerant. Look at the diversity of plant and animal species which exist in the world in a complimentary way. Look at the diversity of chemicals and minerals in the world, many of which can be combined in a complimentary fashion. We humans are unusual in the animal kingdom in our willingness to dominate and exterminate members of our own species.

Often intolerance stems from the human desire to escape from unavoidable, necessary pain. It is painful and difficult to see how others can be so different and yet OK. It is easier to stick with the limited social practices of one small group and call all other practices "bad" or "wrong" or "inferior." It is easier to consider a different gender, race, religion or culture inferior and therefore worthy of dominance or extinction. When we can accept the pain of recognizing our own limited thinking and limited experience, we can grow in tolerance. Brains which have been "hijacked" by fear and intolerance are not functioning well. People with such brains have been traumatized by great losses, or they would be capable of more patience and understanding. (See Appendix 1.)

Self-exploratory question: When was I last the most intolerant? When most tolerant?

Affirmation: Today I am practicing tolerance and am open to the pain of recognizing my own limited thinking and limited experience.

Principle: Letting go and detaching with love transform fear, resentment and forced solutions.

Perennial Wisdom Quote: "By yielding you may obtain victory." -- Ovid

Discussion: Letting go of resentments and criticism involves a certain surrendering of ego. Barriers to this surrender include grandiosity and a mistaken belief that surrender means weakening oneself. Quite the opposite! This kind of surrender strengthens a person. The strength gained from ego surrender is a lot like the strength gained from making love to a spouse. In love making one surrenders his or her body to the pleasure given to and received from one's partner. In love making one is rewarded with intimacy, relaxation and a deep sense of wellbeing through being connected harmoniously with another.

In surrendering our resentments and criticisms we let go of anger and tension and are more connected to ourselves and others. We can see more clearly. In this process we gain emotional strength and resilience, no matter what is happening with the persons whom we formerly resented. We also can see more clearly our own part in any difficulty and begin to correct it.

In democracies it is important to elect leaders who understand how to transform their fears and resentments and not act them out in anger. In this way they can work in teams together.

Self-exploratory Question: What current resentment or criticism can I benefit from relinquishing?

Affirmation: Today I am letting go of my resentments and focusing on improving myself rather than criticizing others.

Principle: Resentments destroy our own hearts and spirits without helping others.

Perennial Wisdom Quote: "Resolve to be tender with the young, compassionate with the aged, sympathetic with the striving, and tolerant with the weak and the wrong. Sometime in life you will have been all of these." –Lloyd Shearer

Discussion: Lewis Andrews, Ph.D., in *Growing Wiser* points out that one "reason why it's so difficult to forgive is that many of us become attached to our resentments. Angry feelings give us a charge of adrenaline and an emotional boost, so it is easy to become psychologically dependent on them." If we pay attention and don't immediately verbalize or act out our angry resentments, we can more easily get in touch with the hurts, sadness, fears, regrets, insecurities, and unmet needs which underlie our resentments. Once we can identify them, we can take responsibility for them and find productive, independent ways through which we can heal them. This way we don't give our emotional power away to anyone through resentment.

When we resent others, we unrealistically empower them and shirk responsibility for areas of self-empowerment. Dropping resentments is very satisfying because, thereby, we can see more clearly and empower ourselves more completely. Rejecting, resentful thoughts and behaviors actually empower others to be rejecting and resentful in response, which ultimately is harder on us. Catch resentful thoughts quickly and replace them with self-responsible actions, such as politely asking for what you need. Notice how much stronger and happier you feel.

Self-exploratory Question: What weakening yet emotionally gratifying pay-offs do I get from hanging on to my current resentments?

Affirmation: Today I am strengthening myself by letting go of resentments.

February 9   **Freedom from Self-**
righteousness

Principle: Self-knowledge transforms self-righteousness, self-pity and pride.

Perennial Wisdom Quote: "Moral indignation is in most cases 2% moral, 48% indignation, and 50% envy." -- Vittorio De Sica, *The Observer,* 1961

Discussion: Have you ever noticed how individuals who speak for the "right" or the "godly" or even God himself often suffer from a lack of humility and self-awareness? When the urge arises to speak for the "right," the "proper" or some divine authority, it's best to pray for humility and guidance and focus on quieting one's own mind rather than trying to silence the minds or words of others.

Self-righteousness is, unfortunately, a plant which readily grows in the soil of religiosity, watered by a desire for social approval. Religious leaders who feel dis-empowered and resentful of the political power and/or decisions of others can easily fall into self-righteousness. Charles Kimball, in *When Religion Becomes Evil (2003),* discusses how dangers abound when people make absolute truth claims based on personal interpretations of small pieces of scripture, or on blind obedience to a leader who claims to speak for "God" or "Allah." This is why members of Happiness Support Groups (as well as members of other 12 Step self-help programs) emphasize their own personal relationships with a Higher Power as they personally understand such a Higher Power. This understanding is not dictated by any outer authority.

Self-exploratory Question: What personal practices currently help me to avoid self-righteousness?

Affirmation: Today I humbly commit to avoiding self-righteous behaviors.

Principle: Self-pity is transformed by self-knowledge, self-respect and non-violent action to correct injustice.

Perennial Wisdom Quote: "Self-pity is one of the most unhappy and consuming defects that we know. It is a bar to all spiritual progress and can cut off all effective communication with our fellows because of its inordinate demands for attention and sympathy." -- Bill Wilson, *As Bill Sees It*

Discussion: Self-pity is an escape from reality, often covering up underlying anger and a collapse of healthy self-improvement. Self-pity is a false and premature surrender of responsibility. It is a resistance to taking responsibility for our own personal experiences. Self-pity can be overcome by self-knowledge, self-respect and non-violent action to correct injustice. When we engage in non-violent attempts to become part of the solution to injustice, rather than part of the problem which perpetuates injustice, we always gain in self-respect. We also empower ourselves by strengthening personal skills, rather than bemoaning personal weaknesses. We stand up for our right to current respect, no matter what our personal past mistakes might have been.

Nature herself is very forgiving. Life, in plants and animals and even rocks and minerals, goes on finding new ways to thrive even after natural catastrophes. We humans have brains large enough to study nature's ways and learn from her lessons. She never pities herself. She always moves on toward renewed life. We need to do the same.

Self-exploratory Question: What helps me the most to overcome my self-pity?

Affirmation: Today I am substituting self-knowledge, self-respect and non-violent action for self-pity.

February 11   **Acceptance of**
Disappointments

Principle: Acceptance of disappointment transforms expectations, resentful anger and blame.

Perennial Wisdom Quote: "The secret of perpetual youth is already known to me. Accept with philosophic calm whatever fate may be." -- Ma-tzu-lau

Discussion: When we don't accept disappointments and instead react to them chronically with anger or blame, we undermine our personal emotional stability and unbalance our brain chemistry. The fundamental causes of personality disorders are not yet known to modern science, but likely they have something to do with early childhood trauma and also the individual's inability to accept disappointment. Likely this process imbalances the healthy development of brain tissue and handicaps the child in the development of a healthy personality.

We can't control what others do, but we can control how we react to what others do. Some individuals have been terribly abused as children and yet have developed healthy personalities and healthy adult relationships. Other individuals have been terribly abused, traumatized or neglected as children and yet have gradually developed personality disorders which prevented them from establishing satisfying adult relationships.

How we respond to disappointments makes a great deal of difference. Responding with resentful anger and blame just upsets our own nervous systems and further alienates us from others. Responding with acceptance and gaining independence from those who have disappointed us is what leads to later satisfaction.

Self-exploratory Question: How can I improve my ability to accept disappointments?

Affirmation: When I can do nothing to prevent a disappointment, I accept it calmly and protect myself from resentment and blame.

February 12   **Freedom from Unhealthy Expectations and Bitterness**

Principle: Expectations for others to fulfill our adult emotional needs usually leads to disappointment and bitterness.

Perennial Wisdom Quote: "Better not to do kindness at all than to do it in the hope of recompense." -- Lao-Tze

Discussion: "If you love me, you would…." is a terribly manipulative way of thinking, which tends to destroy loving relationships. Love does not come with strings attached. Love unconditionally hopes for the best for the loved one and does not ask for recompense.

Unfortunately, often people treat loving relationships like business contracts. They believe that if they give so much the other should give an equal amount. This is unrealistic because each of us has different abilities and ways of giving at different times. Therefore, it is necessary for the giver not to give with expectations of return, but rather from the joy of giving. This involves also setting limits on the time, attention, and gifts shared with a loved one, so there is no risk of forming resentments or being emotionally or physically abused.

When a person forms a resentment, it is his or her responsibility to heal it, not the person being resented. It is a responsibility to make the changes necessary to drop the resentment. The solutions are internal, not external. It might involve asking for another person to make changes and informing another person about one's harm. But we cannot demand changes of another adult. That just furthers resentment. Overcoming a resentment might involve letting go of an unfulfilling relationship, but the letting go can be done respectfully, without shame and blame.

Self-exploratory Question: How do I take responsibility for modifying my own behavior so I don't develop resentment and bitterness?

Affirmation: Today I am taking responsibility for modifying my own behavior so that I don't develop resentments, even when I am disappointed.

Principle: Optimism can be learned and can lengthen our lives.

Perennial Wisdom Quote: "Human beings by changing the inner attitudes of their minds can change the outer aspects of their lives." -- William James

Discussion: When we mentally focus on something, we amplify it in our awareness. Therefore, focusing on our own and others' shortcomings simply amplify them. Focusing on our own strengths and others' strengths also amplify them. So, when we feel discouraged, we need to consciously look for what is going well, what we are doing well, and what we appreciate in others.

Rest and emotional self-care is important. When one is Hungry, Angry, Lonely or Tired one must H.A.L.T. before attempting to do anything else. Take time to eat, if you are hungry. Take Adult Time Out, if you are angry. Call a friend, if you are lonely. Get some rest if you are tired. Then return to the question or concern about which you were feeling negative and notice how different the issue can look, and how much more hope fills your heart.

Martin Seligman, Ph.D. has written two excellent books about optimism: *Learned Optimism* and *The Optimistic Child.* He cites much modern research which confirms that optimistic people are healthier, do better financially, and live longer. He also has developed scientifically tested ways to become more optimistic. Visit his website (www.authentichappiness.org) for more information.

Self-exploratory Question: How can I become more optimistic?

Affirmation: Today, whenever I feel hungry, angry, lonely or tired, I practice the H.A.L.T. formula and take personal responsibility for developing an optimistic attitude.

February 14
Faith

Principle: Faith transforms negative attitudes

Perennial Wisdom Quote: "True faith is not a momentary feeling but a struggle against the discouragement that threatens us every time we meet with resistance." -- Bakole wa Ilunga

Discussion: Process definitions of faith are more helpful than content definitions -- the "how's" of faith, rather than the "whats." Fai'sth means living in each present breath, not worrying about your next breath. Faith means focusing on continuing to breathe and to give of one's self -- not focusing on what others are giving or not giving to us. Faith involves positive psychology. Faith is peaceful, calm and self-reliant. It focuses on what one can give to oneself and to others simply by loving and breathing. Faith involves learning how to soothe one's self and others emotionally. Faith is identifying with the ongoing, loving, rebirthing flow of life and trusting in it and finding joy and peace in it. Faith embraces hope. Faith heals traumatized brains.

   To grow in faith, we need to be awed by nature and the universe and open our hearts to other living beings. Faith involves accepting the limitations of our individual wills. Faith involves trusting that there are natural principles operating in life which will bring satisfaction to our lives if we align ourselves with them. As we grow in maturity we can progress from simple, childlike punishment and reward reasoning all the way to understanding universal ethical principles. This can unite us with others who also practice universal ethical principles.

Self-exploratory Question: How can I more faithfully seek to understand the universal principles which support life?

Affirmation: Today I have faith that, as long as I align myself with universal principles which support life, my life will be fulfilling.

February 15
Visualizations

Principle: Clear, positive visualizations can transform negativity and indecisiveness.

Perennial Wisdom Quote: "Far away there in the sunshine are my highest aspirations. I may not reach them, but I can look up and see their beauty, believe in them, and try to follow where they lead." -- Louisa May Alcott

Discussion: Visualizations are images we consciously create to inspire and soothe us. They can help us to slow down our breathing and our heart rate and become more relaxed and less fearful and anxious. For example, if we have difficulty with impulsive explosions of anger, we can visualize steam blowing out of the top of our heads and escaping upward, causing no damage, rather than coming out of our dragon-like nostrils to scorch an opponent. Or we can visualize ourselves quietly leaving the anger-provoking scene and taking a quiet, solitary walk by a calm sea, feeling the sand between our toes and listening to the soothing sound of the waves. Of course, we need to avoid visualizations of graphic revenge and violence. That will only increase our heart and breathing rates and make it more likely that we will act out our anger in punishing ways which will only boomerang back on us.

Visualizations can also be used to clarify our intentions and our hopes. For example, if a person is lonely and wanting a relationship, he or she can visualize becoming so contented and affectionate that a contented and affectionate partner is attracted. Needy people don't attract others. Contented and affectionate people attract everyone.

Self-exploratory Question: What do I visualize and tend to attract to myself?

Affirmation: Today I am using visualizations to calm, soothe and inspire myself.

February 16
Affirmations

Principle: Conscious affirmations can transform negativity and indecisiveness.

Perennial Wisdom Quote: "Thought is creative action. It is neither good nor bad. However, the thoughts that you dwell on determine what you will possess or not possess. What you think about is what you will become…There is an intelligence and a power in all of nature that is creative and responsive. This intelligence is amenable to suggestion from us." -- Wayne Dyer, Ph.D., *Manifest Your Destiny*

Discussion: An affirmation involves making an intention "firm." There are three essential elements to an effective affirmation:

1) It is in the present tense, e.g. "I am…." or "I can..."

2) It is always affirmative rather than negative. e.g. "I am capable and competent."

3) It is always declarative, rather than hopeful. e.g. " I <u>am</u>…." rather than "I'll try…." or "I

should…." or "I want to be…." or "I will…."

Here are a few examples: "I can express my feelings effectively." "I can kindly disagree." "I love my body." "I am agreeable and non-critical." "I can be powerful and still have needs." "I can think before I make someone else's reality my own."

Notice how you feel when you read these affirmations or make up your own affirmations.

Self-exploratory Question: How can I use affirmations to positively direct my mind, emotions and behaviors?

Affirmation: I am becoming more skillful in using affirmations to enhance my life.

February 17
Hope

Principle: Hope can transform fear and despair.

Perennial Wisdom Quote: "To live gloriously, we need hope, not security, the freedom not only to succeed, but to fail and come back. The tragedy of life lies not in failing to reach our goals, but having no hope and thus no goals to reach. -- Dr. Henry Viscardi, founder of the National Center for Disabilities Services

Discussion: Maurice Lamm in *The Power of Hope* wrote that "Hope is power based on yourself -- and it gives you the energy and strength to fight back when adversity strikes." Emily Dickinson poetically described hope as "the thing with feathers that perches in the soul and sings the tune without words and never stops at all." Both authors emphasized internal resources and perseverance.

When most of us lose hope, it is because we are erroneously placing it on other people, places or things. Hope needs a foundation of personal commitment to productively use whatever strengths we have without doing damage to anyone else. Hope also needs a foundation of trust in a power greater than self. This Higher Power can be defined in any way which is most meaningful to you. You can use a concept of "God" or "Goddess." Or you can use a concept of natural universal principles, or of Mother Nature, or of the power of a loving group of people. What is fundamental is that your hope is not based just on ego-defined successes in the external world.

To hope for material riches is premature if we have not yet developed internal riches. We might win a big lottery and end up being miserable and fearful about securing new wealth. Internal riches include self-confidence in one's own ability to make good choices, which will lead to happiness.

Self-exploratory Question: What helps me the most to maintain hopefulness?

Affirmation: Today I am placing my hope on my increased understanding of how to make healthy choices and maintain conscious contact with my Higher Power.

February 18   **Ego-integration**

Principle: Ego-integration and hope transform fear and despair.

Perennial Wisdom Quote: "In the depth of winter, I finally learned that within me there lay an invincible summer." -- Albert Camus

Discussion: Ego integration is recognized by a state of inner peace and deep personal self-responsibility and self-acceptance. It is the result of years of emotional, attitudinal and spiritual maturation which have allowed guidance from a Higher Power and from an Observing Self to create a compassionate and humble Ego Self. Many people take 45-65 years to fully "integrate" their egos, i.e. their healthy senses of self. Some people work hard at it early in life and reach it before age 45. Some people never reach it.

Ego-integration involves discovering our own personal truths on the basis of our own personal experiences and our observations of how our behaviors and other peoples' behaviors interact. People with ego-integration have learned how to eat and exercise in a healthy way. They have learned how to "parent" themselves effectively so they are not dependent on the directions and admonitions of others. They have learned how to moderate their e motions. They have developed a satisfying sense of a Higher Power. They live their lives assertively in line with their own conscious contact with this Higher Power. They engage in love-based, rather than fear-based, behaviors. They are self-disciplined and accepting of appropriate guidelines for respecting others. They know and respect who they are.

Self-exploratory Question: How can I become more and more ego-integrated?

Affirmation: Today I am integrating my ego in healthy, honest and respectful ways.

52

February 19
Contentment

Principle: Contentment transforms criticism, judgment, complaints and comparisons.

Perennial Wisdom Quote: "Most folks are as happy as they make up their minds to be." -- Abraham Lincoln

Discussion: As Lisa Engelhardt puts it in her delightful little book, *Acceptance Therapy:* "Contentment doesn't mean getting all you want, but enjoying what you have." If we focus primarily on satisfying our mental desires for rewards from our external world, we will likely never find real contentment. It is the nature of the mind to always be grasping for "more and more" from our external world. What brings contentment is focusing on our internal world of self-care and principled choices. When we are contented with ourselves, we can lovingly take care of ourselves without hurting anyone else. When we know that we are following our highest inner principles, we experience some contentment no matter what is going on outside of us.

Abraham Lincoln experienced many moments of personal depression and lived in an age of great national and personal tragedy (his own and the nation's civil war). Yet President Lincoln had such great ego strength and hope for his nation and himself personally that he made up his mind to be happy and was able to lead his nation out of chaos and into peaceful restoration. Many religious leaders such as Buddha and Jesus and Muhammad were also revered for their moments of deep contentment. Of course, they were also able to be angry at injustices and hypocrisies around them. But this periodic discontent with what they saw outside of them did not destroy their ability to restore inner contentment and thereby be an inspiration to millions of people.

Self-exploratory Question: What helps me the most to create contentment in my life?

Affirmation: Today I am contented with myself and my choices to follow my inner principles to the best of my ability.

February 20
Cheerfulness

Principle: Cheerfulness transforms criticism, judgments of others, complaints and comparisons.

Perennial Wisdom Quote: "He who rebukes the world is rebuked by the world." -- Rudyard Kipling, *The Second Jungle Book, The Undertakers*

Discussion: On September 14, 2003, *The Los Angeles Times* printed an article with this title: "Germs Just Love Grumps." It summarized the recent scientific discoveries that being "sociable, agreeable, having friends, all of that hug-y, have-a-really-nice-day, you're-looking-great stuff leads to better health." Sheldon Cohen, a psychologist at Carnegie Mellon University in Pittsburgh, scientifically has shown how the most agreeable people are more immune to infection. Cheerfulness pays off.

The Native Americans have this cheerful, ancient chant: "Beauty above me. Beauty below me. Beauty in front of me. Beauty behind me. Beauty all around me." The American *Course in Miracles* teaches, "It will be given you to see your brother's worth when all you want from him is peace. And what you want from him you will receive."

Cheerfulness is contagious, just as is grumpiness. We get to choose what we want to spread around, inside of us, as well as outside of us. If we can't do this on our own, we can consider an anti-depressant medication, psychotherapy and/or a support group.

Self-exploratory Question: What helps me the most to maintain cheerfulness?

Affirmation: Today I am making a choice to be cheerful and boost my own immune system as well as my spirits.

Principle: Clarifying preferences transforms emotion-backed demands and power dynamics.

Perennial Wisdom Quote: "Keep the other person's well-being in mind when you feel an attack of soul-purging truth coming on." -- Betty White

Discussion: Criticisms, judgments, complaints and comparisons usually involve emotion-backed demands for another to be different. They focus, not on one's own internal unmet needs, but on what is perceived to be wrong with another. They are controlling and self-righteous. They are disrespectful to the other and also to one's own trust in a Higher Power.

Clarifying our own preferences is a good substitute for "soul-purging truth" attacks. Rather than saying something like, "Stop being so critical of me," we can say, "I emotionally withdraw from you when I experience you as being critical. Could you please say that more respectfully?" Rather than saying, "Try to behave like your older sister," we can say, "I don't like your behavior right now. Please wait until I finish what I have to say." When others are acting disrespectfully, we need to respectfully clarify the substitute behavior which we would prefer. This polite request for a change of behavior can lovingly connect us to others, rather than push others away.

Self-exploratory Question: When did I last respectfully clarify my preferences, rather than disrespectfully criticize another?

Affirmation: Today I am respectfully clarifying my preferences whenever I feel mistreated.

February 22   **Accepting Different**
Temperaments

Principle: Accepting different temperaments transforms emotion-backed demands and power dynamics.

Perennial Wisdom Quote: "Truly loving relationships, like transcendent experiences, are always a widening of focus of attention, a detachment rather than an attachment." -- Ralph Metner

Discussion: Different people have different temperaments and different ways of experiencing reality and relating to others. When we are unaware of these differences and expect everyone to be like ourselves, we are disrespectful and create confusion and misunderstanding. We are not only disrespectful to other people but also to the Higher Power which creates so much diversity in the world.

The Meyers-Briggs Temperament Inventory (based on Carl Jung's teachings) identifies different temperament continuums: introvert/extrovert, feeling/thinking, sensation/intuition, judging/perceiving. Some people are gratified more by many social contacts. Others prefer more time alone and less social contact. Some people organize their experiences more by feelings and others more by thoughts. Some people rely more on their senses for information, and others rely more on their intuition. Some people organize their experiences more with internal judgments and others more with perception and senses.

If we are irritated or confused by another's behavior, it is likely because we have different temperaments. By trying to understand and accept another's temperament, conflicts can be resolved. It's worth taking time to learn this practice.

Self-exploratory Question: When did I last accept another's different temperament?

Affirmation: Today I am understanding and accepting others' different temperaments.

February 23
Calmness

Principle: Calmness transforms irritability, drama and impetuousness.

Perennial Wisdom Quote: "You must learn to be still in the midst of activity, and to be vibrantly alive in repose." -- Indira Gandhi

Discussion: Irritability usually happens when our beliefs suit our minds, but not our external situations. It happens when we are blaming others for our feelings, when we are stressed, hormonally challenged, light deprived, tired, hungry or lonely. Irritability and drama thrive where there is insecurity and competition for leadership and control.

Calmness thrives when we take regular time for quiet space and meditation. This means turning off the TV and reading an inspirational or meditative book, or closing one's eyes and quietly watching one's thoughts slow down as one breathes more deeply and pulls awareness away from the outer world.

Nature gives us sleep to restore our bodies and minds. We also need periodic, wakeful moments of quietness and calm in order to stay emotionally centered through the day, avoiding mood swings and over-reactions to external stimulation. Each of us is responsible for creating such quiet moments for ourselves on a regular basis, even if this means just retreating occasionally to a private bathroom which is peaceful and soothing. If you have no other private space, put some meditative aids in your bathroom and keep it simple, clean and quiet. Retreat there, or to some other calming place on a regular basis. Use visualizations, if a suitable outer location isn't readily available. As Mark Twain said, "Calmness is a language that the deaf can hear and the blind can read." It's good for the body and the mind, yours as well as others'.

Self-exploratory Question: How can I create space and time for calmness?

Affirmation: Today I am creating periodic time for internal peace and calmness.

February 24
Serenity

Principle: Serenity transforms irritability, drama and impetuousness.

Perennial Wisdom Quote: "You cannot perceive beauty but with a serene mind." -- Henry David Thoreau

Discussion: The well-known "Serenity Prayer" reads: "God, grant me the serenity to accept the things I cannot change, the courage to change the things I can, and the wisdom to know the difference." Serenity involves acceptance, courage and wisdom. People who put a lot of energy into trying to make other people behave the way they want them to usually are not very serene people. We cannot control other people, places and things. When we attach to trying to do so, we become irritable and unpleasant. We strain our relationships, and others start avoiding us.

When we focus on observing our own thoughts, emotions and behaviors and doing our best to align them with wise principles, life becomes much more satisfying. We also start feeling much more self-empowered, as well as positively related to others.

Practicing silence, unless we have something really important to say, is also an important aid to developing serenity. When we fill our minds with constant chatter, it is difficult to focus on vital self-care. Practicing ongoing self-awareness, both of our inner self-talk and of the results of our outer actions takes energy and attention, especially if we want to align this self-talk and behavior with healthy life principles. The effort promotes serenity and is very rewarding.

Self-exploratory Question: What helps me most to experience serenity?

Affirmation: Today I am practicing behaviors and self-talk which promote serenity.

February 25
Compassion

Principle: Compassion transforms selfishness, indifference, cruelty and abuse.

Perennial Wisdom Quote: "Once when I was going through a very difficult time, my husband touched his fingers to the tears winding down my face, then touched his wet finger to his own cheek. His gesture spoke volumes to me. It said: 'Your tears run down _my_ face, too. Your suffering aches inside _my_ heart as well. I share your wounded place.'"-- Sue Monk Kidd, _Communion, Community, Commoweal,_ John Mogabgab, Ed.

Discussion: When we are being compassionate, we are not being critical or judgmental of another Instead, we are recognizing that the other is doing the best he or she can within the limits of his or her current beliefs and capabilities. As Dan Millman suggests in his _The Laws of Spirit,_ we can all learn compassion by studying the Earth herself. We tread on her skin. We cut and burn her trees. We exploit her wealth without thinking of asking permission or giving thanks and yet, Mother Earth continues to offer up her great beauty and bounty to us. She has the energy to keep showing us, through her own example, how to live bountifully upon her great lap.

Acceptance of ourselves and of others is foundational to compassion. Then comes understanding. Then comes love and compassion. When we are not being treated compassionately by others, it is likely because they are self-rejecting and also have not learned how to understand others. They dwell in ignorance and emotional darkness. To reduce the violence and abuse in the world, we need to help turn on the lights, not fight with the darkness.

Self-exploratory Question: When was I last able to respond to another with compassion, even when I was being unfairly treated?

Affirmation: Today I choose to respond to others with respect and compassion, even when I see myself as being mistreated.

Principle: Step Two of the Wise Ways Happiness Program is: "We become willing to accept reality and to surrender our ego-minds to love, not to fear."

Perennial Wisdom Quote: "But I say to you who hear, love your enemies. Do good to those who hate you." -- Jesus, *The Bible,* Luke 6:27

Discussion: Happiness Step Two involves learning to practice love rather than attachment and hatred. What causes attachment and hatred and gets in the way of genuine love more than anything else is fear. Fear is a mental creation of the "low brain." (See Appendix 1.)

When the low brain's amygdala becomes excited, the message is sent to the heart to beat faster and blood flows away from our feet and hands, towards the heart, chest and pelvic areas, facilitating a fight or flight response. When this is going on in our bodies, but we are facing no real physical danger, our bodies are stressed for no reason and our mind's judgment abilities are short circuited in the brain. If we have trained our minds to attach to fearful thoughts and expectations about others, there is little room for the growth of real love.

Love requires a brain functioning well in its "higher centers" not just in its lower limbic centers. When the higher centers of our brain are not functioning well because our low brains are so excited, fear tends to escalate easily into anger and the anger tends to get acted out. We become blind to the grief and loss which underlies our fear. Our problem-solving skills disappear. Rather than thinking, "How can I heal this grief and loss?" we think, "How can I change or punish this person?" Love then disappears.

Self-exploratory Question: When did I last experience love overcoming fear?

Affirmation: Today I am practicing accepting reality and opening my mind to love.

February 27   **Happiness Groups' Tradition Two: Anonymity &
Confidentiality**

Principle: Tradition Two is: "Personal anonymity and confidentiality (use of first names only at meetings, and respect for confidential sharing) are the foundation of trust in the Wise Ways Happiness Program."

Perennial Wisdom Quote: "Never spend time with people who don't respect you." -- Maori saying

Discussion: Tradition Two of the Wise Ways Happiness Program focuses on respect and trust. To help ourselves and each other we must respect ourselves and each other, as well as trust ourselves and each other. In group meetings we introduce ourselves by our first names only. If there is more than one John or Mary in a group, we add our last initials. Sharing of phone numbers or e-mail addresses is completely voluntary, as is socializing with each other outside of meetings. We also don't gossip about each other or share outside of meetings who said what. "What we say here, let it stay here," is posted at all our meetings. This tradition allows each member to feel completely comfortable, if he or she so chooses, to talk about intimate problems and situations. None of us want our private experiences shared with strangers. We need to be able to share our life stories and challenges without worrying who else, other than those in the room, will hear about them.

We are, of course, free to share with others the principles which we talk about in our meetings. We just don't reveal personal material which is shared in meetings. In this way we learn how to be more respectful and trusting of ourselves, as well as others.

Self-exploratory Question: How can I better practice respect for others' privacy and anonymity?

Affirmation: Today I am trustworthy and respectful in all my communications.

February 28
Gentleness

Principle: Gentleness transforms selfishness, indifference, cruelty and abuse.

Perennial Wisdom Quote: "The softest things in the world overcome the hardest things in the world." -- Lao Tze, *The Way of Lao Tze*

Discussion: Gently flowing water, over time, carves out rock. Lapping waves break down stones into sand. A gentle parent's soothing voice and body allows a child to yield angry, harsh words. Flowers, soft flute music, and gentle stroking can open hard human hearts. The violence which occurs in the world springs from unhealed past trauma or deprivation. Gentleness usually accompanies acceptance and understanding.

Try envisioning an enemy hurt and in the arms of a parent or another loved one. Try imagining the trauma or loss which has hardened your enemy's heart. Do you experience your own heart softening some and your own thoughts becoming gentler?

As a leading psychologist said to a recent audience, "We are all Bozos on the same bus." Identifying with others and experiencing our common humanity usually promotes gentleness. Of course, we first need to be gentle with ourselves.

Self-exploratory Question: When did I last experience giving or receiving gentle touch or words?

Affirmation: Today I am practicing gentleness of mind, heart and action.

(The February 29th reading for leap year is placed after the Dec. 31ˢᵗ reading.)

March 1
Kindness

Principle: Kindness transforms selfishness, indifference, cruelty and abuse.

Perennial Wisdom Quote: "My religion is kindness." -- The Dalai Lama, *Ethics For A New Millennium*

Discussion: In order to express kindness, we need to accept differences and accept responsibility for managing our own fears. Most acts of cruelty and selfishness stem from fear and intolerance of differences. When we are frozen in fear or overwhelmed with greed or envy, we can not experience kindness. When we are afraid, our observing ego capacities shrink, and our minds become absorbed in protecting ourselves from pain, both emotional and physical. This is unpreventable when we are in immediate physical danger. Our restless minds can imagine all sorts of dangers which block our willingness to offer acts of kindness.

We all need to practice daily acts of kindness as much as we all need to earn a daily living. If we don't express kindness, how can we possibly expect others to do so? As Bylle Avery, founder of the National Black Women's Health Project, once said, "Practicing the Golden Rule is not a sacrifice; it's an investment." Sonya Lyubomirsky, a Professor of Psychology at Stanford, did research in 2004 which established that asking people to daily do five random acts of kindness reliably increased their level of positive emotion. Kindness benefit's the giver, not just the receiver.

Self-exploratory Question: When did I last experience giving or receiving an act of kindness?

Affirmation: Today I look for opportunities to be kind.

March 2   **Fair-**
mindedness

Principle: Fair-mindedness transforms indifference and injustice.

Perennial Wisdom Quote: "None of you is a believer until you like for others what you like for yourself." -- Muhammad, *The Hadith*

Discussion: If a person has a history of lots of hurt and trauma, hyper-vigilant self-protection often over-rides fair-mindedness. "Do to others the same damage they have done to you" revengeful thinking can easily replace the Golden Rule of doing unto others what you would want done unto you. All the major world religions were founded by teachers of some version of the Golden Rule.

Fair-mindedness requires a calm and knowledgeable mind and a loving heart. Such a mind and heart can usually see that, "What goes around, comes around." In Hinduism and Buddhism, this is referred to as "karma." The kind of actions we take towards others will eventually come back to us or to our descendants. Christianity bases its teaching of fair-mindedness on the love ethic: "This is my commandment, that you love one another as I have loved you." (Jesus in *The Bible,* John 15:12) Muhammad stated clearly that all true believers in God "like for others" what they like for themselves.

Whatever our religious orientation, to be fair-minded requires respect for others and also a belief that fair-mindedness is somehow rewarded, if not in one's life, at least in the "hereafter" or in the lives of one's descendants.

Self-exploratory Question: What most supports me in maintaining fair-mindedness?

Affirmation: Today I am practicing fair-mindedness in all my interactions.

Selfishness

Principle: Selfishness is transformed when the heart opens to compassion and kindness.

Perennial Wisdom Quote: "All the joy the world contains has come through wishing happiness for others. All the misery the world contains has come through wanting pleasure for oneself." -- Shantideva, *The Way of the Bodhisattva*

Discussion: Addiction promotes selfishness. One's entire energy becomes focused on getting what one wants -- be it a drug, money, power, or whatever. To be free from selfishness one needs to be free from addiction. To be free from selfishness a person also needs to know the difference between self-care and selfishness. Self-care involves taking the necessary time and energy to be sure one's own body, mind and spirit are sustained and replenished. Without this kind of self-care none of us can effectively be helpful to another. Selfishness involves grasping, attachment, addiction and obsessively focusing on personal pleasures or power. It involves a lack of empathy for others and a lack of belief that "What goes around comes around."

To be free from selfishness we have to be individuated enough to practice good self-care and also empathic enough to be kind and compassionate toward others. It is a day by day, hour by hour challenge to raise mental energy above our primitive, clutching low brains, up into higher areas of our brains where causes and effects can be comprehended and wise choices made.

Self-exploratory Question: How do I seek to free myself from selfishness?

Affirmation: Today I am focusing on substituting kindness and compassion for selfishness.

March 4
Humor

Principle: Healthy humor transforms over-seriousness, hostile teasing and sarcasm.

Perennial Wisdom Quote: "In laughter there is always a kind of joyousness that is incompatible with contempt or indignation." -- Voltaire

Discussion: True humor is identifiable by the belly laughs which erupt in both the jokester and the listener. Norman Cousins in 1976 wrote *Anatomy of An Illness* in which he told of his discovering that ten minutes of solid belly laughter would give him two hours of pain-free sleep. He was suffering from severe inflammation of his spine and joints. It was painful even to turn over in bed. He was given a very poor prognosis for recovery. Rather than staying in a hospital he checked himself into a hotel, located hours of comedy videos and laughed himself to sleep and eventually back to health. Humor is healing!

Seriousness sometimes masks arrogance, fear or self-righteousness. Humor is the best medicine for curing these ailments. This is why many cultures have used clowns as a way to create joy and irreverence to balance the sacredness of ceremony. Many Native American cultures have "sacred clowns." These clowns have arduous preparation, to cleanse them of their own "un-harnessed forces," i.e., ego issues. Then they have the tasks of teaching children by acting out bad example, and by mocking adults who are too pompous during the community rituals. Their job is to point out the need for order and respect for others by showing, in culturally acceptable ways, the results of disorder and of egotism. Sanctioned community clowning prevents leaders from becoming dictatorial and out of touch with their people. Perhaps cartoonists and late-night comedy TV shows are modern sacred clowns.

Self-exploratory Question: How can I bring more laughter and healthy humor into my personal and community life?

Affirmation: Today I am making time for humor and my own form of "sacred clowning."

Principle: Sarcasm is transformed by healthy humor and playfulness.

Perennial Wisdom Quote: "Humor simultaneously wounds and heals, indicts and pardons, diminishes and enlarges; it constitutes inner growth at the expense of outer gain, and those who possess and honestly practice it make themselves more through a willingness to make themselves less." -- Louis Kronenberger

Discussion: Sarcasm is not healthy humor. The root meaning of the word "sarcasm" literally means "the tearing of flesh." Sarcasm's intention is usually to put another person down, rather than to lighten up a stressful situation. Healthy humor may involve poking fun at one's self or another, but the intention is always to heal, enlarge, grow and pardon. In sarcasm the intention is to tear down, not facilitate healthy change.

If a person is subjected to sarcasm by an intimate other, the best way to respond is to be direct with a statement like, "I don't feel deserving of that put-down" or "Are you having a bad day? Do you mean to be putting me down?" Assertively confronting the aggressive sarcasm can begin to heal the conflict, if both people are motivated to stay intimate. With strangers, however, usually just ignoring the sarcasm and walking away is the best policy, especially if you can choose to have no further dealings with the person.

Self-exploratory Question: What helps me the most to avoid sarcasm?

Affirmation: Today I choose to engage in only healthy humor, not sarcasm.

March 6
Gratitude

Principle: Gratitude transforms self-pity and victim attitude.

Perennial Wisdom Quote: "Life's under no obligation to give us what we expect. We take what we get and are thankful it's no worse than it is." -- Margaret Mitchell

Discussion: Gratitude is the willingness to be thankful for what already is. Gratitude helps us to stay focused on what we are receiving in the present, rather than focusing on what we didn't receive in the past. The Polish say, "The giver should forget, but the receiver should remember forever." Since our objects of focus are magnified by attention, this kind of focusing brings more and more joy to our hearts, and tends to attract other joyful people.

When counting your blessings, include anything which has brought joy to your heart, lightened your burdens, increased your endurance, expanded your understanding, increased your compassion, tested your strength, forced you to grow, or reminded you to treasure your relations and your life. Obviously, some of these things might not have been pleasant when you went through them, but, nevertheless, you can be grateful for what you learned in the process.

People who have little gratitude are usually people who are not learning from their experiences. They are dependent people who rely on others to gratify their needs, and then are resentful when they don't get what they want. Such people are hurtful to healthy people, so healthy people tend to avoid them. In order to have satisfying adult relationships, we have to learn independence and gratitude. Once we have developed these traits, others are more attracted to us and are more available to help us.

Self-exploratory Question: How can I develop more gratitude in my heart and mind?

Affirmation: Today I am filling my heart and mind with gratitude for what already is.

Principle: A victim attitude is transformed by gratitude and understanding.

Perennial Wisdom Quote: "Some people are profoundly unhappy because they have lost a sense of gratitude. They can speak only of rights. No gifts can bring joy to one who has a right to everything." -- Paul Tourier, *The Meaning of Gifts*

Discussion: Gratefulness can be learned and is the only appropriate attitude toward life. Gratefulness dissolves impatience and irritability. It helps us to detach from what is out of our control. Gratefulness is a "Yes" to life which dissolves victim attitude. It accepts the fact that life is a gift, not a right or a privilege. If we accept life each day, each hour, as a gift, we can focus on all the blessings in it, even if we are surrounded by sorrow and pain.

When we begin to take life for granted and expect others to make it worthwhile for us, we remain emotional children. Emotional adulthood means taking responsibility for our own physical, financial, spiritual and emotional needs. Emotional childhood means expecting others to take care of them for us. Emotional adulthood means doing our share of the subsistence work if we are part of a family. Responsible subsistence work needs to start when we are little children and gradually grow with our physical strength and mental abilities. Young adults need to accept the responsibilities which go along with the freedoms of adulthood. Spouses need to assume responsibility for being functional adults and not make a partner into a parent or a child. When all this happens, we all are happier and more peaceful.

Self-exploratory Question: How can I avoid having a victim attitude?

Affirmation: Today I am freeing myself from any victim attitude.

Principle: The Third Step of the Wise Ways Happiness Program is "We decide to trust a Higher Power or energy of our own understanding, one which supports life, love, nature, beauty, harmony, freedom and diversity."

Perennial Wisdom Quote: "Always in observing nature look at one and every creature; nothing's outside that's not within. For nature has no heart or skin. All at once that way you'll see the sacred open mystery. True seeing is the joy it gives, the joy of serious playing. Nothing is single if it lives, but multiple is its being." -- Goethe, *Epirrhema*

Discussion: The view that we are all separate is an illusion. The deeper we look into the natural world, the more we see how interconnected everything is. We literally breathe in and swallow new cells which have formerly been part of other persons, plants and animals. How we behave affects, not only ourselves, but others as well as the plants, animals, minerals and space around us. Trusting in these interconnections and the principles which sustain them is a big part of trusting in a Higher Power. When we don't have this trust, we tend to fall into the illusion of separateness and become self-centered, angry and controlling. When we have this trust, we become interested in and generous towards all that exists seemingly around us, but which is also in us.

We can accept our own chosen religion's definition of a Higher Power, or we can define our own. We can even be agnostic or atheistic and do this. What is important is that we recognize that there are energies and wisdoms greater than our own.

Self-exploratory Question: How can I expand my trust in a Higher Power of my own understanding?

Affirmation: Today I am trusting in a Higher Power of my own understanding.

March 9   Happiness Program Tradition Three: Clear Purpose and Mutual Support

Principle: The Third Tradition of the Happiness Program is: "The primary purpose of Happiness Support Group meetings is to study this *365 Wise Ways to Happiness* book and to support each other in the practice of the Wise Ways Happiness Program."

Perennial Wisdom Quote: "Vision without action is a daydream. Action without vision is a nightmare." -- Japanese proverb

Discussion: Groups can be either healthy or destructive. When a group's purpose is clear and positive and its members stay focused on it, individuals' energies are magnified and grow geometrically. When a group's purpose is virtuous self-education and mutual support, hearts as well as minds grow. The resulting positive changes can seem miraculous.

The Wise Ways slogans, "How important is it?" and "Principles, not personalities" can be helpful. Group members can even dislike one another and yet benefit from each other's presence in a meeting, by listening and accepting. Since Happiness Support groups don't have leadership hierarchy, there is no need to argue over privilege or territory. Since Happiness Support groups own no property and each group is self-supporting, there is no need for individuals or groups to become competitive. Staying away from gossip, from giving direct feedback to others during meetings, and from talking about other group members, allows plenty of time to stay focused on studying the Wise Ways Happiness principles. By sharing stories of success and struggle in applying the principles of the Program, everyone learns and benefits.

Self-exploratory Question: When I participate in groups, do I stay focused on the group's primary purpose and offer support to others?

Affirmation: When I participate in a group meeting, I stay focused on clear purpose and mutual support.

March 10   **Freedom from False Pride &**
Narcissism

Principle: Arrogance and false pride are transformed by humility.

Perennial Wisdom Quote: "If you do good, keep it a secret; if you receive good, make it known." -- Lebanese proverb

Discussion: When we reject the shadowy parts of ourselves and mentally separate ourselves from others, our minds tend to tell us that we are better than others, or at least more important than others. Humility is a very important part of emotional self-care. Humility is the healthy middle point on the continuum between feelings of unworthiness and feelings of prideful entitlement. When a person has healthy self-pride, he or she is self-confident, but can also maintain a "beginner's mind" in terms of confronting new experiences and new people. This means being open to new learning and not assuming superior knowledge to others. Wise people accept the limitations of their knowledge and they also do not compare themselves to others. They just keep humbly learning from each new experience.

Narcissism is a Freudian term drawn from the Greek myth of Narcissus, a man who fell in love with his own reflection. It is used to describe a person who is very self-absorbed, harboring an exaggerated sense of his own importance and uniqueness. A person with these problems tends to lack empathy for others and to take advantage of others in the interest of self-promotion. Narcissistic attitudes actually grow out of emotional insecurity. Emotionally secure people tend to be naturally empathic with others and naturally interested in others. In order to avoid narcissism, if we are disappointed in relationships, we need to look inside ourselves for ways to change our choices so that our relationships can become more satisfying.

Self-exploratory Question: How can I stay free of arrogance and false pride?

Affirmation: Today I am practicing humility and "beginner's mind" along with empathy for others.

March 11   **Freedom from Self-destructive, Impulsive**
Behavior

Principle: Avoiding impulsive behavior ourselves, and not rescuing others from theirs, brings true independence.

Perennial Wisdom Quote: "Contracts break rescues." – Bruce Bibee, Counselor

Discussion: Rescuing others from the negative consequences of their impulsive behaviors is always a mistake. Instead contract with impulsive loved-ones so as to discourage their self-destructive behaviors.

Impulsive, acting-out behaviors are the result of unresolved emotional dependency issues. The impulsive individual imagines that the drinking, drug-using, over-eating, over-spending, power-hungry, stealing, lying or reckless sexual or driving behavior will establish independence from constraints created by others. This is common adolescent reasoning, but it is faulty reasoning. The constraints are not created by others. They are created by physical, adult, emotional or financial realities which are impossible to escape.

True adult independence only comes from recognizing and accepting the above physical, emotional and financial realities. It comes from recognizing that impulsive choices and rescuing choices are usually self-sabotaging choices which lead, not to adult independence, but rather to child-like dependence.

Self-exploratory Question: When have my impulsive or rescuing behaviors sabotaged my adult independence or the independence of others?

Affirmation: I avoid impulsive and rescuing behaviors so as to remain truly independent.

March 12
Moderation

Principle: Moderation creates freedom and satisfaction.

Perennial Wisdom Quote: "Happiness is found in the golden middle of two extremes." -- Aristotle

Discussion: Ancient philosophers have written a lot about the merits of moderation. Publilius Syrus said, "No pleasure lasts long unless there is variety in it." Homer said, "Too much rest itself becomes a pain." Aristotle actually defined virtue as "the mean by reference to two vices: the one of excess and the other of deficiency." Epictetus said, "All philosophy lies in two words, sustain and abstain."

Many proverbs speak to the same theme: "Sorrow doesn't kill. Reckless joy does." (West African) "Don't sail out further than you can row back." (Danish) "Even God can't make two mountains without a valley in between." (Gaelic)

So why is moderation so difficult in the modern world? Likely it has always been difficult, but modern technology and the great economic divides between the rich and the poor make it easier for some to be excessive and greedy.

The antidote is a clear understanding of how real happiness can only exist when we are aligning our choices with the balances inherent in the natural world. If we imbalance our bodies or our minds and our planet with greedy grasping, the result is always suffering. If we balance our bodies and our minds and our planet with humility, empathy for others, and acceptance of nature's limits, we thrive.

Self-exploratory Question: How can I practice more moderation in my life?

Affirmation: Today I am practicing moderation in all things.

March 13
Balance

Principle: Balance transforms addiction, obsession, greed and escapes from reality.

Perennial Wisdom Quote: "..for all objects and experiences there is a quantity that has optimum value. Above that quantity, the variable becomes toxic. To fall below that value is to be deprived." -- Gregory Bateson, *Mind and Nature*

Discussion: It is vital to realize that pleasure and pain exist on a continuum and that excesses on both ends of the continuum need to be avoided. This lesson is everywhere in nature, but it still seems difficult for the willful human mind to grasp. Recent human brain research shows when the pleasure-producing chemicals of the brain are over- produced, there is an inevitable later swing towards a depletion of these chemicals. The result is depression. This is why cocaine and heroin and other "street" drugs are so dangerous. Fermented sugars creating alcohol are also dangerous because, when used in small amounts, they cause an inhibition of anxiety, but when used in large amounts, they cause chemical depression in the brain. Other pleasures such as sex and food are healthy for the body when experienced moderately

When indulged in excessively to escape depression or anxiety, they also can become dangerous. There is no escaping the need for balance in all aspects of life. It is built into our very cells and life maintenance processes.

Humble minds which accept this principle can create happiness and serenity. Willful minds which try to be superhuman and defy these natural balances eventually self-destruct.

Self-exploratory Question: How can I create balance in all aspects of my life?

Affirmation: Today I am creating more and more joyful balance in my life.

March 14   Non-
possessiveness

Principle: Non-possessiveness leads to tranquility.

Perennial Wisdom Quote: "Those who want much are always much in need."--
Horace

Discussion: The world's literature has many references to the virtues of voluntary simplicity and non-possessiveness. Now that the planet's growing human population and the use of fossil fuels is threatening to destroy the ecosystem, the need for voluntary simplicity isn't just preferential; it's a matter of planetary survival. Great disparity between the "haves" and the "have-nots" is also the breeding ground for violence. Modern weaponry threatens the survival of the human species, especially when huge inequities exist between nations. Therefore, learning to distinguish between needs and wants and generously sharing whatever excess resources we have is the modern world's best defense against terrorism and best assurance for security.

Siddhartha Gotama (The Buddha) was born a wealthy prince in India and yet, once he learned about the suffering and poverty of others, he gave up his material wealth and spent his life teaching about the dangers of attachment to material possessions. Islam and Christianity also teach about the importance of generosity and the spiritual difficulties which riches bestow.

Martin Seligman, Ph.D., positive psychology's pioneering researcher, found that wealth has a surprisingly low correlation with happiness levels. So next time you consider buying something in an attempt to make yourself happy, ask yourself, "Do I really need this?"

Self-exploratory Question: How can I reduce my possessions and lead a simpler life?

Affirmation: Today I am buying only what I need. I am practicing non-possessiveness.

Principle: Freedom from greed is true freedom, indeed.

Perennial Wisdom Quote: "A man builds a fine house, and now he has a master, and a task for life; he has to furnish, watch, show it, and keep it in repair the rest of his days." -- R.W. Emerson, *Society and Solitude*

Discussion: Alexis de Tocqueville, the famous 19th century Frenchman who wrote *Democracy in America,* commented about the United States, "I know of no country, indeed where the love of money has taken a stronger hold on the affections of men." Soon after, Charles Alexander Eastman (Ohiyesa), a Santee Sioux physician who was instrumental in founding the Boy Scouts and the Campfire Girls, wrote, "It was our belief that the love of possessions is a weakness to be overcome."

In the modern world today extreme greed and extreme generosity live side by side. But the extreme greed side of modern Western culture is what is most visible to the rest of the world. Corporations, undisciplined by appropriate governmental legislation, are unabashedly greedy. This is a major social challenge in the 21st century. Each of us in the modern Western world need to be part of the solution to this problem by seeing amassing material possessions as a "weakness", not as a sign of "success." We also need to be willing to elect governmental representatives who are willing to represent common people, not just large corporations and rich individuals who donate money for political campaigns. We need to enact election reforms which make this possible.

Self-exploratory Question: How can I better overcome personal as well as corporate and governmental greed?

Affirmation: Today I am prioritizing personal freedom over material wealth.

March 16
Simplicity

Principle: Simplicity breeds greatness and joy.

Perennial Wisdom Quote: "All the big people are simple, as simple as the unexplored wilderness. They love the universal things that are free to everybody. Light and air and food and love and some work are enough. In the varying phases of these cheap and common things the great lives have found their joy." -- Carl Sandburg

Discussion: Simplicity comes from finding joy in everything which has no price tag on it -- sunshine, trees, flowers, loving hearts, clear air breezes, white sand beaches. When we don't know how to bring these sustaining experiences into our lives, we become workaholic and materialistically greedy. Possessions weigh us down. We can't move into new joyous experiences nearly as readily when we are preoccupied with securing and maintaining possessions. And what is most satisfying to most people is change and loving connection to others. The Shakers put it this way is their song, "Simple Gifts": "When true simplicity is gained, to bow and to bend we shall not be ashamed; to turn, to turn will be our delight, 'til by turning, turning we come round right."

Modern psychological studies have shown that most people in the United States who make a moderate middle income are just as happy as most millionaires. Happiness is correlated more with gratitude, emotional intelligence, good social support networks and spirituality than it is correlated with wealth.

Self-exploration Question: How can I simplify my life and make it more satisfying?

Affirmation: Today I am prioritizing simplicity and inner satisfaction.

Principle: The "4 R's" of Planetary Competency are: Reduce, Reuse, Recycle and Redesign.

Perennial Wisdom Quote: "The frog does not drink up the pond in which he lives." -- Sioux proverb

Discussion: The human population has grown more since 1950 than it did during the previous four million years. At the current human population growth level, starvation will become a common human problem. The development of energy sources which don't pollute our planet is happening in some areas, but it is not nearly widespread enough. Many governments are still dependent on fossil fuel consumption. Many citizen voters still do not believe in the seriousness of our environmental pollution problems. Industries which recycle our waste still do not receive enough governmental support. Non-polluting public transportation is still not sufficiently supported by the public. The building of simpler, smaller, less costly, more energy efficient houses, condos and apartments is still not given priority.

If each of us is not a part of the solution to these problems, each of us become part of the problem. At the community and individual level some progress is being made but, at national levels still there is much denial and avoidance of these essential challenges.

Self-discovery Question: What am I doing to Reduce, Reuse, Recycle and Redesign in my life?

Affirmation: Today I am reducing my consumption, reusing consumables, recycling waste, and redesigning my life so as to heal our planet.

Principle: Coveting and stealing lead to dissatisfaction and unhappiness.

Perennial Wisdom Quote: "Every man takes care that his neighbor shall not cheat him. But a day comes when he begins to care that he does not cheat his neighbor. Then all goes well. He has changed his market cart into a chariot of the sun." -- R.W. Emerson

Discussion: One of the Hindu "yamas" (moral constraints) translates as "non-stealing." This involves not only abstaining from taking what does not belong to us, but also abstaining from coveting more than what is necessary for basic living.

"Coveting" is an old-fashioned word originally meaning wanting the possessions or experiences of others. It can also be defined as desiring more than one's fair share of the world's natural resources, and more than what one really needs for simple living.

All forms of modern advertising promote this kind of coveting. We are encouraged by modern informational technology and corporate power to be always shopping. So how can we utilize the benefits of this technology and personal spending power to lead a simple, non-consumer-oriented life? The task is daunting.

We need to take personal responsibility, somehow, for not allowing advertising to cause us to buy things which we really don't need. We can share what we can with others, those of us with money to spend after we have secured our basic needs, can find ways to use our extra money to help relieve others' suffering. As our population grows there will be more and more of it. We can learn to take as much pleasure in giving as in receiving. We can begin to see our tax money as our sharing money, our governments as our collective consumers. We can vote so as to keep our government's spending according to healthy collective values. We can maintain healthy personal lives and also healthy national infrastructures. We can be respectful of ourselves as well as other human beings.

Self-exploratory Question: How can I abstain from coveting and stealing? How can I help my government to support healthy common values?

Affirmation: Today I am abstaining both from stealing and coveting. I am valuing giving as much as receiving.

Principle: Perfectionism is transformed by fluidity of action and flexibility of thought.

Perennial Wisdom Quote: "The willows bend and do not break. The lesson is -- rigidity will bring defeat." *Mother Nature Is Our Teacher, a* Yakima Indian Nation Museum publication

Discussion: Perfectionism can become an obsessive addiction, just as food or drugs can become an addiction. In perfectionism there is a self-righteous drive to always excel in one's own and others' eyes. Since we all learn from making mistakes and each individual has unique strengths and shortcomings, reaching for perfection creates frustration and alienation. It also blocks creative learning. When perfectionistic people suffer an emotional pain or limitation, rather than listening to that pain so that it becomes a gain, they see it as a loss and run away from it. They shame themselves whenever the results of their efforts do not meet their expectations.

        Emotionally free people know how to detach from the outcomes of their behaviors. They are principled people who do their best to meet daily challenges, but they do not set idealistic goals and then chastise themselves when they are not met. Instead they focus on their daily intentions, following them to the best of their abilities and then accepting whatever happens. They also do not lay idealistic expectations on their loved ones. They choose principled, honest, and companionable friends, and they accept their shortcomings along with their strengths. They do not criticize others. Rather they notice others' strengths and comment on them with appreciation. They do not expect approval and praise, and they find joy in life's natural pleasures. Being emotionally free in this way is much better than being perfect.

Self-exploratory Question: How can I free myself from perfectionistic ideals? How can I accept my disappointments without being self-critical?

Affirmation: Today I am replacing perfectionistic ideals with realistic intentions.

Principle: Obsessions are transformed by fluidity and flexibility of thought and by balanced brains.

Perennial Wisdom Quote: "To be elated at success and disappointed at failure is to be a child of circumstances; how can such a one be called a master of himself?" -- Chinese proverb

  Discussion: When we give ourselves permission only to be elated at outer success, when we are disappointed with failure, we set ourselves up for trying to control the uncontrollable. When we persist in impossible efforts to control externals, we create painful obsessions. The obsessive behaviors themselves create pain, and yet we delude ourselves into thinking they will remove the pain.

  Obsessions are ways to escape really feeling the pain of life. We distract ourselves so we don't have to feel painful emotions. What we don't feel, we can't heal, so our avoidant behavior just becomes more intense. Depression is the inevitable result. Fortunately, psychotherapy, healthy support groups and certain medications (such as the serotonin reuptake inhibitors) all are helpful in recovering from obsessions. But before we can cure our obsessions, we must recognize them and get help.

  Striving for riches, fame and power, cleanliness and approval, are all socially sanctioned efforts, but they can become harmful obsessions. Prioritizing inner peace, balance and health in our lives can help bring enough humility to seek help for damaging obsessions.

Self-exploratory Question: How can I free my life from damaging obsessions?

Affirmation: Today I am balancing my life with fluid and flexible thoughts.

March 21
Flexibility

Principle: Flexibility transforms obsessiveness and perfectionism.

Perennial Wisdom Quote: "…'flow' is the period in the creative process when self-consciousness disappears, time vanishes or becomes full, and there is total absorption in the activity. There is an intense clarity about the moment and a sense of clear movement, and there is little or no concern for failure." -- John Briggs and David Peat, *Seven Life Lessons of Chaos*

Discussion: Obsessions and perfectionism are about the fear of letting go, of deeply experiencing and accepting the flow of life. This fear blocks the creative process. Creativity requires flexibility. It requires the acceptance of change and movement. It requires total absorption in a creative process, rather than self-absorption and attachment to some mental concept of success or perfection. Here are seven steps which can help to break out of avoidance and rigidity: 1) Recognize and accept your present feeling experience; 2) Breathe deeply and relax your muscles; 3) Shift your focus from your mind to your heart and concentrate on sending your breath to your heart for at least ten seconds; 4) Recall a time, situation and place in which you felt loved and peaceful; 5) Let go of your previous obsessive thoughts, accepting them as simply escapes from your feelings; 6) Experience whatever is with you in the moment, accepting it; 7) If you can't do the above six things, seek help from a mental health specialist.

Self-exploratory Question: How can a practice more "flow" in my life?

Affirmation: Today I am flowing with my present experience, without resistance.

March 22
Happiness

Principle: Happiness is an inside job.

Perennial Wisdom Quote: "Happiness does not depend on external or physical comforts or pleasures, but proper moral conduct and related self-satisfaction." -- Socrates

Discussion: Short cuts to happiness through relationships, adventure, food, drugs, alcohol, etc., just don't work. Taking the principled, internal path to happiness, though it may be long, is the only path that really gets us there.

There are many ancient philosophies which teach that being "mindful" rather than "willful" is what really brings happiness. Part of this is accepting both pain and pleasure without willfully attaching to one or the other. Another part is really learning to trust and respect ourselves and others. Martin Seligman, Ph.D., in *Authentic Happiness,* describes recent research which concludes that "flow" (absorption and engagement happiness) and meaning and service-based happiness are more satisfying types of happiness than pleasure-based happiness. His website (www.authentichappiness.org) has many self-report inventories which can help to discover our strengths and best avenues to happiness. (Also see Appendix 3.) The Christian New Testament (*Matthew 5:3-12*) has taught these truths for centuries, emphasizing how those who are humble, pure in heart, peaceful, and merciful are the most blessed with happiness. Other great religions teach similar values.

Self-exploratory Quote: How can I create more absorption, engagement, meaning and service-based happiness in my life?

Affirmation: Today I am creating more "flow," meaning and service-based happiness in my life.

Principle: The foundation of self-esteem is "The 3 R's of Maturity:" 1) Respect for Self, 2) Respect for Others, 3) Responsibility for all your actions.

Perennial Wisdom Quote: "You must be the change you wish to see in the world." - - Mahatma Gandhi

Discussion: Self-esteem grows through the gradual accomplishment of what Erik Erikson (famous developmental psychologist) called essential life tasks, the development of 1) trust, 2) autonomy, 3) initiative, 4) industry, 5) identity, 6) intimacy, 7) generativity (the voluntary ability to creatively care for others), and 8) ego integrity.

Self-esteeming children and adults somehow find a way to allow their lives to further the development of these qualities. They might have had very dysfunctional parents and impoverished environments, and yet somehow these young people find people they can trust. They choose behaviors which allow them to be more autonomous and take more initiative, be more industrious, and have loving, intimate relationships. They learn to creatively care for others, and they find meaning and purpose in their lives. Being whole-heartedly engaged in this maturation process builds self-esteem. Seeking personal pleasure for its own sake does not build self-esteem and happiness. Neither does building power and prestige.

Self-esteem and happiness come through gradual increases in respect for self, respect for others, and responsibility for all one's own actions. Self-esteem must be earned through adherence to healthy personal values.

Self-exploratory Question: How can I strengthen my self-esteem?

Affirmation: Today I am strengthening my self-esteem by respecting myself and others and by taking responsibility for all my actions.

Principle: Being pro-active involves being self-caring and self-responsible.

Perennial Wisdom Quote: "If a man carries his own lantern, he need not fear darkness." -- Hasidic saying

Discussion: To be pro-active rather than reactive, it is vital to avoid fear-based behaviors. Fear always pushes us into reactivity. This may be fear for ourselves or fear for others. The opposite of fear-based action is love-based action. When we choose to act out of love rather than fear, we become pro-active. Fear primarily arises in the mind. Love primarily arises in the heart. Real freedom comes from loving action stimulated by the heart and accepted by the mind. This can only happen when we are paying attention. Boredom and inattention keep us dangling at the edge of unconsciousness. From this cliff it is very easy to fall into fear-based reactivity.

We need to be pro-active with inner work as well as outer work in order not to fall into reactivity and emotional unconsciousness. This inner work involves learning awareness of our feelings, acceptance of our emotional needs, and skill in expressing our feelings and finding ways to meet our emotional needs without harming others. This often involves learning to work through inner and outer conflicts peacefully. Focusing on pro-activity can displace reactivity.

Self-exploratory Question: How can I replace my reactive behaviors with pro-active behaviors?

Affirmation: Today I am making responsible, self-caring, love-based, pro-active choices.

Principle: Reactive, fearful reasoning just strengthens fear and dependency.

Perennial Wisdom Quote: "It is better to light a candle than to curse the darkness. -- Chinese proverb

Discussion: Unfortunately, many people make decisions when their brains are anxious, agitated and overly stimulated in their emotional (limbic, "low brain") centers (See Appendix 1.) Their "high brains" are not adequately engaged to result in clear thinking. Fearful, anxious thinking usually results in flight or fight reactions which do not promote adult independence and well-being. Fearful reasoning usually results in addictive and dysfunctional behavior. Often the fearful reasoning is so hidden underneath rage and adrenaline surging that the person can't even see it. This is why it is so important to keep one's brain free of alcohol and other drug poisoning, as well as sugar highs or lows and adrenaline rushes. Behavioral decisions need to be made by calm minds in order to be self-caring and wise. Fearful states need to be calmly observed until they pass. Here are some suggestions for overcoming reactive behaviors:

1) Don't make assumptions about what others are feeling and thinking;

2) check out your perceptions;

3) respect others' opinions;

4) when disagreeing, do so respectfully;

5) disengage from an argument if the other person is demanding agreement;

6) explore your own inner complexities which are beyond another's perceptions;

7) stay in touch with your own feelings, while also accepting the feelings of others;

8) learn to wonder about and respect others, even when they are being disrespectful;

9) remember that when another is unconsciously projecting an inner conflict onto you, it

   is best to disengage respectfully.

Self-exploratory Question: How can I avoid fearful reasoning and impulsive behavior?

Affirmation: I keep my mind calm and clear and make wise decisions which promote my well-being.

Principle: Avoiding emotional issues always makes them worse.

Perennial Wisdom Quote: "Life truly lived is a risky business and if one puts up too many fences against risk one ends by shutting out life itself." -- Kenneth S. Davis

Discussion: When dealing with emotional issues timing is important, but complete avoidance never pays off. Good timing involves being ready to clarify your own emotions and your own needs, and also being ready to engage in caring, respectful dialogue.

The spark which ignites unconscious arguments is usually one or more person's unconscious desire to avoid feelings. When we can allow ourselves to feel our feelings and responsibly acknowledge them, usually destructive arguments do not occur. Most arguments get started because at least one person can't clarify his or her own feelings and needs and/or isn't ready to engage in a caring, respectful dialogue. Usually there is some underlying fear, hidden underneath anger, and the argumentative person is unconsciously attempting to get the other person to fix the fear. In such a state of emotional unconsciousness, usually the attempt is controlling or manipulative and doesn't achieve the desired reduction of fear. Instead, often the person who is being unconsciously confronted just gets angry and distances himself or herself in self-defense. This just aggravates the argumentative person's initial, unconscious fear, such that he or she just becomes angrier. Recognizing one's own avoidance patterns and replacing them with responsible Adult Time Out and Time In behaviors heal relationships and boosts self-esteem. (See Jan. 16, 17 & 18 readings on Adult Time Out.)

Self-exploratory Question: In what areas of my life am I the most avoidant?

Affirmation: Today I experience all my feelings and process them responsibly. When I am angry, I look for any underlying fear and take responsibility for it.

March 27
Authenticity

Principle: Authenticity transforms avoidance and insincerity.

Perennial Wisdom Quote: "True gold fears not the fire." -- Confucius

Discussion: When a gem is authentic, it is "real," "genuine." It is what it is labeled and perceived to be. Sometimes human beings hide behind "personas" (emotional masks), which don't reveal genuine feelings and emotional needs. "Personas" are ways of presenting ourselves to others so as to be seen how we want to be seen. When we hide genuine feelings and emotional needs in order to keep up some sort of "persona", everyone suffers. This is a form of dishonesty easily engaged in for financial profit or political benefit. It is always destructive in the long run, because no one can hold up a false mask forever.

Eventually our true feelings and emotional needs will come out. This is because it is unhealthy for the human organism to repress emotions. Such repression will eventually lead to some form of emotional or physical illness. To stay well and to establish healthy relationships, we have to be authentic. Even if we make mistakes, we need to be honest and real about them, or eventually we will damage ourselves even more than others. We need to remember this for ourselves, as well as when we are voting for our leaders.

Self-exploratory Questions: In what areas of my life am I most authentic? Where most inauthentic?

Affirmation: Today I am presenting myself to others authentically and honestly.

March 28
Sincerity

Principle: Sincerity is the best policy.

Perennial Wisdom Quote: "Nothing is more disgraceful than insincerity." -- Cicero

Discussion: It is customary in Western society to end letters with the words "sincerely" or "sincerely yours," unless the word "love" feels appropriate. Why is this? Likely it is because all of us want our words to be perceived as genuine and honest. When our faces can't be seen so that the listener can determine sincerity based on non-verbal signals, then we need to signal the listener that we are sincere -- we mean what we say; we aren't just putting on a drama or a scam.

If we are internally conflicted over a matter, it is almost impossible to be sincere. At best we have to admit that we are torn, conflicted, and ambivalent. If we are divided and dishonest with ourselves internally, there is usually little we can effectively do externally until we heal our inner conflict. Therefore, when we are sincere, we are usually also not internally divided. We feel whole and in harmony inside. In such a harmonious state we can then make a sincere request of others, or share a sincere opinion or feeling.

Sincerity requires inner harmony as well as a willingness to reveal one's true feelings, needs or opinions to others. To maintain sincerity takes effort and clear intention. It's worth the work, because caring others are drawn to it.

Self-exploratory Questions: Where in my life am I the most sincere? Where the most insincere?

Affirmation: Today I am being sincere in all my words and actions.

March 29
Integrity

Principle: Integrity requires being completely honest with one's self, as well as with others.

Perennial Wisdom Quote: "This above all: to thine own self be true, And it must follow, as the night the day: Thou canst not then be false to any man." --- William Shakespeare, *Hamlet*, Act I, Sc. 3

Discussion: Integrity is based on congruence and consistency between one's values and one's actions. Its Latin root word, "integritas" means wholeness. When we act against our best values, we lose integrity. We become less than whole. When we act based on our best values, we build integrity.

Integrity involves aligning thought, speech and action in all that one does. The English word "integrity" comes from the Latin words meaning "in truth." The emphasis is on internal, inside truth. A person with integrity has learned how to take time to check with an internal ethical code before taking action. This internal ethical code says keeping internal peacefulness and internal honesty is more important than controlling external situations. A person with integrity is more afraid of internal punishment from an internal conscience (i.e., an ethical inner voice) than external punishment from others. He or she values internal peace.

When a person has integrity, he or she can be trusted. Such a person cannot use rationales and justifications for untruthful or disrespectful behavior. People with integrity are trusted by others and also have trustworthy friends and associates. They realize that when they are trustworthy themselves, they will attract and maintain trustworthy friends. They also realize that, if they violate their personal integrity, they will lose both internal peace and the trust of others. They are not willing to take this risk.

Self-exploratory Question: In what areas of my life do I have the most integrity? In what, the least integrity?

Affirmation: Today I value my integrity and choose not to do anything to violate it.

Principle: Always observe your thoughts, sight, word and deeds to avoid evil.

Perennial Wisdom Quote: "See no, hear no, speak no evil." -- Ancient Chinese saying

Discussion: In Asian gift shops you can find three little carved monkeys, one with hands over his eyes, another with hands over his ears, and the third with hands over his mouth. They symbolize the ancient Chinese teaching to "See no, hear no, speak no evil." Evil is defined in the dictionary as a noun or an adjective meaning immoral, harmful behavior, or the cause of suffering. Evil can also be thought of as a verb, as "live" spelled backwards. Evil acts are acts which humiliate or destroy life. Evil acts are committed when a person loses integrity. Peterson and Seligman (*Character Strengths and Virtues,* 2004) defines integrity as not only a regular pattern of behavior that is consistent with espoused values, but also public acknowledgment of moral convictions, even if those convictions are not popular, and also sensitivity to the needs of others. Integrity is a strength that motivates social action. Evil acts break down society.

It is important to avoid using the word "evil" as an adjective applying to another human being. History is full of wars in which whole nations declared the "enemy" "evil" and therefore justified atrocities against them. Actions can be evil, but not total human beings. To judge another human being as "evil" or a whole nation as "evil" denies the capacity for good which resides in every human brain. Such judgments can lead the judger to drop attempts to understand "the enemy" and to thereby commit evil acts himself or herself.

Ancient Chinese sages saw evil as darkness and taught that darkness cannot exist without light also existing. They taught the importance of looking for the light in darkness and the darkness in light. When we have integrity, we look for the goodness even in those who threaten our security. We don't give in to the urge to commit evil acts ourselves. Instead we strive to defeat "enemies" with understanding.

Self-exploratory Question: Where have I seen, heard, done or spoken evil?

Affirmation: Today I choose to see, hear, do and speak no evil.

Principle: Personal integrity goes along with a genuine interest in others.

Perennial Wisdom Quote: "The ultimate measure of a man is not where he stands in moments of comfort and convenience, but where he stands at times of challenge and controversy." -- Martin Luther King, Jr.

Discussion: People with integrity have learned to take a genuine interest in others. They realize that they cannot live isolated lives and be happy. They realize that happiness is built on a foundation of mutually satisfying relationships. Therefore, when challenges come up in their relationships, they rise to the challenges and struggle with them until a mutually acceptable resolution is determined. They don't run away from conflict, either through avoidance or through attempts to dominate others.

People with integrity realize that at some level all life is interdependent so that, when they are of service to others, they are indirectly being of service to themselves. They can offer this service without need for reward other than their own satisfaction from having rendered service. Such people are genuinely curious about others and enjoy different stories and experiences. They do not need others to be similar to them in order to feel validated. They know they are OK, and they can see others as both being OK as well as different.

Self-exploratory Question: How can I take a genuine, enjoyable interest in others?

Affirmation: Today I am taking a genuine interest in others and enjoying differences. I can respect people with different opinions.

Principle: Self-responsibility transforms dependency and irresponsibility.

Perennial Wisdom Quote: "The greatest griefs are those we cause ourselves." --
Sophocles, *Oedipus Rex*

Discussion: Our most important confrontations are with our own weaknesses and
limitations. We must be comfortable confronting ourselves first, before we become
very effective in confronting others. Being responsible means being capable of wise
responses to situations and having the ability to effectively respond, not just to react.
Being responsible obviously requires awareness and adequate knowledge. A
responsible person doesn't choose to diminish his or her own response capability.
He or she cherishes this capacity. Therefore, he or she chooses not to drive too fast
or not to drink and drive, or not to get intoxicated, because all of these choices
reduce response capacity.

A self-responsible person doesn't choose to run away from awareness.
Awareness is accepted, even painful awareness. Other people, even loved ones,
frequently don't respond in ways we want them to respond. Nature's balancing
energies sometimes bring floods, droughts, fires, earthquakes and hurricanes. The
self-responsible person accepts these realities and makes choices to protect himself
or herself against them. He or she does not bemoan others' choices or nature's
energies. He or she accepts the limitations of self-will and, at the same time,
exercises that will as beneficially as possible. He or she does not expect others to
rescue him or her from mistakes.

Self-exploratory Question: How can I become more self-responsible?

Affirmation: Today I choose, moment by moment, to be self-responsible.

Principle: Taking responsibility for our moods is vital in building character.

Perennial Wisdom Quote: "Character building begins in our infancy and continues until death." -- Eleanor Roosevelt

Discussion: Here are a few effective mood management techniques:

• Become a good observer of your own moods and take responsibility for them.

• Avoid blaming others and outside circumstances for your bad moods.

• Eat healthy food throughout the day and get adequate sleep.

• Abstain from nicotine, barbiturates, cocaine, amphetamines, and narcotics.

• Use alcohol, caffeine and sugar only in moderation and not as mood medicine.

• Allocate at least one hour each day for your own self-care and pleasure.

• Avoid serious problem solving when you are tired.

• Address your Hunger, Anger, Loneliness and Tiredness (H.A.L.T.) issues internally before trying to problem-solve with another.

• Practice active mood elevating strategies such as relaxation, exercise, meditation, prayer, yoga, positive affirmations, and wise readings on a regular basis.

• Use pleasure and distraction strategies such as social support and activities, sports, dancing, creative outlets, hobbies and humor.

• If necessary, consult with a therapist about medication for serious mood swings.

Self-exploratory Quote: What areas of self-discipline and mood management can I improve upon in my life?

Affirmation: Today I am taking responsibility for managing my moods.

Principle: Self-discipline is the foundation of a happy, satisfying life.

Perennial Wisdom Quote: "There is perhaps no psychological skill more fundamental than resisting impulse. It is the root of all emotional self-control, since all emotions, by their very nature, lead to one or another impulse to act." -- Daniel Goleman, Ph.D.

Discussion: The word "discipline" comes from the same root as "disciple" and means the capacity to learn. Disciplined people go on learning their whole lives. They go into things less afraid than undisciplined people because they can rely on themselves to do their best. They are willing to risk making mistakes because they can trust themselves not to shame themselves for their mistakes and instead to learn from them. Disciplined people know why they are doing what they do and how to do it. They combine knowledge, skill and desire.

Undisciplined people are unwilling to pursue knowledge and skill in order to fulfill their desires. They want to impulsively and quickly fulfill their desires and unrealistically jump ahead, causing their own failures. They aren't trustworthy.

Self-discipline is about the ability to observe one's own thoughts and emotions and behaviors and monitor them so as to lead to optimal results. Being able to direct one's mind to go where you want it to go, when you want it to go there is a big part of self-discipline, and it takes practice. Our minds are like monkeys and need to be disciplined by our hearts and spirits. We are not our minds. We are that which watches and directs our minds. When we identify with our minds and just react to our environments in monkey-like fashion, we don't use our whole selves, and we cause our own suffering.

Self-discipline helps us to own our higher selves and create meaning and joy in life.

Self-exploratory Question: How can I be more self-disciplined so as to learn more and to experience more joy in my life?

Affirmation: Today I am using self-discipline and prioritizing self-care and education.

Principle: Positive habits build self-discipline and character.

Perennial Wisdom Quote: "Our characters, basically are a composite of our habits…. Habits are powerful factors in our lives. Because they are consistent, often unconscious patterns, they constantly, daily, express our character and produce our effectiveness…or ineffectiveness." -- Stephen Covey, Ph.D.

Discussion: Paramahansa Yogananda, a noted yogi and lecturer of the 20th century, said, "Weaken a bad habit by avoiding everything that occasioned it or stimulated it, without concentrating upon it in your zeal to avoid it. Then divert your mind to some good habit and steadily cultivate it until it becomes a dependable part of you."

Modern psychological research has validated the merit of his words. For example, if you have established a habit of going to a favorite bar every day and drinking too much, it is important to avoid that bar and substitute some non-drinking, relaxing activity every day such as taking a walk or a hot tub bath. If you have a habit of overeating refined sugar at home and in restaurants, you can buy more fruits and go to restaurants which specialize in interesting spices, not sweets. (Study the Self-inventory in Appendix 3 for "life enhancing" habits which can be substituted for "life-defeating" habits.)

Self-exploratory Question: What positive habit can I substitute for a negative one?

Affirmation: Today I am focusing on establishing positive habits.

April 5
Purposefulness

Principle: Purposefulness overcomes avoidance.

Perennial Wisdom Quote: "There is a law in psychology that if you form a picture in your mind of what you would like to be, and you keep and hold that picture there long enough, you will soon become exactly as you have been thinking." -- William James

Discussion: Avoidance is likely the most frequently practiced emotional defense and perhaps the most important one to overcome. Many great teachers have written about the importance of substituting clear intentions and purposefulness for avoidance.

Clear intentions focus on our own attitudes and behaviors. They do not focus on external goals. For example, it is more productive to form a clear intention to prepare to do the best in one's ability in a musical performance, than to focus on a desire to get tremendous audience applause. Factors other than your performance may influence the audience's response. But if my purpose is to prepare for the performance to the best of my ability, when I do so, my self-esteem will be enhanced and the likelihood of a good audience response will also be enhanced.

Effective purposefulness focuses on one's own behavior, not on others' behaviors. It removes unnecessary dependency on others. Modern brain research will likely soon show how purposeful thoughts strengthen pre-frontal cortex functioning and quiet over-activity in the emotional amygdala. (See Appendix 1.) If you have trouble forming clear intentions, consider reading Gendlin's book, *Focusing,* and also Gail Sheehy's book, *Pathfinders*.

Self-exploratory Question: In what areas of my life do I need to be more purposeful?

Affirmation: Today I am holding a picture in my mind of the person I want to be.

Principle: Ambivalence undermines effective action.

Perennial Wisdom Quote: "Even if you're on the right track, you'll get run over if you just sit there." -- Will Rogers

Discussion: Ambivalence usually results from the avoidance of inner feelings and outer information. It is also usually fear-based. If I am ambivalent about applying for a new job, it's likely because I'm afraid of change, not because I'm very satisfied with my current job. If I am ambivalent about staying in a marriage, it's likely because I fear I won't be able to get my emotional needs met in it, but I also am afraid I won't get my emotional needs met out of it. Extended ambivalence can lead to mental illness. Don't wallow in it. Get help.

       The way out of ambivalence is to squarely face our inner conflicts, make friends with both sides of our inner arguments, and take a first, small step which will help to gather more information and lead to the next small step. Psychotherapy can help in this process. So can a good support group. With support we can more easily accept all our emotions, and make small changes. Learning to be honest, direct and respectful toward ourselves can help us to work through our inner conflicts and also be more honest, direct and respectful toward others.

Self-exploratory Question: How can I reduce ambivalence in my life?

Affirmation: Today I am working through my ambivalences and taking action.

Principle: Honest self-assessment is the foundation of personal change. Wise Ways Happiness Step 4 reads, "We make honest assessments of our assets and our shortcomings."

Perennial Wisdom Quote: "If you like things easy, you'll have difficulties; if you like problems, you'll succeed." -- Laotian saying

Discussion: Self-examination isn't easy. All of us have blind spots in our self-awareness. None of us enjoys examining his or her shortcomings but, how can we purposefully replace our shortcomings with assets when we don't fully know the nature of our shortcomings?

The 4th step in the Wise Ways Happiness Program involves inventorying our own characters, both our shortcomings and our assets, then writing down this inventory in preparation for reviewing it with a trusted other who will keep it confidential. Step 4 can be done with a therapist or a good friend. The important thing is complete self-honesty and willingness to look at and accept both one's assets and shortcomings.

Step 5 (which is discussed more in a May reading) involves the confidential sharing of this written material. "Getting things off our chests" can strengthen us. Spending time defining our assets which we can build upon is also strengthening. Like any good exercise, doing the 4th step takes some time and energy, and it also has a great deal of benefits. (Appendix 3 might be helpful in doing Step 4.)

Self-exploratory Question: Am I ready to write down a searching self-inventory?

Affirmation: Today I am doing some 4th Step work, no matter how brief or challenging.

April 8
Groups

Tradition 4: Autonomous Support

Principle: Tradition Four reads, "Each Happiness Support Group is autonomous.

Perennial Wisdom Quote: "We increase our ability and stability when we increase our sense of accountability and responsibility." -- Curtis Mayfield

Discussion: Every Wise Ways Happiness Support Group is primarily responsible to its own members. Group decisions which best serve the emotional, mental and spiritual growth of all group members are the best decisions. Each group, as a group, is financially independent, although, if it is facilitated by a professional therapist, fees for the therapist's time may be paid. Each group commits to following the 12 Traditions of the Happiness Support Group Program to the best of its ability. Each group is responsible for interpreting the 12 Steps and Traditions for themselves, with the help of this book. (See Appendix 4.)

Some Happiness Support Groups can form like book clubs spontaneously by friends who are using this book. Some Happiness Support Groups can be formed in Mental Health Community Centers or substance abuse treatment centers or in correctional facilities. This author only asks that the Guidelines for maintaining these groups follow the suggestions in Appendix 4 and that this author be informed if groups are to advertised.

Self-exploratory Question: If I am in a Happiness Support Group, do I understand and practice the 12 Traditions of this Happiness Program?

Affirmation: Today I commit to supporting the health of my Happiness Support Group by following the 12 Support Group Traditions.

April 9
Industry

Principle: Industry builds self-esteem and reduces dependency.

Perennial Wisdom Quote: "The busy man is troubled with but one devil, the idle man by a thousand." -- Spanish proverb

Discussion: Erik Erikson, famous American developmental psychologist, defined learning "industry" as one of the primary tasks of childhood. Industry is defined by Webster as "earnest steady effort, intelligent work, systematic work." Erikson saw this developmental task as following the tasks of "trust" and "autonomy." Unfortunately, when a child hasn't been able to develop trust in others and some emotional and financial autonomy from others, it is difficult for him or her to develop industry. The child might be handicapped in some way or suffering from abuse and loss. Such a child has to first address his or her handicap, abuse or loss issues, before successfully becoming industrious.

Prisons are full of individuals who were unable to become successfully industrious because of unresolved handicaps, abuses or losses. An industrious society strives to give opportunity for ALL persons to become industrious in some satisfying and socially productive way. When we take responsibility, not only for our personal industry but also for supporting an employed, industrious society, social happiness will grow proportionately and prison populations will shrink. To feel worthwhile, people need a sense of connecting to and contributing to others. When these opportunities are limited, everyone suffers. Politicians need to be reminded of these realities in order to make correctional facilities truly correctional. Giving former inmates the vote, after they have served their time is a step in this direction.

Self-exploratory Question: How can I be more industrious and also contribute to an industrious society?

Affirmation: Today I am engaging in intelligent, steady, systematic effort for myself and also to benefit others.

April 10
Persistence

Principle: Persistence is necessary to achieve most worthwhile goals.

Perennial Wisdom Quote: "Just don't give up trying to do what you really want to do. Where there is love and inspiration, I don't think you can go wrong. " -- Ella Fitzgerald

Discussion: Persistence usually requires self-respect and hope. If we don't respect ourselves and we don't feel deserving we aren't likely to persist with behaviors which will improve our life situation. If persistence is a problem for you, you may also need to take a look at improving your self-respect and your hopefulness. (See February 17 and April 19 readings.) As the Japanese say, "Beginning is easy, continuing is hard."

To persist in a behavior, we usually also need to believe that the effort will be rewarded. Many people make the mistake, however, of relying on rewards from external sources, and when these don't materialize, they lose motivation to persist. When we can turn inward for our reward systems, rewards become much more reliable. When we can reward ourselves for persisting with some behavior which we see as of some merit and/or service, we are much more likely to continue until some positive results are observable. This is why internalized value and reward systems are so important. Outside people cannot be relied upon to always be sufficiently knowledgeable and motivated to distribute just rewards. We need to count on ourselves for doing this.

Self-exploratory Question: How can I reward myself more effectively for positive, persistent behaviors?

Affirmation: Today I am rewarding myself for positive, persistent effort.

April 11
Resourcefulness

Principle: Personal success requires resourcefulness

Perennial Wisdom Quote: "I am a great believer in luck, and I find the harder I work, the more luck I have." -- Thomas Jefferson

Discussion: Great periods in history are usually characterized by resourceful leaders. Thomas Jefferson and other writers of the United States Declaration of Independence and Constitution were resourceful people. They read about others' successes and failures, and learned from them. They knew how to charismatically gather support from surrounding communities. They knew how to address common concerns and represent them in political settings. They knew how to reward individuals who had demonstrated resourcefulness and courage. Of course, they were also limited by the time in which they lived. In that time, slavery was still legal and women and unpropertied men and African Americans couldn't vote.

Now that the Earth's human population has exploded so phenomenally, human resources are more available, but challenges to coordinate these resources and to treat everyone are daunting. To be truly resourceful modern individuals need to understand the importance of international cooperation, global conservation of physical resources, and global cooperation in the just use of human resources so as to reduce pollution and global warming.

Whether they are practicing simple, agricultural living in the "heartland" of the United States, or working through the United Nations to reduce global poverty and starvation, resourceful people utilize what they have for the benefit of others, as well as themselves.

Self-exploratory Question: How can I better utilize what I have for my own benefit as well as for the benefit of others?

Affirmation: Today I choose to use all my skills and assets resourcefully.

April 12
Promptness

Principle: Promptness is a by-product of respect and clarity of purpose.

Perennial Wisdom Quote: "Successful people are seldom people who dilly-dally, who postpone action, or who cannot make up their minds. Get into the habit of answering letters immediately, of paying bills promptly, of repairing what needs to be repaired at once. One usually saves time, money, and energy by responding quickly to all demands which daily living makes upon us." -- Johannes A. Gaertner

Discussion: William Shakespeare in *The Merry Wives of Windsor* wrote "Better three hours too soon than a minute too late." Sometimes delay simply causes us to "miss the boat" entirely. Abraham Lincoln offered good advice when he suggested that it is best to "deliberate slowly, but execute promptly." It is all too easy to deliberate quickly and still execute slowly. It's important to take time to think things through sufficiently, but ruminating like the stomach of a cow over what is to be done about a problem usually doesn't help.

In many work and social matters promptness is a matter of courtesy, a matter of respect for other's time. People who hate to wait themselves often are late and consciously or unconsciously disrespectful to others. Cultural standards of promptness vary, but being respectful of others' time is always important.

Self-exploratory Question: How can I be more prompt in all my affairs?

Affirmation: Today I am practicing promptness and respect for others' time.

April 13
Purity

Principle: Purity of heart and mind brings peacefulness.

Perennial Wisdom Quote: "Blessed are the pure in heart for they shall see God." -- Jesus in *The Bible Matthew 5:8*

Discussion: *The Upanishads* of ancient India advised, "Let us therefore keep the mind pure, for what a man thinks, that he becomes." All the great world religions addressed the importance of "purity" in mind and in heart, and yet in modern times the concept is mostly used in relationship to minerals, chemicals and colors. Why is this so? Have we become so skeptical about the possibility of a "pure" mind and heart that we can no longer even speak about it conceptually? Most colors, minerals and chemicals aren't totally "pure", and yet we find it helpful to promote movement toward the concept of purity. Can't we also promote this movement in our minds and hearts without being perfectionistic? We can also remember that the brightest day will also inevitably move toward darkness, and that at the darkest hour the light is nearest. We can know that this same natural movement is also present in human minds and hearts.

The Sanskrit word *saucha* translates as purity and cleanliness. To be pure in the sense of *saucha* is to be simple, unmixed, absolutely ourselves. "Purity" essentially means uncontaminated, wholly of one essence. It is a state of mind and of heart which can be realized, one moment at a time, with great joy. We don't have to be rigidly moralistic to seek for "purity." We can simply be dedicated to resolving our inner conflicts and ambivalences.

Self-exploratory Question: How can I become purer of heart and mind?

Affirmation: Today I am keeping my mind and heart focused on my essence of love.

April 14
Cleanliness

Principle: Cleanliness of body and mind help to create a good spirit.

Perennial Wisdom Quote: "Better keep yourself clean and bright; you are the window through which you must see the world." -- George Bernard Shaw

Discussion: Nature isn't clean in a compulsive way. But it is clean and pure in a simple, beautiful, life-promoting way. Most wise teachers promote this same kind of cleanliness for their students. They recognize that dirt itself isn't bad. Actually, soil is as valuable as air or water. But dirtiness of body, clothes, surroundings and mind involve accumulated inattention to promoting personal health and more pleasant interactions with others.

Surrounding ourselves with simple, clean, natural beauty and attempting to mirror this simple, clean, natural beauty in our minds and our hearts is what the Hindus call *saucha.* It is considered an important spiritual practice. Moses, Buddha, Jesus, Muhammad, and other great spiritual teachers also emphasized the importance of this kind of simple, cleanliness. They all taught the importance of this quality on anyone's path to happiness.

Self-exploratory Question: How can I promote more cleanliness in my heart, mind and surroundings?

Affirmation: Today I am keeping my body, mind, and surroundings simple and clean.

April 15
Thrift

Principle: Thrift allows us the pleasure of doing more with the money we have.

Perennial Wisdom Quote: "If you want to know whether you are destined to be a success or failure in life, you can easily find out. One test is simple and infallible. Are you able to save money?" -- James J. Hill

Discussion: Thrift means frugality as a means to thriving prosperity. It involves not spending more than you have and using what money and resources you have wisely. Thrift also involves impulse control and thoughtfulness of others. Thrifty people usually realize that they are happiest when in community with others and they are aware of other people's needs in addition to their own. They don't want to waste any extra resources because they are aware that these resources can also be useful to others.

Thrifty people are not usually greedy people. Greedy people tend more to live beyond their means and be unconscious to the needs of others. Thriftiness in past centuries was very esteemed by the common person because poverty was the common order.

Poverty is still the common order among much of the world's peoples, in the United States as well as elsewhere. Yet many wealthy individuals, corporations and countries only feel concerned about themselves. This self-centeredness promotes anger, humiliation and envy, and these emotions lead to conflict and war. Thrift, along with generosity, is also a means to personal safety, national and international peace.

Self-exploratory Question: How can I be more thrifty with my resources?

Affirmation: Today I am only buying what I need, and sharing my extra resources.

April 16   **Freedom from Compulsive Spending**

Principle: Compulsive spending is impoverishing more than satisfying.

Perennial Wisdom Quote: "What maintains one vice would bring up two children." -- Benjamin Franklin

Discussion: Any form of compulsion is usually an escape from some awareness. Unhappy and depressed people often use compulsive spending as a way to try to escape their unhappiness. Because the mind is insatiable in its desire for new objects and pleasures, usually the shopping brings only brief relief from unhappiness and then goes on to create more unhappiness, due to financial problems and/or guilt.

The way to escape compulsive spending is to seriously address what is causing the original unhappiness, and to become aware that lasting happiness is an inside job. Giving to others, service and kindness to others gives much more lasting happiness than accumulating material goods.

Often compulsive spending happens in an attempt to escape loneliness. But the loneliness returns soon after the shopping spree. When a person suffers from compulsive spending habits, it is best to avoid shopping areas as much as possible and substitute activities, such as exercise, relaxation and socializing, which offer much more lasting relief from unhappiness.

Self-exploratory Question: How can I avoid compulsive shopping and spending?

Affirmations: Today I am buying only what I need. I am avoiding compulsive shopping.

April 17   **Learning from**
Mistakes

Principle: Learning from mistakes helps to develop mastery.

Perennial Wisdom Quote: "Face your deficiencies and acknowledge them; but do not let them master you. Let them teach you patience, sweetness, insight. When we do the best we can, we never know what miracle is wrought in our life, or in the life of another." -- Helen Keller

Discussion: Helen Keller was born deaf and blind. Nevertheless, she became a noted speaker and teacher. She serves as a tremendous example, not only to the physically handicapped, but also to those who make mistakes, which is all of us.

Cicero outlined the following six common mistakes. Even though he lived thousands of years ago, notice how relevant these mistakes still are in modern times.

- The delusion that personal gain is made by crushing others.

- The tendency to worry about things that cannot be changed or corrected.

- Insisting that a thing is impossible because we cannot accomplish it.

- Refusing to set aside trivial preferences.

- Neglecting development and refinement of the mind, and not acquiring the habit of reading and studying.

- Attempting to compel others to believe and live as we do.

Self-exploratory Question: Which of Cicero's "mistakes" do you most practice?

Affirmation: Today I am learning from my mistakes and not repeating them.

April 18
Mastery

Principle: Practice and learning from mistakes develops mastery.

Perennial Wisdom Quote: "Practice is the best of all instructors." -- Publilius Syrus

Discussion: Mastery, like freedom, is an inside job. Mastering something means becoming really, really good at it. Practice creates mastery, not just mental knowledge.

"Masters" are mentors of living -- people who have focused so deeply on self-awareness, awareness of others, and on their part of the universe that they can teach both from knowledge and from experience. Such persons may be honored in history books and scriptures or they may be quietly living next door.

As the Native Americans recognized so well, mentors may even reside in the buffalo or the fox or the deer, eagle or beaver, not just in human forms. Whoever can teach by example and from experience -- even without words -- is a "Master." Masters prioritize what is most important to them and commit their time accordingly. When they have become skillful, they teach through example. Seeking out such teachers and learning from their wisdom and knowledge is important for all of us.

Self-exploratory Questions: From what "masters" have I learned? What skills have I personally mastered?

Affirmation: Today I am working on mastering at least one positive skill.

Principle: Self-respect overcomes self-neglect.

Perennial Wisdom Quote: "Self-respect is the fruit of discipline; the sense of dignity grows with the ability to say no to oneself." -- Abraham Heschel

Discussion: Everyone wants respect from others, but are we willing to pay the price? The price involves self-discipline. When we might avoid punishment by telling a lie, we need to tell the truth. When we might rather not make the effort to be of service to someone who is needy, we make the effort. When we might rather pursue random pleasures, we refine our talents and find meaningful work for ourselves. When we might rather spend some time sleeping, we get up to care for a sick child. When we might rather break our parents' house rules, we choose to be respectful of them and thereby earn their respect.

This kind of self-discipline is what builds self-confidence and self- respect. We choose to honor our own principles even when it would be easier to not do so. Our principles are not only respectful of ourselves, but also respectful of others, so we do not get into trouble with others when we are taking care of ourselves. Because we can say "no" to ourselves when our desires lead us into trouble, we stay out of trouble and earn both the liking and the respect of others.

This kind of self-respect is worth more than money. Money cannot buy it, it comes only with consistent self- discipline and effort. We can also take time, of course, to have fun. Our sources of fun are creative and good for us and others. They involve laughter and playfulness. Our humor is not at anyone else's expense. We laugh with others, but not at them. In addition, these choices leave us feeling good about ourselves and others.

Self-exploratory Question: What choices cause me to have the most self-respect?

Affirmation: Today I am only making choices which enhance my self-respect.

Principle: As an adult, we are most responsible for taking care of ourselves.

Perennial Wisdom Quote: "Nothing may be more important than being gentle with ourselves…. We learn the value of recognizing our limits, forgiving ourselves our bouts of impatience or guilt, acknowledging our own needs. We see that to have compassion for others we must have compassion for ourselves." -- Ram Dass

Discussion: Have you learned how to soothe yourself when you are emotionally upset? Have you learned how to rest when you are tired? Have you learned how to eat only when you are hungry and stop with you are full? Have you learned either to use alcohol moderately only in social situations or not at all? Have you learned to exercise at least four times a week? Do you abstain from all illegal drugs? Have you learned how to make and keep at least a few friends? Have you learned how to give to others as much as they give to you? Do you know how to manage your moods so as not to get very depressed or overly excited? Have you learned how to have fun without being hurtful to yourself or others? Have you learned how to educate yourself about matters which are important to you? Have you learned how to keep respectful relationships with your friends and family? Have you learned how to settle disputes non-violently? Can you say both "yes" and "no" when you need to? Do you get annual checkups with your doctor? Do you wear your seat belt in a car?

All these behaviors are necessary for good self-care. No one can do them for you the way you need to do them for yourself.

Self-exploratory Question: If you answered any of these questions "no," what do you need to do so as to be able to start answering them all "yes"?

Affirmation: Today I am taking full responsibility for taking care of myself.

Principle: Life is more satisfying when we identify and use our talents and strengths.

Perennial Wisdom Quote: "Be true to yourselves; cherish whatever talent you possess, and in using it faithfully for the good of others, you will most assuredly find happiness for yourself, and make of life no failure, but a beautiful success." -- Louisa May Alcott

Discussion: A person's outer world is usually a mirror of his or her own inner world. So, if we want to change our outer world, we have to begin with changing our inner world. One of the best ways to do this is by identifying our personal strengths and talents. If you go to Dr. Seligman's website (www.authentichappiness.org) or read his book, *Authentic Happiness,* you will find many helpful suggestions and self-inventories for discovering your strengths. There is also a self-inventory in the Appendix in this book.

   You can also ask yourself what you love to do the most and ask yourself how to use this love in service to others. This, along with talking to a career counselor who can give you the Strong Campbell Interest Inventory and some aptitude tests, can help you to develop your talents in such a way as to make them into a satisfying career. Going on-line for information from the Occupational Outlook Handbook maintained by the U.S. government can be helpful. Hobbies and volunteer work can utilize talents in a satisfying way. Everyone, no matter how handicapped, has some unique talent which can be used in a satisfying, service-oriented way.

Self-exploratory Question: How can I use my talents more fully?

Affirmation: Today I am using my talents to the best of my abilities.

Principle: Over-indulgence in harmful pleasures destroys self-respect.

Perennial Wisdom Quote: "You must structure your world so that you are constantly reminded of who you are." -- Na'im Akbar

Discussion: When we over indulge in meeting our desires, no matter what harm we do to ourselves or others, we forget who we are. The ancient Hawaiians said we are all "bowls of light" and when "stones" get in the way of our "light" all we have to do is dump them out. This is easier said than done. Have you ever eaten so much that you feel bloated and heavy? Have you ever been intoxicated to the point that you don't know what you are doing, and you get yourself in trouble? Have you ever indulged in a temper tantrum to the point of alienating a friend or a family member or landing in prison?

All these harmful behaviors happen because we forget who we are. We see ourselves as unimportant, unhappy victims of others around us. We forget that all the biggest "stones" in our life are of our own creation. We block our own "light" out of fear -- fear of our inner resources, our inner beauty, or fear that this beauty won't be recognized by others. But we have to recognize this beauty ourselves before others can recognize it. This is what the Hawaiians meant by "light". It comes from a source deep within us which we have to access though our own choices and our own self-discipline. If we lazily allow "stones" to fall into our "bowls of light" by forgetting whom we really are, our light becomes blocked by our own choices. Claiming our own "light" is a personal responsibility. No one can do this for us.

Self-exploratory Question: How can I stop dropping "stones" into my "bowl of light?"

Affirmation: Today I am recognizing the light within me and resisting over-indulgences.

April 23
Solitude

Principle: Some solitude and some time with Nature are necessary to see our own light.

Perennial Wisdom Quote: "Every now and again take a look at something not made with hands -- a mountain, a star, a turn of a stream. There will come to you a wisdom and patience and solace and, above all, the assurance that you are not alone in the world." -- Sidney Lovett

Discussion: It seems paradoxical that people who do not know how to provide themselves with enough solitude tend to feel alone in the world. They connect to others, but not deeply enough to feel real community; they feel alone. It takes knowing ourselves well to know others well.

If we run away from our inner selves through always staying busy with chores or contact with others or digital escapes, we lose contact with our innermost source of strength and light. All the great teachers of the world took time for solitude. They learned how to be deeply compassionate and of service to others, through also learning how to be alone with themselves and Nature and how to feel revived and supported through that contact.

Too much solitude, of course, can be as harmful as too much constant social contact. We need to relate to other human beings. But our ways of relating need to be compassionate and supportive. If we cannot be compassionate and supportive of ourselves when in solitude, we will not be able to do it when we are relating to others. People are social beings, and they are also beings in need of inner inspiration and quiet contemplation.

Self-exploratory Question: Do I take regular time for quiet solitude and contemplation?

Affirmation: Today I am making time for solitude and quiet time with Nature.

Principle: Emotional support from others is also necessary to see our own light.

Perennial Wisdom Quote: "When someone tells you the truth, let's you think for yourself, experience your own emotions, he is treating you as a true equal -- as a friend." -- Whitney Otto

Discussion: Self-discipline is necessary to support ourselves adequately. Emotional support from others is also necessary to see our own light. Self-disciplined people know this and take time to make and sustain stable friendships, family connections and support groups. There are times when all of us are confused or despairing, and at such times we all need the helpful comfort of people who love us and accept us despite our weaknesses and times of confusion. If no such people exist in our birth families, we can create such relationships with friends. This takes time and commitment and a willingness to give as much as we receive.

Giving to others raises us out of our self-absorption and gives us perspective, even on the gravest of losses. Modern economics often require housing or job changes, but this does not mean we have to let go of current friends. We can stay in touch by e-mail, postal mail, the phone and visits whenever possible. Prioritizing such contact is what is vital. Sometimes we have to go the extra mile for a friend, literally or figuratively, in order to have a friend who will go that extra mile for us, and we should drop any score cards. Sometimes we give to one person, and receive back from another. What is vital is to give what we can of ourselves and what we have. It always comes back multifold from somewhere.

Self-exploratory Question: Do I both give and ask for stable, emotional support?

Affirmation: Today I am both giving and asking for emotional support when needed.

April 25
Lonesomeness

Principle: Paradoxically when we are no longer afraid to be alone, that's when we are free from lonesomeness.

Perennial Wisdom Quote: "Solitude is one thing and loneliness [lonesomeness] is another." -- May Sarton

Discussion: Webster's Dictionary defines "loneliness" as a "feeling of being without company, of being in solitude." "Lonesome" is defined as "conscious of solitude, depressed by solitude." These definitions suggest that there is a difference between experiencing "loneliness" and "being lonesome." Somehow "being lonesome" suggests being depressed by solitude. Loneliness, according to Webster, doesn't necessarily suggest this. Loneliness is a statement of fact and being lonesome is a statement of mood, an attitude of loss and depression, a resistance to what is. May Sarton was really talking about "lonesomeness" when she pointed out how "solitude" is different.

James Hillman reminds us in his book, *The Soul's Code*, that there are other sources of comfort than human company, and letting go of our desires is a big part of receiving what we need. When our mind is fixed on wanting to be with a certain person or persons, we cannot relax and enjoy our solitude, or seek out new company. Instead we fall into lonesomeness. But we are in charge of our moods, and we are also capable of reaching out for new sources of emotional support. The choice is ours.

Self-exploratory Question: How do I allow myself to fall into lonesomeness?

Affirmation: Today I take responsibility for avoiding lonesomeness.

Principle: Anxiety signals a need for some healing change.

Perennial Wisdom Quote: "A panic attack is the most common advanced warning system for an emerging healing process." -- Bruce Bibee

Discussion: Panic attacks have a biological component which sometimes requires medicine to heal, but they also signal the importance of behavioral change. Sometimes it is not obvious what behavioral change is being called up. Sometimes it is very obvious. If we are in panic over the idea of leaving the house, we clearly need to leave the house to find a therapist who can help us confront the fears which we cannot confront alone. If we are anxious about performing in a concert or making a speech, we are being signaled to practice speaking or performing in front of small groups of trusted others, until we can feel more comfortable in front of strangers. If we are anxious about a sexual encounter, we need to ask ourselves if we are afraid of judgment, rejection, abuse or whatever. We need to choose a partner carefully, and talk about our fears ahead of time until we are sure that none of these responses will happen.

Several of the modern anti-depressant medications are very helpful for safely reducing anxiety but, they are not sufficient in and of themselves. Some of the modern anti-anxiety medications are very addictive and should be used very cautiously. Someone who suffers from anxiety needs behavioral changes, not just medicine to become really free.

Self-exploratory Question: How can I reduce anxiety in my life?

Affirmation: Today I am doing all I can to reduce my anxiety and to experience joy.

April 27
Strength

Principle: Strength comes from knowing yourself and having compassion for others.

Perennial Wisdom Quote: "There are two ways of exerting one's strength: one is pushing down, the other is pulling up." -- Booker T. Washington

Discussion: Have you heard the analogy between human strength and sticks? One stick alone is easily broken, but a bundle of sticks is very strong. It also matters how this strength and union are built. If strength is built through intimidation and domination, it doesn't stay strong indefinitely. Human social history shows how it takes knowing yourself and having patience and compassion for others to build and maintain true strength.

Martial artists are very familiar with how it takes calmness, balance, concentration and flexibility to develop strong self-defense. Out-of-control anger is a sign of emotional weakness and usually damages self, more than others. To be strong in asserting one's needs a person also has to be aware of the needs of others and find a way to respect them at the same time that he or she is getting personal needs met. Otherwise, If a person's needs are met by force or dishonesty, he or she will just inspire oppositional strength in those who were previously dominated.

Societies which democratically allow free elections, and freedom of speech, press and religion are automatically stronger than autocratic societies because they are based on strength which comes from union and pulling others up, not pushing others down.

Self-exploratory Question: How would you define your strengths?

Affirmation: Today I am exercising strength by knowing myself and having compassion for others.

Principle: Being honorable means holding oneself to a standard of ethical and respectful conduct.

Perennial Wisdom Quote: "He has honor if he holds himself to an ideal of conduct though it is inconvenient, unprofitable, or dangerous to do so." -- Walter Lippman

Discussion: In many diverse cultures the standard of honor is some form of the "Golden Rule." Six hundred years before Jesus, the Greek Pittacus wrote, "Do not that to thy neighbor that thou wouldst not suffer from him." Five hundred years before Jesus, the Buddha said, "Hurt not others with that which pains yourself." Three hundred years before Jesus Christ, a Hindu epic poem, *The Mahabharata,* included these words, "This is the sum of all true righteousness: deal with others as thou would thyself be dealt by. Do nothing to thy neighbor which thou would not have him do to thee hereafter." Confucius in China and Jewish writers also included their own renditions of "The Golden Rule." Jesus Christ said, "Do unto others as you would have them do unto you." Over five hundred years after the death of Jesus, Mohammad said, "Do not unto others what you would not they should do unto you."

In the 18th century the German philosopher Kant offered a secular, philosophical version of the Golden Rule: "Act so that the maxim (principle) of your action can be willed as universal law." Many ethical principles since Kant's time have been based on this fundamental teaching. To be honorable, following some version of this principle is necessary. Without this principle many unethical behaviors can be rationalized as means to some desired end, especially if these behaviors are presented as protecting one's own group or nation.

Self-exploratory Question: Are all your behaviors based on honorable principles?

Affirmation: Today I am following the Golden Rule and making only honorable choices.

Principle: Courage involves the willingness to do the right thing despite fear.

Perennial Wisdom Quote: "If we take the generally accepted definition of bravery as a quality which knows no fear, I have never seen a brave man. All men are frightened. The more intelligent they are, the more they are frightened."--General George Patton, Jr.

Discussion: The American Indian symbol for courage is the eagle. The eagle has sharp vision, defies fear, swoops down to capture his food, builds his nest in high places, breathes fresh air and has free movement through shadow as well as light. Human courage takes the strength of an eagle and also human wisdom.

Mark Twain observed, "Courage is resilience to fear, mastery of fear, not absence of fear." James Liszka, Ph.D., in *Moral Competence,* defines courage as "the willingness to do the right thing despite serious pain, significant harm, or risk to one's well-being or even to one's life. In other words, fear may be present, but action is still performed for noble and collective reasons. Selfish courage is impossible; it is simply strong self-defense." Strong self-defense is often mistaken for courage, especially among the young.

Maturity brings more understanding about courage. Courage may involve some self-defense, but it also needs to involve respect for others. It needs to be principled. Take for example, the young African-Americans who first entered mandated, desegregated schools in the United States. They were defending their personal right to an "equal" education, and they were also defending all African-Americans' right to an "equal" education. Practicing this kind of courage takes well-integrated, well-functioning brains.

Self-exploratory Question: How can I practice courage rather than just self-defense?

Affirmation: Today I am facing all my challenges with real courage.

Principle: Death is only a transition and survived by love.

Perennial Wisdom Quote: "In nature, there is less death and destruction than death and transmutation. " -- Edwin Way Teale in *Circle of the Seasons*

Discussion: The Chinese have a saying, "The brave person regards dying as a going home." Many teachers write and speak about how death is just a part of the circle of seasons of life. Many sages teach about the power of love to transcend death. When we love others and are loved by others, when our bodies die, the love we have helped to create goes on. This love, being our truest essence, is our link with immortality.

Loving people don't usually fear death. They are too busy living their lives fully to worry about death. They have learned to accept loss as a part of life while their bodies are still alive, so they approach death as a loss of the senses, but not a loss of all the love which has surrounded them. They don't fear pain so much because they know they will have support in facing it. They gratefully live each moment until they die. They don't carry regrets. They quickly make amends for mistakes. They ask for what they want and need, and take action to thoughtfully give it to themselves. Such a life is to be celebrated.

Self-exploratory Questions: Am I afraid of dying? If so, how does it affect my life?

Affirmation: Today I am living each moment fully, without fearing death.

May 1   **Freedom from Fear of**
Death

Principle: When we live in each present moment, fear of death vanishes.

Perennial Wisdom Quote: "My concern is not what will happen to me when this life ends. My concern is, can there be a dying to resentments and grudges? What he did or what she did to me - can we die to that? Be done with it? Maybe there was anger a moment ago. Can that anger end, be finished and not carried over in the mind? Can we die to each moment so there is a freshness of living that is not possible if we keep carrying around everything that has happened?" -- Toni Packer in interview with William Elliott in *Tying Rocks to Clouds*

Discussion: How we perceive death influences greatly how we live. Is death an end, a beginning, both, something else? Finding some meaning in death is important for all of us in order to overcome the fear of it. Richard Nelson, in *The Island Within,* writes that "there can be no final death, only a transmutation of life, a flowing through, a constantly changing participation in the living community. The fate of all living things is an earthbound immortality. During these moments, a profound comfort spreads through me, as I look at the island, the forest and the stream, realizing I can never be separated from them, can never be alone, can never fall away."

Self-exploratory Question: What meaning does death give to my life?

Affirmation: Today I am identifying with life beyond myself and letting go of fear.

May 2
Friendship

Principle: Friendship is a gift, both to the giver and the receiver.

Perennial Wisdom Quote: "A true friend knows your weaknesses but shows you your strengths; feels your fears but fortifies your faith; sees your anxieties but frees your spirit; recognizes our disabilities but emphasizes your possibilities." -- William A. Ward

Discussion: The following beautiful description of friendship was given by an anonymous Shoshone Native American to Kent Nerburn and Louise Mengelkoch who included it in *Native American Wisdom:* "Oh, the comfort, the inexpressible comfort of feeling safe with a person, having neither to weigh thought nor measure words, but pouring them all right out, just as they are, chaff and grain together, certain that a fruitful hand will take and sift them, keep what is worth keeping and, with a breath of kindness, blow the rest away."

This kind of safe presence is the product of unconditional love for another. This love can grow over time, or it can form suddenly. It can be offered to a limited few or to a great many. Wherever it is offered, it is of great service to anyone receiving it. Friends know how to accept weaknesses, forgive mistakes. They value another beyond any material limitations of time and space. Friendship can exist between family members, or not. Friendship is always a choice made within the heart of the giver. It can never be bought or even earned. It is a voluntary gift. It can, however, be lost by neglect, dishonesty, disloyalty and meanness, just as any gift can be broken or tarnished. Friendship is a gift which enlightens the heart of the giver, as well as the receiver.

Self-exploratory Question: How do I choose to give and receive friendship?

Affirmation: Today I am reaching out both to give and to receive friendship.

Principle: Friendship transforms isolation, arrogance and fear.

Perennial Wisdom Quote: "No person is your friend who demands your silence, or denies your right to grow." -- Alice Walker

Discussion: Isolation is usually created by anger, shame and fear. To make things worse, shame and fear continue to grow in isolation. Mental illness is the inevitable result of long periods of extreme isolation, especially if no uplifting reading or healthy, human communication is available. Ideally prison isolation cells would have sound systems playing calming music and provide self-improvement literature twelve hours a day. Otherwise it is too easy for an inmate to just play his or her own thinking errors over and over in his or her isolated head, worsening whatever problem led to the isolation punishment.

Any of us can create our own prisons by isolating ourselves because of self-pity, shame and fear. Finding healthy company is a responsibility, neglected at a great price.

Healthy company does not demand silence. It encourages us to grow emotionally. Human beings have a natural drive for companionship, as well as personal maturation. Both need to be satisfied. There is a wide range of difference among individuals as to how many friends and how much social contact they enjoy. Nevertheless, everyone suffers from isolation. When we are emotionally isolated it is difficult to experience ourselves completely. Instead there is a tendency to avoid parts of ourselves which we judge negatively and to fool ourselves into thinking there is nothing at all destructive in our own minds and hearts.

When we isolate, we tend to see our misery as being caused by others. These errors can be overcome by healthy friendship and group participation.

Self-exploratory Question: How do I reach out best for healthy company?

Affirmation: Today I am both offering and looking for healthy company.

May 4
Respect

Principle: Everyone is worthy of respect, even when he or she makes mistakes.

Perennial Wisdom Quote: "There are two things over which you have complete dominion, authority and control -- your mind and your mouth." -- Molefi Asante

Discussion: It is easiest to become disrespectful of another when we are somehow mentally insufficiently autonomous from the other. When we become contentious (prone to argument), we are always somehow enmeshed with another in an unsatisfying way. Therefore, when we feel the urge to say or do something disrespectful to another, the best substitute behavior is to determine how we can become more emotionally independent from this other person. Once we can establish this independence, it is usually easier to detach from the other in a respectful way.

Let's look at "road rage" as an example of disrespectful behavior. When we notice another driver doing something unsafe, the best response is to quickly and calmly drive more defensively ourselves. If we allow ourselves to become enraged with another driver, our own perceptions narrow, and we become dangerous ourselves to others on the road. Similarly, in any situation in which we become contentious or enraged, our vision usually narrows and, while seeking to punish another, we actually endanger ourselves and others. When we cannot offer positive help, it is best to detach.

Self-exploratory Question: Do I rationalize being disrespectful to others when I judge them to be somehow in the wrong?

Affirmation: I choose to treat everyone as worthy of respect, even when they make mistakes.

May 5
Courtesy

Principle: Courtesy shows the worth of the giver more than the worth of the receiver.

Perennial Wisdom Quote: "To speak ill of anyone is to speak ill of yourself." -- Afghan saying

Discussion: It is sometime necessary to point out another's mistaken behavior. It is never necessary to speak ill of the complete person. To speak ill of another person, rather than just respectfully pointing out behavioral errors, is to judge that person incapable of change. To judge another incapable of change is to ultimately endanger ourselves, not just the other.

Somehow this principle is easily forgotten when another person commits a terrible crime. It is very easy to sink to the level of error and mental violence of someone who perpetrates a crime against us. Most crimes are justified somehow as retaliation in the mind of him or her who commits the crime. This is especially true when the crimes are committed on the part of governments in the form of warfare.

When courtesy is only given when we believe others to be "deserving," it is easy to justify many acts of discourtesy, disrespect and even violence. Courtesy has to be given on the basis of the giver's and receiver's humanity, not on the basis of the receiver's deservedness.

Self-exploratory Question: Do I offer courtesy to others based on their humanity?

Affirmation: Today I choose to speak ill only of erroneous acts, not whole persons.

Principle: Step 5 reads, "We share our self-inventories with our own Higher Powers, and confidentially with a loving, accepting other, without self-recrimination or shame."

Perennial Wisdom Quote: "Where love rules, there is no will to power; and where power predominates, there love is lacking. The one is the shadow of the other." -- Carl Jung

Discussion: Most of what blocks honest, open self-disclosure is fear of another person using that self-disclosure against us. We want to maintain self-empowerment. We do not want to be controlled by others. This is natural and, to a certain degree, even wise.

In some circumstances others actually have the power to harm us with disclosed information, and they might choose to do so. Therefore, it is wise to be thoughtful about to whom we choose to self-disclose. There are times when silence, or even securing an attorney before speaking, is wise. However, it is vital that when we do self-disclose, it is honest. It is also vital that when we self-disclose, our innermost thoughts and feelings will be respected by the listener. In some instances, it is also vital that our self-disclosures will be held in confidence by the listener.

All the 12 Step programs stemming from the Alcoholics Anonymous program's original 12 Steps include a Step providing a safe place for self-disclosure. This is true for our Wise Ways Happiness Program, as well. Self-disclosure is the 5th Step, after the 4th Step's self-assessment. Self-disclosure, to a respectful other, helps to release shame and self-rejection. Shame and self-rejection block emotional health and growth. Everyone who has made mistakes (which is everyone) needs a safe place to confess these mistakes, to receive respectful listening despite these mistakes, and to receive encouragement to make changes preventing the reoccurrence of these mistakes. Even the worst of criminals deserves such a safe place.

Self-exploratory Question: Am I ready to share my self-inventory with a safe listener?

Affirmation: Today I am readying myself for honest, and safe self-disclosures.

May 7   Happiness Group Tradition Five: Group Leaders Are Trusted Servants

Principle: The Happiness Group Tradition 5 reads, "Our leaders are but trusted servants. They do not govern, nor have more status than any other group member."

Perennial Wisdom Quote: "One leg cannot dance alone." -- East African saying

Discussion: In Wise Ways Happiness Support Groups, as in all 12 Step fellowships modeled after Alcoholics Anonymous, decisions are made from the bottom up, not the top down. Groups are autonomous. Group decisions are made by group consensus at open business meetings calling for "a group conscience" on any question. Service work, such as chairing meetings, are opportunities for individual growth. Individuals have both ultimate freedom and ultimate responsibility in Happiness Support Groups. No one person is allowed to dominate group decisions or discussions.

Happiness Support Groups decide when and where to meet by group consensus. They may agree just on a certain number of meetings and then to disband. Or the group may decide to continue on an open-ended basis. If groups are meeting in the building of an agency, a staff member may be assigned to open and close the meeting room, or to distribute loaner books, but, as much as possible, it is best for that staff member to ask for volunteer chairpersons to open and close the meetings and to suggest a topic for reading and sharing from this book.

Self-exploratory Question: Do I understand the Happiness Support Group Traditions?

Affirmation: Today I see volunteering to chair meetings and select group topics as an opportunity for service.

Principle: Opening the heart in safe places transforms fear and lack of attachment.

Perennial Wisdom Quote: "Love is attraction, connection, coherence; it is a place to belong, a series of intersecting circles that extend out from each individual to include everyone else in varying degrees of closeness." -- David Suzuki, *Sacred Balance*

Discussion: Daniel Siegel, M.D., a pediatric neuropsychiatrist, in *Healing Trauma* and in *Parenting From The Inside Out,* discusses his brain research findings about the power of attachment. As children, if we form positive emotional attachments, our brains literally develop in a more complete, healthier way than if we did not form such attachments. If we were traumatized as children and not able to form such attachments, the good news is that in most cases the damage is repairable, if the individual is motivated and able to discover reliable, healthy people with whom to emotionally attach.

When we take the risk to trust life and trust others who have proven their healthy concern for us, we not only "open our hearts" we also literally build healthier, more functional brains.

When looking for people to trust, choose people who are honest, respectful, genuinely interested in you, willing to be of service for their own betterment, and knowledgeable about emotional boundaries

Self-exploratory Question: Where and when can I most safely open my heart?

Affirmation: Today, to further my growth, I am opening my heart in safe ways.

May 9
Innocence

Principle: The "innocence" of childhood is also a receptivity of brain and heart.

Perennial Wisdom Quote: "If you would live long, open your heart." -- Bulgarian saying

Discussion: The "open heart" is usually associated with the innocence of childhood. At the same time the Bulgarians talk about opening one's heart in order to have a long life.

Why is this? Doesn't an open heart increase the risk of being disappointed and betrayed? Yes, but only if we make poor choices in whom to trust. An open heart also increases our positive emotional connections to others. Modern research has found that this promotes happiness and longevity.

Being "innocent" doesn't have to mean being "naïve." Being "innocent" means not having dishonesty and cruelty in one's mind or actions, and being open to the discovery of love and connection with others. As we grow in experience, we also grow in our ability to judge trustworthiness in others. We can exercise this ability and still maintain "innocence."

Jesus Christ spoke about people coming to him "as little children" in order to gain "the kingdom of heaven." He was asking people to open their hearts, knowing that attitude toward life is the path to happiness. Modern psychological research has verified this ancient teaching. This same teaching is also taught by the founders of other world religions. When we close down our minds because of past traumas, we also eliminate the option of healing our brains and hearts. Mental and physical illness is inevitably the result of a closed heart.

Self-exploratory Question: How can I maintain a more open heart?

Affirmation: Today I have both an "innocent" mind and an open heart.

May 10
Love

Principle: Love is the inner essence of life.

Perennial Wisdom Quote: "The love we desire is already within us." -- *A Course in Miracles*

Discussion: Many teachers have agreed with Nelson Mandela that "Our deepest fear is not that we are inadequate. Our deepest fear is that we are powerful beyond measure. It is our light, not our darkness, that most frightens us." We are scared to own the love and light which is our gift at birth. We look for it outside of ourselves when it resides inside all along. Once we claim our inside love, we begin to attract others who can also claim their inside love.

Jesus taught that God is love and that the kingdom of God is within us. This means that our very essence is love. In *The Bible* in the First Book of John (4:17), it reads, "In love there can be no fear, but fear is driven out by perfect love: because to fear is to expect punishment, and anyone who is afraid is still imperfect in love."

The Buddha taught that, "Hatred does not cease through hatred at any time. Hatred ceases through love. This is an unalterable law." Hating and fighting evil does not make it go away. Loving and educating those who have chosen evil ways is what reduces evil.

Some ancient spiritual teachers see love as having 5 aspects: 1) loving-kindness (the ability to bring joy & happiness to others), 2) understanding (deep-looking to understand others' deepest troubles & aspirations), 3) compassion (the ability to ease another's pain & look deeply into another's heart), 4) joy, & 5) equanimity or freedom (offering freedom to the persons you love).

Self-exploratory Question: How do I practice the 5 aspects of love in my life?

Affirmation: Today I am owning my inside love, sharing it, and attracting others to me.

Principle: Hatred tightens the heart, restricts breathing and promotes ill health.

Perennial Wisdom Quote: "…and then the day came when the risk to remain tight in a bud was more painful than the risk it took to blossom." -- Anais Nin

Discussion: Many writers speak poetically of the pain of hatred. James Baldwin in *Nothing Personal* wrote, "The moment we cease to hold each other, the moment we break faith with one another, the sea engulfs us and the light goes out." George Bernard Shaw in *Major Barbara* wrote, "Hate is the coward's revenge for being humiliated." Tacitus in *Life of Agriola* wrote, "It is human to hate those whom we have injured."

Hate is a hostile connection. It is dualistic, based on black and white thinking. It is an energy which binds us to the hated person. It is love soured by dependency, demands, and conditions. We can let go of hate when we can accept that sometimes connection to a specific person isn't possible because of some limitation in ourselves or in the other person. When there is acceptance of limitations, acceptance without judgment, there is a letting go of hatred. A person might still avoid contact with someone, but that avoidance is based on the knowledge of one's own limitations, not just the limitations of another.

Great teachers such as Jesus Christ were criticized for associating with "sinners," "tax collectors" and "harlots." He didn't reject or hate people because of their pasts. He accepted anyone with an open heart, anyone willing to learn and change. He saw that potential in everyone. Other great teachers have done the same. All of us, perhaps, can't be so generous, but we can reach in that direction.

Self-exploratory Question: How can I better let go of hatred in my life?

Affirmation: Today I am making only loving choices.

May 12
Loyalty

Principle: Loyalty builds self-esteem and sustains friendship and family.

Perennial Wisdom Quote: "Hear me! A single twig breaks, but the bundle of twigs is strong." -- Tecumseh (Shawnee)

Discussion: Loyalty requires both loyalty to one's own integrity and loyalty to friends and family. Sometimes these two loyalties seem in conflict. What if a friend asks me to lie or do something illegal? Is such a person a trustworthy friend or family member?

We must be loyal first to our own ethical principles. Healthy friends and family members will respect this and not ask us to go against our principles. They will not ask us to lie for them or engage in illegal and unhealthy behaviors with them. If they do so, we can decline respectfully.

People who "betray" us usually feel they themselves have been betrayed by us. Sometimes this may be true, but sometimes it is because we are operating under different principles.

When a friend or family member is operating under unhealthy principles, all we can do is respectfully point that out to him or her and then refuse to join in the misguided behavior. This is being loyal to one's self and also loyal to the higher self of the friend or family member. Even though he or she might not see it, we would just be hurting that person, if we joined in unhealthy and/or dishonest behavior.

Self-exploratory Question: How can I be loyal to my own principles and also to my friends and family members?

Affirmation: Today I choose loyalty to my friends and family, as long as I can also be loyal to my own highest principles.

Principle: When we can't change another's self-destructive behavior, it is best to detach with love.

Perennial Wisdom Quote: "The secret of happiness is realizing some things can be controlled and some cannot." -- Epictetus, *The Art of Living*

Discussion: Detachment does not imply judgment or criticism of the person or situation from which we are detaching. It does involve separating ourselves from the negative effects another's behaviors could have on our lives. When we see someone we love engaging in self-destructive behavior such as alcohol, some other substance abuse or destructive behavior, it is easy to become over-responsible and try to control another adult's behavior. This only causes us to experience disappointment and retaliation. Instead we can lovingly detach and examine our own behavior to see if we can change anything which has been enabling the other's self-destruction. For example, we can refuse to give this person money, we can refuse to drink alcohol or use drugs with this person, we can refuse to be around this person when he or she is engaging in shaming or self-destructive behavior, etc. All of this involves detachment, but not punishment or rejection.

If we have difficulty detaching, we can go to a support group such as Al-Anon or Alateen to find emotional support for ourselves. If there is no such group in our community, we can start such a group, using available literature. Similarly, if a loved one has a mental illness and refuses to take appropriate medication, we can withdraw financial support, and even take time out from personal contact with this person, until he or she agrees to again follow medical advice. We cannot force another adult to engage in appropriate self-care, but we can be sure we do not enable another adult to be self-destructive.

Self-exploratory Question: How can I be sure I am not enabling another's self-destruction?

Affirmation: Today I am detaching from destructive people and situations which I cannot change.

Principle: Abstaining from personalizing another's self-destructive behavior is important self-care.

Perennial Wisdom Quote: "The indestructible hall of human memory contains two keys. One is made of iron and is called Attachment, the other is made of gold and is called Detachment. The iron key opens the door of the house to lower life. The golden key opens the door of the house to higher life." -- Sri Ananda Acharya, *Yoga of Conquest*

Discussion: When we personalize another's behavior, we see that behavior as somehow attached to us. Our mental connections with this other person cause us to feel responsible for his or her feelings and/or behaviors. Personalization robs another of respect and responsibility. Personalization is an over-responsible process. It is the result of emotional enmeshment with another.

Often people who personalize are well meaning, sensitive people. But, they haven't yet learned how to develop good emotional boundaries, so it is easy for them to inappropriately try to control another's behavior. They haven't learned how to say, "I don't like this behavior," instead of "You are hurting my feelings." Freeing ourselves from personalization also helps to free ourselves from shame and blame.

Self-exploratory Question: How do I personalize others' feelings and behaviors?

Affirmation: Today I choose not to personalize anyone else's behaviors.

Principle: Jealousy is a personal problem; it isn't created by someone else's behavior. It is a response for which we need to take responsibility.

Perennial Wisdom Quote: "For if we try to keep for our own private, personal aggrandizement - no matter how subtly - the love of others, then jealousy, tyranny and all manner of suffering will result." -- Glenn Clark, *Windows of Heaven*

Discussion: Jealousy usually involves fear, attachment and projection overcoming love. When we truly love someone, we want them to be appreciated by others and be free to grow emotionally and socially. We are honest and open with them and trust that they are honest and open with us. We are keeping our commitments to them, and we have confidence that they are honoring commitments to us. We are not afraid of betrayal.

When we are emotionally attached to someone, but not truly loving, we treat that person more like an object of gratification rather than a whole person. We are attached to being gratified in certain ways, and we expect the person to gratify us in certain ways. If he or she is not doing so, we become angry, withdrawn, jealous, and possibly even violent. When this happens, we need to work on learning how to truly love, rather than just attaching to another.

Often psychotherapy is necessary. Sometimes self-help reading and/or a spiritual, support group is sufficient. In any case, we need to take responsibility for our own jealousy and get help with it, not make it the responsibility of the object of our jealousy.

Self-exploratory Question: How can I take more responsibility for my jealousies?

Affirmation: Today I am taking complete responsibility for my jealousies and working on healing them.

Principle: I am not responsible for anyone else's feelings or behaviors.

Perennial Wisdom Quote: "Men are disturbed not by things that happen, but by their opinion of the things that happen." -- Karlfried Gaf Von Durckheim, *Hara, The Vital Centre of Man*

Discussion: When a person becomes over-responsible, he or she falls into these traps: suffering because of the actions or reactions of other people; allowing oneself to be used or abused; doing for others what they could do for themselves; manipulating situations so others will eat, go to bed, get up, pay bills, not drink, etc.; covering up for someone's mistakes; creating a crisis or preventing a crisis if it is in the natural course of another's behavior.

To prevent over-responsibility, it is important to remember that we are responsible for our own feelings and behaviors, not anyone else's. This is true even if the other person is a family member. Legally, we may be responsible for a spouse's bills, unless we inform the creditor that we refuse responsibility and/or get a divorce. But we are certainly not emotionally responsible for a spouse's addictions, betrayals, or indulgences. If we are in a situation wherein a spouse or an adult child or sibling or parent is engaging in self-destructive behavior, our challenge is to detach with love and not enable that person's irresponsibility by being over-responsible ourselves.

Self-exploratory Question: In what relationships do I tend to become over-responsible?

Affirmation: Today I am taking responsibility for myself, not other adults.

May 17
Confidence

Principle: Confidence transforms avoidance and non-confrontation.

Perennial Wisdom Quote: "No one tests the depth of a river with both feet." -- Ashanti African proverb

Discussion: Confidence is the product of good self-care and confrontational skills. Confident people have good emotional boundaries, so they do not personalize others' experiences, nor become enmeshed in other persons' problems. They know what they have control over and what they do not. They know how to detach from what they can't control, and they know how to manage their own feelings and behaviors.

When another person slights them, they know how to respectfully request more appropriate behavior. If another person persists in disrespectful behavior, they know how to detach and protect themselves emotionally and physically from abuse.

While developing self-confidence, it is helpful to practice self-confrontation for a while before attempting a lot of confrontation of others. Ask yourself, "What conflicts or discrepancies in myself can I confront? How can I remove these conflicts between my own ideal behavior and my actual behavior?"

Become successful in improving yourself before you ask for improvement from others. Then, when you are ready to ask for improvement in another, that person will likely be aware of your own commitment to self-improvement and will likely be more willing to work on personal change. Also, you will have a much better understanding of how difficult personal change can be.

Self-exploratory Question: How can I become more self-confident?

Affirmation: Today I am focusing on self-improvement, not on controlling others.

May 18
Confrontation

Principle: Effective communication is honest, respectful, behaviorally specific and kind.

Perennial Wisdom Quote: "When competition becomes combat, it loses its power to inspire, and becomes instead a form of pressure which creates disharmony in our minds and senses, upsetting the natural balance of our lives." -- Tarthang Tulku, *Skillful Means*

Discussion: Dennis D. Adams, M.A., a marriage and family therapist in Los Angeles, has written a valuable little book called *Honest, Direct, Respectful.* In it he describes two communication styles to avoid: "passive" and "reactive." Passive communicators don't like conflict and give in for the sake of peace and harmony. Reactive communicators don't want to feel bad alone so they blow off steam to try to feel better. They want others to see things their way.

Effective communicators are "Honest, Direct and Respectful (HDR)." These HDR guidelines are included in part of the vision plan of the Partnership Health Plan of California and are used by many employees of the Kaiser Permanente Tri-Central Services Area of California. It's important to use these guidelines at home as well as at work.

When we are unhappy with the behavior of someone we care about, we need to be able to confront that person respectfully and kindly, specifically describing how his or her behavior causes harm and then making a clear request for a substitute behavior which is respectful to both parties. (See January 18th, The "Anger Formula.)

Self-exploratory Question: How can I improve on my confrontation skills?

Affirmation: Today I choose only to deliver respectful, kind, behaviorally specific confrontations. I don't call people names nor shame them.

May 19
Forgiveness

Principle: Forgiveness transforms blame, resentment and rejection.

Perennial Wisdom Quote: "He who requires much from himself and little from others will keep himself from being the object of resentment." -- Confucius

Discussion: One way to define "forgiveness" is "for-giving-away-resentments" or "letting go." When we hang onto resentments, we burden ourselves, not the person we are resenting. Forgiveness is not approving or condoning another's behavior. Forgiveness is acknowledging and accepting another's behavior, because we realize it is out of our control.

We do not have to have contact with someone we are forgiving. Forgiveness is a shift in our own hearts away from bitterness, blame and resentment into acceptance. Blame, revenge, and resentment are ways to react to negativity with negativity. They can lead to scapegoating and bitterness. Forgiveness is a way to respond to negativity with acceptance of the humanity of the person and a recognition of another's limitations.

When we forgive, we can still affirm that the other's behavior was hurtful and wrong. We can even take Adult Time Out from contact the other, until we can be assured that the other is capable of improved behavior. We can describe the damage done to us and ask the other to repent and change his or her behavior. We can wait for a response and give ourselves time to rebuild trust. All these steps are a part of the forgiveness process. Forgiveness involves humbly recognizing that we ourselves are not perfect and others also can make mistakes and still change.

Self-exploratory Question: Where do I need to work on forgiveness in my life?

Affirmation: Today I choose to move towards forgiveness and away from resentment.

Principle: When we point at another there are usually three fingers pointing back at ourselves.

Perennial Wisdom Quote: "Take your life in your own hands, and what happens? A terrible thing: no one is to blame." -- Erica Jong

Discussion: People who tend to blame others usually are trying to avoid blaming themselves, because they would do so harshly and without self-forgiveness. They don't know how to take responsibility for their mistakes without shaming themselves and feeling unworthy of love.

We need to teach our children how to recognize their mistakes, how not to judge themselves harshly, how to accept themselves, acknowledge their mistakes, and move into speedy correction. If as adults we haven't learned how to do this, we need to take responsibility for learning.

Some people compulsively blame others in a retaliatory fashion because they expect to be unfairly blamed and punished themselves. If this has been your history, do your best to surround yourself with adults who will not do this to you, and don't treat them that way yourself.

Underneath blame is usually shame. Shame is energy which puts down the essence, the humanity of the person being shamed. Shame is not corrective, behaviorally specific feedback. It is damaging both to the giver and the receiver. Shame causes the giver to disconnect and isolate. Shame causes the receiver to withdraw or personalize. When we feel the urge to blame another, it is best to first take responsibility for our own part in the matter, and avoid confronting the other until we can do so respectfully.

Self-exploratory Question: How can I take more responsibility for my own mistakes?

Affirmation: I take responsibility for my mistakes, even when others are also mistaken.

Principle: No one deserves negative judgment.

Perennial Wisdom Quote: "Keep the other person's well-being in mind when you feel an attack of soul-purging truth coming on." -- Betty White

Discussion: Judgment can be used both positively and negatively. Negative judgment is when we use our discerning capacities to purposefully criticize, wound or hurt ourselves or someone else. Positive judgment is when we use our discerning capacities to evaluate ourselves or others for the purpose of offering loving assistance.

When we offer positive judgment, it is always important to clarify our loving intent, especially if the receiver may erroneously perceive the words as intending harm or devaluation.

In some situations, such as parenting a child, teaching a student or evaluating an employee, we are sometimes called upon to correct another's behavior. In such circumstances, pointing out an incorrect answer or an unproductive behavior might be necessary. However, in these circumstances it is always best to give the corrective feedback in a kind way, including positive comments on the others' productive behaviors. When giving corrective feedback, it is vital to focus on the other's mistaken behavior and not on the other's personality or core self.

All beings are worthy of respect and kindness. What we give to others is usually what we end up receiving back.

Self-exploratory Question: In what situations am I prone to negative judgment?

Affirmation: Today I am treating everyone with respect and kindness.

May 22   **Freedom from**
Rejection

Principle: Respecting loved ones' privacy reduces feelings of rejection.

Perennial Wisdom Quote: "For a love to grow through the tests of everyday living, one must respect that zone of privacy where one retires to relate to the inside instead of the outside." -- Kahil Gibran, *The Prophet*

Discussion: Some people are so insecure that they cannot give their loved ones zones of privacy. When people do not have private space and time, they can neither replenish inner reserves nor maintain loving, open hearts. When we resent our loved ones' time away from us and attempt to confine them, we reduce the likelihood of their being able to sustain loving, open hearts towards us. This kind of behavior stems from attachment, fear and insecurity, not love.

When we have fearful thoughts about our loved one's absences, it may be OK to ask for reassurance, but it is not OK to demand increased attention. Demanding attention rarely results in loving attention. Requesting more time with a loved one might be appropriate, as long as it is done in a kind, respectful way. What is to be avoided is clinging criticism.

When we receive a kind request for more time from a loved one, it is best to honor its positive intention to deepen and enrich the relationship. Perhaps we have been preoccupied and not available enough to a loved one. Maybe the loved one is having a particularly difficult time and needing temporary, additional attention. Even when we can't immediately make more time available for a loved one, we can take a few moments to honor the request and the loving intent behind it.

Self-exploratory Questions: How can I take and give private time with loved ones without feeling rejected? How can I also make and honor requests for more contact?

Affirmation: Today I choose to give my loved ones private time, and also attention.

Principle: Empathic listening is usually more helpful than giving advice.

Perennial Wisdom Quote: "Having two ears and one tongue, we should listen twice as much as we speak." -- Turkish saying

Discussion: James Jakob Liszka, Ph.D. in *Moral Competence* defines empathy as "the native ability to read the emotional state of feelings of others as based on past experience or the experience of one's own feelings, emotional states and sufferings." Empathy is frequently confused with sympathy, which he defines as "the feeling of distress, sadness or joy that may occur when we understand the emotional state of another. "

Empathy requires a certain resonance of emotional experience between two people. It also occurs in a more detached consciousness. The empathic person does not take on the mood or opinions or feelings of the other. A sympathetic person has less clear emotional boundaries and has a tendency to take on the mood, opinions or feelings of another.

Sympathy can, unfortunately, sometimes promote a victim attitude in the listener. Empathy doesn't do this. Empathic listening gives more room to the speaker to explore his or her own experience without attending to the listener's experience. An empathetic listener can even be silent most of the time. Empathic listening is heart to heart, and sometimes doesn't even require language. Empathy involves being able to see things from another's perspective without also losing your own perspective. Empathic listening requires dropping judgment, blame and criticism and being completely emotionally present with another person. It's not about problem-solving or fixing things for others, and yet it is very helpful, as it facilitates the speaker's discovering his or her own solutions.

Self-exploratory Question: How can I improve my empathic listening skills?

Affirmation: Today I am doing my best to empathically listen to those I love.

Principle: Simply attaching to others can never make us feel whole.

Perennial Wisdom Quote: "Rejection is only damaging when you start out believing you are not complete…If you understand that you can only draw to yourself what you already are, you can see rejection in another light." -- Iyanla Vanzant, *Acts of Faith*

Discussion: When we believe that we are incomplete within ourselves and must attach to another to be complete, we set ourselves up for rejection. This belief in our own incompleteness is what needs to change in order to be able to truly love another. If we are presently burdened with this limiting belief, it is our personal responsibility to find ways to make ourselves feel whole. This may mean clarifying our personal talents and strengths and building on them. It may mean examining our spiritual lives to create more meaning for our place in the larger universe. It may mean joining into some community activities in which we can be of service. Whatever it takes, it is a personal responsibility.

Romantic fantasies tend to suggest that another human being, if we can just find the "right" one, can make us feel complete. This is not the case. Yes, finding a compatible partner can greatly enrich life, but this is because it is a mutual enrichment process. We must also have a whole self to offer a partner, in order to attract and keep a partner with a whole self. There are no shortcuts to self-realization. Spiritual support groups can help, but ultimately the work must be done by the individual, not by a help-mate.

Self-exploratory Question: Where and when do I feel incomplete?

Affirmation: Today I am a complete and worthy human being.

Principle: We can't please anyone all of the time, or everyone some of the time.

Perennial Wisdom Quote: "Loving someone and pleasing someone are two different things." -- Jerry Jampolski

Discussion: Some people confuse approval with love and disapproval with rejection. Love is not about approval or disapproval. Love is about kind acceptance and a desire for the best for another. It is a decision to do our best not to harm another. It is a decision to open one's heart to another. This does not necessarily mean approving of all of another's behavior, or having all of our own behavior approved. Therefore, learning to accept kind, negative feedback, (appropriate admonition) even from loved ones is an important skill, as is learning to give it.

We need to recognize that we don't have to agree with the admonition, we just need to respectfully accept it, rather than seeing it as hostile criticism. Criticism is hostile judgment and rejection of a whole person. It demands agreement. This kind of criticism needs to be ignored. Kind admonition, on the other hand, involves respectfully telling another what behavior seem to be destructive, or at least non-productive. It does not demand agreement. (Also see Sept. 5th reading.)

When giving kind, negative feedback, clearly describe the behavior which you perceive as producing non-productive ends, and then make a positive request for a productive replacement behavior. For example, "When you yell at me, I just shut down. If you want me to listen, please use a normal tone." This indicates to the receiver that your intent is not rejection, but instead the healing of a broken interaction.

Self-exploratory Question: How can I effectively give and receive kind admonition?

Affirmation: I choose to accept kind admonition and detach from shaming criticism.

Principle: Argument is a waste of time.

Perennial Wisdom Quote: "The sage does not talk; the talented ones talk; the stupid ones argue." -- Chinese proverb

Discussion: The March 26th reading discussed the connection between emotional avoidance and argument. Today let's consider how arguments are kept going and how to stop them. Arguments are kept going when we buy into needing to feel "right" when someone else sees us as "wrong", or when we feel we have to prove someone else to be "wrong."

We can't control others' opinions and conclusions. We can control our own behaviors which can calmly focus on expressing our own views, without demanding that anyone else thinks we are "right" and without proving that someone else is "wrong." We can "agree to disagree." We can still be friends or family members with someone and disagree in many areas of our lives.

Love does not demand agreement. Love involves acceptance and letting go of differences. When love "gets the last word in," it's an apology, even if the other person has not apologized. Arguing is always the result of power and ego demands, and both of these tend to shut down the loving heart. Loving hearts are open to disagreement. They love whole persons and see opinions as transitory and not worth argument. Loving hearts know how to love those who are in disagreement with them. They value heart connection even more than mind connection or approval.

Self-exploratory Question: In what situations am I most prone to argument?

Affirmation: Today I choose not to waste my time in argument.

Principle: Listening carefully to another and validating his or her feelings is always a valuable gift, even when we may disagree with another.

Perennial Wisdom Quote: "The reason why so few people are agreeable in conversation, is that each is thinking more of what he is intending to say, than of what others are saying; and we never listen when we are planning to speak." -- Francois La Rochefoucauld

Discussion: Safe people know how to accept and validate others' feelings. They listen, hear and make eye contact. They are direct, loyal, supportive and authentic. They know the difference between validating another's feelings and approving of another's behavior. If they disagree with some choice you are considering, they can accept and understand your feelings and also indicate that your choice may not be in your own best interests, or at least might not be a choice they would make themselves. They are respectful.

People who can validate feelings can distinguish their own feelings from others' feelings. When listening to others, they don't take over and shift the focus onto their own experience. Instead they listen carefully, consider what others are saying, recognize the feelings being expressed and accept and respect them.

Many suffering people need simple validation of their feelings more than they need assistance. They want to be heard, accepted and understood, not fixed. This is the basis of emotional intimacy. This skill is especially important between spouses.

Self-exploratory Question: How can I improve on my ability to validate others' feelings?

Affirmation: Today I choose to validate my own and others' feelings.

May 28
Differentiation

Principle: Differentiation transforms enmeshment and jealousy.

Perennial Wisdom Quote: "Let there be spaces in our togetherness." -- Kahil Gibran, *The Prophet*

Discussion: Here are several definitions of differentiation:

- "a balance between self-regulation and connection" (Noel Larson, Ph.D., 2003 lecture)

- "the ability to differentiate your thoughts, feelings, actions, issues and problems from other people's thoughts, feelings, actions, issues and problems." (Vonda Olson Long, *Facilitating Personal Growth in Self and Others*)

- "standing up for what you believe. Calming yourself down, not letting your anxiety run away with you, and not getting over reactive. Not caving in to pressure to conform...." (David Schnarch, *Passionate Marriage)* Dr. Schnarch asserts that differentiation involves the ability: 1) to maintain a clear sense of self in proximity to others, 2) to regulate one's own anxiety (to self soothe), 3) to maintain a non-anxious presence when another is anxious, and 4) to tolerate emotional pain for emotional growth.

Self-exploratory Question: How can I be more differentiated in my relationships?

Affirmation: I am able to differentiate my own thoughts, feelings, actions, issues and problems from those which belong to others.

Principle: Clear emotional boundaries facilitate healthy relationships.

Perennial Wisdom Quote: "Good fences make good neighbors." -- Robert Frost

Discussion: In order for back yard fences to be "good", people on both sides of them need to agree to their existence, their size and their purpose. Good fences mark areas of ownership respectfully and clearly and prevent unwanted intrusions into private space. The same is true for emotional boundaries. Individuals "own" their own emotions and bodies and need to protect them from unwanted intrusion from others. This is not to push people away, but rather to make "good fences" so as to keep "good emotional neighbors." This is especially true in marriages, families and friendships.

       The emotionally closer the relationship, the more challenging are the emotional boundaries. When establishing good emotional boundaries, both sides need to start out by agreeing that verbal abuse, physical abuse and sexual abuse are unacceptable. Verbal abuse is clarified to include blaming, shaming, yelling, name calling, and verbal put- downs. Physical abuse includes shoving, pushing, slapping, and hitting. Sexual abuse includes sexual touch between adults and children and sexual touch between non-consenting adults. Both sides also need to agree that if one person, in a state of distress, violates these boundaries, the other person rightfully removes himself or herself from contact with the other, at least temporarily. (See January 19th on "Adult Time Out.")

Self-exploratory Question: How can I establish better emotional boundaries?

Affirmation: Today I am keeping good emotional boundaries with others.

Principle: Emotional enmeshment leads to increased shame and blame.

Perennial Wisdom Quote: "Always remember there are two types of people in this world. Those who come into a room and say, 'Well, here I am!' and those who come in and say, 'Ah, there you are!'" -- Frederick L. Collins

Discussion: Emotional enmeshment comes from personal insecurity, self-consciousness, and difficulty loving others without becoming overly dependent on them. Loving adult hearts and minds accept primary responsibility for self-care and their love overflows freely without entrapping their loved ones. All adults need their own independent adult, support circle of friends and family members, so as not to become overly emotionally dependent on just one individual. That kind of dependence smothers and eventually kills true love.

      Enmeshed people tend to confuse empathy with sympathy. Bruce Bibee, a therapist, distinguishes the two with this analogy: "There is a person at the bottom of a deep hole and you are standing at the top. If you jump in and share the pain, that's sympathy. If, on the other hand, you offer to drop them down a ladder so they can get out, that's empathy." If you experience yourself jumping into holes with people, you are experiencing enmeshment.

Self-exploratory Question: Where do I experience emotional enmeshment?

Affirmation: Today I am practicing empathy, and avoiding enmeshment.

Principle: Self-reliance, along with respect for others' needs, creates personal security.

Perennial Wisdom Quote: "How wrong it is for a woman to expect the man to build the world she wants, rather than set out to create it herself." -- Anais Nin

Discussion: The source of most conflict and anger is unmet security needs. When we can identify these security needs in ourselves and find independent ways to meet them, we contribute less to conflict and anger. When we depend primarily on other people to meet our security needs, we set ourselves up for anger and conflict.

To be secure ourselves, we must respect the security needs of others. This is true on the personal level, the family level, the national level and the international level. Insecure people easily project their fear and create many enemies. When we are the recipient of such fear from another, it's important to do our best to discover the source of the other's insecurities and to help the other feel more secure. Just because another sees us as an enemy doesn't mean that we have to see him or her as an enemy. Of course, we need to protect ourselves from immediate violence. However, in the long run the best source of security is living among others who also feel self-secure. This is true between different genders, different nationalities, different religions, and different generations.

In summary, self-security is a two-step process: 1) the ability to rely on one's own resources for self-care, and 2) the ability to respect the security needs of others in order to not threaten them and to help them to feel secure.

Self-exploratory Question: How can I be more successful in both self-security steps?

Affirmation: Today I take responsibility for my own security and for respecting the security needs of others.

Principle: Maintaining a separate sense of self is vital for stable, intimate relationships.

Perennial Wisdom Quote: "Love consists in this, that two solitudes protect a border and salute one another." -- Rainer Maria Rilke

Discussion: A healthy, balanced perceptual/emotional relationship has two-directional energy in it. There is open giving and receiving on the part of both persons. Both people can see themselves and the other clearly and separately. Both people have a clear "sense of self" and respect the other's "sense of self." The giving and receiving is voluntary and from the heart. It is not done out of fear or manipulation. Both people can identify their security needs and feel independently capable of meeting them. What they give is given freely. What they receive is received freely. Love and intimacy can thrive.

When we can't clearly identify our own security needs and we don't feel capable of independently meeting them, a "loss of self" happens. This "loss of self" leads to reactivity to people and events and dependent, unconscious, knee-jerk behaviors. We make assumptions about others based on the past, without really seeing them in the present moment. We project onto new relationships disappointments from past ones and expect repeated losses, or we project onto others possibilities for being rescued from past pain. Either way, by looking outside ourselves for destruction or security, we set ourselves up for disappointment.

It is vital to develop a healthy sense of self before committing to an intimate relationship. Otherwise the relationship becomes an emotional parent/child relationship and both parties suffer.

Self-exploratory Question: How can I avoid losing myself in my relationships?

Affirmation: I am capable of maintaining a strong sense of self in my relationships.

Principle: Projecting our fears onto outside situations and relationships create "paranoid fantasies."

Perennial Wisdom Quote: "The future depends not upon what others decide to do but upon what you decide to become." -- Frank Buchman

Discussion: Intimacy in a free society, unfortunately, tends to create some degree of "paranoid fantasy." When we entrust another with our love and attention, it is only human to have some fears about our love and attention not being honestly reciprocated. This is especially true if our finances and living arrangements and possibly even employment are somehow also connected to a love relationship. When we fear abandonment, rejection or betrayal, it is fundamental to take full responsibility for this fear and not project it onto the other, making it his or her responsibility to fix. What one does with one's fear is always one's own personal responsibility. It is vital not to blame another for being fearful oneself. If the other's behavior does not appear to be trustworthy, we can either choose to leave the relationship or work to rebuild trust in the relationship. Either way it is a personal choice.

       We can request changed behavior from another, but we cannot demand it without damaging the love in the relationship. Love is always a free choice. It cannot be forced. When we try to force love, we destroy it.

Self-exploratory Question: How can I more responsibly own my own "paranoid fantasies" in my most intimate relationship?

Affirmation: Today I choose to own my own "paranoid fantasies" and to heal my fears.

June 3   **Financial**
Responsibility

Principle: Financial responsibility helps to build a strong sense of self.

Perennial Wisdom Quote: "Every man is a consumer, and ought to be a producer. He fails to make his place good in the world, unless he not only pays his debt, but adds something to the common wealth." -- R.W. Emerson

Discussion: In modern economies it is sometimes hard to see whether one is being responsible in creating a balance between "production" and "consumption." True, a person can be sure not to spend more money than he or she earns. But, what about taking out responsible loans to go to college or buying a house or a car? What about paying them back responsibly? When using modern credit systems, the challenge to be financially responsible can be very difficult.

      Here are some simple guidelines for budgeting and using credit: 1) When you leave your parents' home, establish your own checking account and pay your budgeted rent, utilities, child care, transportation, medical and insurance bills promptly by check at the beginning of the month, right after payday, before putting any cash in your pocket for anything else. 2) Budget how much weekly cash you will need to withdraw for food, gas, and recreation and withdraw only that amount from the bank once a week. 3) Don't use a credit card for anything but real emergencies and expenses which can be paid off within six months or less. 4) Don't take out more student loans than you can pay off in ten years. 5) Finish college promptly, figure out a 5-10 year pay-off schedule for your school loans and prioritize those monthly payments as soon as you graduate. 6) Buy a car only if you can pay off the loan in 4 years or pay cash. 7) After paying off college loans, budget and save the maximum amount of money which gives you tax benefits and a retirement plan. 8) Buy real estate only if you have an adequate, steady job and can pay off the mortgage in thirty years.

Self-exploratory Question: How can I be more responsible with my money?

Affirmation: Today I am responsibly earning, budgeting and spending my money.

June 4   **Freedom from Financial Over-**
responsibility

Principle: Enabling another person's financial irresponsibility is not responsible.

Perennial Wisdom Quote: "The white man knows how to make everything, but he does not know how to distribute it." -- Sitting Bull, Lakota Native American Chief, 1885

Discussion: Modern economies make the distribution of money and resources much more complicated than subsistence economies, and yet we can all still learn things from successful subsistence economies. In such economies, individuals were expected to contribute to the community whenever they could do so. Children learned to hunt, farm, sew, gather, cook, and clean as soon as they were physically able to do so. They took a healthy pride in contributing to their families and communities at a young age. Adults, during the prime of their physically productive years, responsibly cared for the basic needs of their families, including their children and their elders. If a child or elder was left resourceless due to a death or illness, he or she was usually "adopted" by productive members of the community, although still given opportunities to contribute.

In modern economies, children and young people need to be given opportunities to be productive and helpful to the community as much as they are physically able. Productive adults need to abstain from being over-responsible for able-bodied young people. Productive spouses need to abstain from being over-responsible for non-productive spouses. Enabling healthy adults to be irresponsible financially is a mistake. Communities need to be responsible to give adults responsible work to do to earn at least subsistence food and shelter, when they are able.

Self-exploratory Question: How can I avoid enabling others' financial irresponsibility?

Affirmation: I am responsibly contributing to my community, without enabling others.

Principle: The Wise Ways Happiness Step Six reads, "We continue strengthening our assets and letting go of our shortcomings."

Perennial Wisdom Quote: "One leg cannot dance alone." -- East African saying

Discussion: All the major world religions and ancient philosophies stress the importance of continued self-examination and ethical conduct. Because self-deception is so easy, most religions and philosophies also stress the importance of seeking assistance for honest self-appraisal and character development. Traditional cultures set up clear guidelines for seeking advice from elders, and often have negative consequences for individuals who refuse to follow elder advice.

   Modern secular societies have less structured and less mandatory guidelines for seeking help with ethic and self-improvement. Adults tend to be given more freedom for choosing their own advisors and times for advisement. Many modern communities could likely benefit from making self-assessment and advisement guidelines more explicit. The Wise Ways Happiness Program seeks to offer self-assessment tools and advisement opportunities to any interested individual. Appendix 3 offers extensive self-inventorying suggestions. Listening to others at Happiness Support Groups can help all of us to use the tools in this book to build on our assets and to let go of life-depleting choices.

Self-exploratory Questions: How am I continuing to let go of my shortcomings?

Affirmation: Today I am strengthening my assets and letting go of my shortcomings.

June 6   **Happiness Support Group Tradition Six: Group Membership**

Principle: The Happiness Support Group Tradition Six reads, "Group membership is based on attendance at Happiness Support Group meetings and on commitment to practicing the Wise Ways Happiness Steps and Traditions."

Perennial Wisdom Quote: "Right protection is something within us rather than something between us and the world, more about finding a place of refuge and strength than finding a hiding place.: -- Rachel Naomi Remen, M.D., *My Grandfather's Blessings*

Discussion: Joining a healthy support group and spiritual community is mostly about internal commitments. The internal commitments need to be 1) to show up at meetings, 2) to be honest, and 3) to seek personal emotional/spiritual growth. In Happiness Support Groups simply attending meetings and studying the Wise Ways principles is enough for membership. After spending some time in a group, service work such as chairing meetings is encouraged, but never required.

No group of people, or group process, is perfect. Individual and group shortcomings need to be acknowledged and worked on. There is a Group Evaluation set of questions in Appendix 2. Everyone in the Happiness Support Groups enjoys equal status. Everyone needs to work on following the Happiness Support Group guidelines in the Appendix.

Self-exploratory Question: Am I ready to form or join a Happiness Support Group?

Affirmation: I am committed to studying Wise Ways Happiness principles and considering joining a group.

Principle: Grief and loss must be faced and healed; otherwise it becomes buried in anger and resentment.

Perennial Wisdom Quote: "Nature is always lovely, invincible, glad, whatever is done and suffered by her creatures. All scars she heals whether in rocks or water or sky or hearts." -- John Muir

Discussion: Scientists have recently learned that there is a natural tranquilizer in tears. When we have suffered a loss or an injury, it is healthy to cry. It is much healthier to cry than to depend on man-made tranquilizers. At times we all need help in becoming more tranquil. This is what tears and grieving are about -- helping ourselves to gradually become more tranquil. If we don't honor and respect our grief, if we just repress it, it usually shows up labeled as anger. Some people have been so shamed for crying as children that they have taught themselves not even to recognize grief or loss. All they are aware of is the anger that results when grief is forced out of awareness. This makes for a great deal of difficulty managing one's anger, because the roots of the anger are pushed out of awareness.

In order to effectively process our anger, we need to know about our losses, as well as what is needed to heal them. When we can't identify these two things, when all we experience is rage and no more information is available, we are in trouble. Adult Time Out is designed to give a person time to get calm, identify unmet needs, and heal losses. (See Jan. 17 & 19 Readings.)

Self-exploratory Question: How can I learn to grieve more effectively?

Affirmation: Today I am facing my losses and not repressing them under anger.

Principle: Effective anger management transforms destructive anger.

Perennial Wisdom Quote: "The more you express your anger, the angrier you become…. The Buddhist attitude is to take care of anger. We don't suppress it. We don't run away from it. We just breathe and hold our anger in our arms with utmost tenderness…. The important thing is to bring out the awareness of your anger in order to protect and sponsor it. Then the anger is no longer alone; it is with your mindfulness…. If you keep breathing on your anger, shining your compassion and understanding on it, your anger will soon crack, and you will be able to look into its depths and see its roots." --Thich Nhat Hanh

Discussion: When we become angry the tendency is to focus all our attention on the object of our anger. In the process we dehumanize others and lose vital awareness of ourselves. Effective anger management involves what is called "mindfulness." Mindfulness includes staying calm enough to watch our own thoughts, emotions and body sensations without acting them out on others. Usually when we become angry, we start breathing more quickly and with less depth, and our hearts start beating more quickly. When you notice these physical sensations accompanying your anger, you can breathe deeply for twenty seconds or more, relax your muscles, especially in your arms and shoulders, and look for fears underneath your anger. If you can identify them and take responsibility for them, this can diffuse your anger, and you won't need to speak in rage.

Far more people use their words as weapons than people use their hands or guns as weapons. For us to learn to have intimate, loving relationships, we need to learn how NOT to use words as weapons of punishment and revenge. Anger is a gift our bodies give us when our needs are not being met. It is energy designed to be used defensively or assertively to create safety. It is not energy designed for punishment and verbal abuse. When anger is used aggressively to punish or act out revenge, it becomes a boomerang which is eventually returned on us or our family or nation in the form of other persons' destructive anger.

Thus, to be free from destructive anger, we need to learn how to observe and express healing anger. Healing anger takes time to observe itself and be compassionate towards itself. Healing anger does not focus on the wrongs of others. It briefly focuses on one's own unmet needs, just long enough to take responsibility for these needs and for expressing them assertively and respectfully.

Self-exploratory Question: How can I be freer from destructive anger?

Affirmation: Today I choose to avoid destructive anger.

Principle: Verbal abuse is aimed at hurting another, rather than at correcting a problem.

Perennial Wisdom Quote: "Many have fallen by the edge of the sword, but more have fallen by the tongue." -- Anonymous

Discussion: Far more people use their words as weapons than use their hands or guns. For us to learn to have intimate, loving relationships, we need to learn how not to use words as weapons of punishment and revenge. Anger is a gift our bodies give us when our needs are not being met. It is energy designed to be used defensively or assertively to create safety. It is not energy designed for punishment and verbal abuse. When anger is used aggressively to punish or act out revenge, it becomes a boomerang which is eventually returned on us or our family or nation in the form of other persons' destructive anger.

Thus, to be free from destructive anger, we need to learn how to observe and express healing anger. Healing anger takes time to observe itself and be compassionate toward itself. Healing anger does not focus on the wrongs of others. It briefly focuses on one's own unmet needs, just long enough to take responsibility for these needs and for expressing them assertively and respectfully.

Self-exploratory Question: How can I be free from destructive anger?

Affirmation: Today I choose to avoid destructive anger.

June 10
Assertiveness

Principle: Being assertive means, not being aggressive or passive; it is presenting one's own needs, feelings and requests, while being respectful of the needs, feelings and requests of others.

Perennial Wisdom Quote: "Power, in the sense of domination over others, is excessive self-assertion [or aggression.] The social structure in which it is exerted most effectively is the hierarchy…. There is another kind of power, one that is more appropriate for the new [deep ecology] paradigm -- power as influence of others. The ideal structure for exerting this kind of power is not the hierarchy but the network, which, as we shall see, is also the central metaphor of ecology." -- Fritjof Capra, *The Web of Life*

Discussion: Violence and aggression don't work because there is always an opposite and equal force to every action. This is a metaphysical truism, just like the similar axiom in physics. When we push someone, that person pushes back, or, if he or she is dis-empowered to push back immediately, the reaction goes underground for a while until it can be acted out later. When we repress emotions, a similar thing happens: the emotion goes underground for a while, but comes out later, often at an inopportune time and in an ineffective way.

Expressing emotions and thoughts assertively, respectfully and with good timing is vital. An effectively assertive person knows when to listen and when and how to speak. Such a person works to find solutions which meet all parties' needs as much as possible. Assertive people know how to network with others to fulfill common goals. As Brooke Astor once said, "Power is the ability to do good things for others."

Self-exploratory Question: How effective are my assertion skills?

Affirmation: Today I am assertively expressing my emotions and thoughts.

Principle: Using preferential language is an important assertion skill.

Perennial Wisdom Quote: "Temperate anger well becomes the wise." -- Philemon

Discussion: Assertive people often use the words, "I would prefer…." This way of introducing one's wishes is respectful to the receiver. These words make it clear that the speaker is not attempting to dominate decision making. The speaker is simply asserting his or her own wishes and placing them side by side with others' wishes, so that an appropriate, democratic decision can be made by all.

Preferential language supports effective networking. As Fritjof Capra in *The Web of Life* said so well (See June 10 reading), networking is "the central metaphor of ecology." The natural world contains massive interacting networks. The world is full of millions of different organisms. Room is made for all of them. If humans can learn to be as accepting and accommodating as other life species, there may be hope for peaceful, human coexistence on a continually thriving planet. We might be able to solve our global warming problems without many, many more species being lost.

Self-exploratory Question: How can I more effectively use preferential language when asserting myself?

Affirmation: Today I am using preferential language when expressing my wishes.

Principle: Aggressive anger hurts the giver as much as the receiver.

Perennial Wisdom Quote: "Those who scored in the upper 20% of hostility when tested 20 years earlier had a 42% increased risk of premature death from all causes combined, including heart disease and cancer, when compared to those who scored in the lower 20% of hostility." -- Dean Ornish, M.D., *Love and Survival*

Discussion: As Booker T. Washington once said, "You can't hold a man down without staying down with him." Recent medical research confirms that this is literally true. When we live a life characterized by lots of hostility, our physical bodies literally suffer. We are not designed to be chronically in a "fight" state. Such states physically wear us down.

Freedom from aggression does not mean complete freedom from anger. It means freedom from inappropriately experienced and expressed anger. When anger is observed in the self with compassion, not dumped on others, and when it is assertively, respectfully expressed using the Anger Formula (See Reading on Jan. 17-18), it creates energy. Eventually serenity and even intimacy are possible. It is just when anger becomes aggression, meaning when it is acted out at the expense of others, that it becomes toxic, both to the receiver and the giver.

When anger is expressed appropriately, it can actually be a gift, because it is meant to heal a rift between people. It is not the anger of rejection or frustration or depression. It is the anger of assertive compassion and potentially laser-like healing.

Self-exploratory Question: How can I express anger without being aggressive?

Affirmation: Today I am freeing myself from aggressive anger.

Principle: Complaints negatively focus on what is missing, rather than positively focusing on the good which exists and how it can be built upon.

Perennial Wisdom Quote: "It is easier to criticize than to do better." -- Swiss saying

Discussion: Excessive complaining is usually the result of ineffective grief processing. Disappointments and losses lead to grief. Grief, when effectively processed, involves accepting the loss, accepting the grief, finding emotional support and taking personal responsibility for recovering from the loss.

This does not mean that grief is quickly forgotten. Grief is not forgotten; it is accepted and carried courageously. The individual might cry loudly with other mourners, or might grieve silently, but he or she does not complain excessively.

Complainers are usually trying to escape from taking personal responsibility for their losses and their grief process. They want to focus on what others are doing wrong. Frequently, they harbor a child-like, dependent attitude toward the world. They expect to be taken care of, and when that doesn't happen, they complain.

Non-complainers, if they have a grievance, assertively present it, along with a clear request for replacement behaviors. They can negotiate with others and seek Win/Win outcomes to disagreements. Complainers seek to control others without taking responsibility themselves for engaging in productive negotiations and repairing behaviors.

Self-exploratory Question: How can I complain less and productively negotiate more?

Affirmation: Today I am presenting my requests specifically and assertively

Principle: Commitment focuses one's energy and facilitates trust in others.

Perennial Wisdom Quote: "Until one is committed, there is hesitancy, the choice to draw back, always ineffectiveness…. Whatever you can do, or dream you can do, begin it. Boldness has genius, power, and magic in it." – Goethe

Discussion: Before making a serious commitment to any adult relationship ask yourself these questions: Is this person honest with me? Is this person self-secure enough to be able to keep confidences? Is this person functioning independently and adequately in his or her own life? Does this person always treat me respectfully? Is this person kind and caring? Does this person know how to ask for emotional support, as well as give it? If the answers are "yes," this is likely an adult person, safe for a loving relationship. As Lewis B. Smedes has said, "To dare to make and care to keep commitments, this is love."

Once a commitment has been made to a relationship (be it a friend, a child, an employee, a lover, or a spouse), it is vital to stay loyal to that commitment, recognizing that the other person will have some imperfections. No one is ever perfect and, as intimacy grows, we learn more and more about the imperfections of others. Ideally, as intimacy grows, we are also learning more and more about our own imperfections and how to make changes which will allow us to be more loving.

This is what intimate relationship is all about -- learning about how to be more loving ourselves. Intimate, committed relationship is not about getting all our needs for intimacy met perfectly from one person. It is about committing to learn more and more about oneself and about another, in a loving, safe, accepting atmosphere. We all need to stay loyal to doing our part to create this kind of atmosphere in our committed relationships.

Self-Exploratory Question: How can I commit to learning more in relationships?

Affirmation: Today I dare to make and I care to keep my commitments.

June 15
Dialogue

Principle: Honest, open dialogue between two people facilitates self-awareness and awareness of others.

Perennial Wisdom Quote: "Life must be lived forwards. But is must be understood backwards." -- Soren Kierkegaard

Discussion: Webster defines "dialogue" as "a conversation between two or more persons or between characters in a novel, drama, etc." or "an exchange of ideas with a view to reaching an amicable agreement." Through dialogue with another we learn whether this is a safe person with whom to commit friendship. Through dialogue we learn more about ourselves and others. Appendix 8 gives helpful guidelines for dialoguing.

Learning to listen, to drop defenses, and to deepen one's understanding of others are the primary goals of dialoguing. There is no need to reach agreement. Dialoguing is not a problem-solving process. (See Appendix 7.) It is a process designed to build mutual understanding between two or more people, not necessarily agreement between these people. Safe relationships offer plenty of room for dialogue and disagreement. If there is an urgent problem which must be solved via a joint agreement, this is handled following a different "Win/Win problem-solving" process. (See the July 12 reading.)

Self-exploratory Question: How can I improve my dialoguing skills?

Affirmation: Today I am practicing effectively dialoguing with others.

Principle: Fear of emotional intimacy can be overcome by reaching out to dialogue with others.

Perennial Wisdom Quote: "The continuity and history of a long-term relationship is the crucible in which we can melt down the lead we carry in our psyches and transform it into the gold of the soul." -- Tian Dayton, Ph.D.

Discussion: Nature has made human hearts and minds inclined towards company and inclined towards healing. Fear of emotional contact and fear of emotional pain is what blocks this healing. Some people are introverts (satisfied and thriving with only a few close friends) and some are extroverts (satisfied and thriving only with many human contacts). No matter which personality style a person has, complete isolation from emotional contact with other humans is mentally damaging. The human brain seems to need healthy relationships in order to grow and thrive. (See Appendix 1.)

Most people who avoid emotionally intimate contact have not yet learned how to determine whether another is emotionally "safe", as well as how to provide emotional "safety" to others. They often jump too quickly into self-disclosure or physical intimacy, not taking the necessary time to establish healthy acquaintance, companionship, and friendship before venturing into deeper emotional or physical commitment. This usually ends in painful abandonment or rejection which promotes fear of future attempts for contact.

The dialoguing practice outlined in Appendix 7 can be very helpful for young people or adults who have not yet learned how to carefully develop healthy emotional intimacy with others.

Self-exploratory Question: How do I practice the development of emotional intimacy?

Affirmation: Today I am thoughtfully, respectfully and honestly connecting to others.

Principle: Mature love involves a conscious choice, made over and over again to be loving and to accept and appreciate differences.

Perennial Wisdom Quote: "Love doesn't just sit there, like a stone. It has to be made like bread: remade all the time, made new." -- Ursula K. LeGuin

Discussion: Perhaps more than any other modern writer, M. Scott Peck, M.D., has written about the distinctions between romantic love and "genuine love." In his beautiful anthology, *Abounding Grace,* he says romantic love is not a "virtue." Instead he describes it as "a wonderfully pleasant feeling, possibly a purely genetic phenomenon, to facilitate mating, but often misleading and inevitably temporary."

"Genuine love," he sees as a virtue, as "the will to extend one's self for the purpose of nurturing one's own and another's spiritual growth." In his popular book, *The Road Less Traveled*, Dr. Peck wrote eloquently about love being a choice, a personal decision each of us makes, or doesn't make, moment by moment in our relationships with ourselves and with others. This kind of "genuine love" is mature love. It can take years to learn how to love in this way. The effort is always worth it. When dying, most people acknowledge that loving relationships have been more valuable to them than any other aspect of life.

Self-exploratory Question: How can I mature in my primary love relationships?

Affirmation: Today I choose love, over and over again, in my primary relationships.

Principle: Immature attachment involves unconscious dependency and manipulation.

Perennial Wisdom Quote: "Love is the child of freedom, never that of domination." -- Erich Fromm, *Escapes From Freedom*

Discussion: Many people confuse "love" and immature attachment. Immature attachment turns to an outer "object" for satisfaction. It tries to make this outer "object" satisfy inner needs. It criticizes the outer "object" when he or she doesn't meet these needs. It throws temper tantrums. It feels helpless and hopeless. It tries to avoid the "purposeful work" of learning how to genuinely love. It clings to childhood dependencies and enmeshment.

Mature love does none of these things. When we make an effort, one day at a time, to grow in our capacity for mature love, we gradually outgrow our immature attachments. These attachments are replaced by the strengthening will to learn, to understand and love others. Immature attachments are replaced by a deep commitment to personal, spiritual growth, the kind of growth that makes life worth living, even when we have suffered great losses. The longing for compassion is replaced by the longing to become more compassionate. The longing to receive love is replaced by the longing to give more love. And gradually trust grows that "as we give, so shall we receive." We learn patience and a broader view of time. Justice is seen as existing in the big picture, not always in the little picture.

Self-exploratory Question: Where do I still suffer the most from immature attachments?

Affirmation: Today I am replacing my immature attachments with mature love.

Principle: Building and maintaining trust is fundamental to a loving relationship.

Perennial Wisdom Quote: "Love, and you shall be loved. All love is mathematically just, as much as the two sides of an algebraic equation." -- R.W. Emerson

Discussion: Trust is defined by child psychologists as the earliest primary, developmental task. When this task cannot be done well in childhood because our care-givers are untrustworthy, it is harder to build trust in adulthood, but it is not impossible. Modern brain research is showing how children <u>and</u> adults are capable of improving the functioning of their own brains, with conscious, careful effort and good guidance. (See <u>Appendix 1</u>.)

Learning to dialogue and share with others in emotionally safe settings is an important aspect of remedial brain development. This can be done with a professional psychotherapist and/or it can be done in a safe dialoguing or group setting. It takes time, effort, and commitment to literally reprogram our brain and nervous systems to know how to trust in appropriate settings and how to detach when emotional contact is being hurtful. The <u>January 19</u>th reading discussed how behavioral techniques such as Adult Time Out can help to build trusting relationships. The <u>July 12</u>th reading will discuss Win/Win problem solving.

For today the focus is on learning to look for and trust the "big pictures" of life, which teach us that there is justice built, long-range, into all of life's principles. These can be observed and trusted if we turn to Nature and long periods of history for the lessons.

Self-exploratory Quote: How can I trust more that "as I give, so shall I receive"?

Affirmation: Today I am trusting that as I love, so shall I be loved.

Principle: Openness in relationship requires overcoming fear of engulfment, of abandonment, of self-awareness and of failure.

Perennial Wisdom Quote: "It is more noble to give yourself completely to one individual than to labor diligently for the salvation of the masses." -- Dag Hammarskjold

Discussion: Fear of intimacy takes many different forms, depending on one's history. If our primary caregivers in childhood were overbearing and intrusive, we can harbor fears of emotional engulfment as an adult. If our primary caregivers were not sufficiently emotionally available, we can harbor fears of abandonment. If we were abused or neglected in childhood, we can repress many feelings and have a fear of emotional expression in general. If we had excessive expectations and rules imposed on us in childhood, we can have fears of failure in adulthood.

The good news is that all these kinds of fears can be overcome, with attention, diligence and determination. The most important thing is to take deep personal responsibility for our fears and not blame them on someone else. A loved one may be making a request, or leaving on a trip, or giving us some undesirable feedback, but this does not make him or her the enemy. The enemy is our own entrenched fear which can be magnified by past emotional stress.

We must learn to separate out what is history and what is present reality. We need to take responsibility for healing our emotional pasts and not blaming our over-reactions on present situations. Often this takes help from a therapist or a support group. Learning to see ourselves through someone else's kind, well-meaning eyes is vital. If we are engaged in an emotional struggle with a loved one, we need to be able to see ourselves clearly, as well as to see the loved one clearly.

Self-exploratory Question: How can I be more emotionally present with others?

Affirmation: I am becoming more open and emotionally intimate with others.

Principle: Secrets are always damaging to a relationship.

Perennial Wisdom Quote: "The earth has been made to take an oath neither to drink blood, nor to keep a secret." -- Lebanese proverb

Discussion: When we have something to hide from others, we are usually also hiding from ourselves. We are ashamed of our own behavior, or else trying to control the behavior of another. The only legitimate reason to control another's behavior is when the other threatens emotional or physical violence. In such cases keeping one's location a secret might be necessary self-protection. In most situations, however, secrets are created to protect one's self from punishment and undesired, behavioral consequences.

This is a form of dishonesty, and secrets rarely stay secrets for long, so the inevitable is usually just postponed.

"Confidentiality" is something different from secret making. Confidentiality is agreed upon ahead of time by <u>both parties</u> and is crucial in many professional settings and at times even between friends. Friends don't "rat" on each other. But they also don't lie to cover up friends' mistakes. They try to help their friends to avoid mistakes. They also avoid "triangulated" communications (see the <u>July 25</u> Reading) and refer questions back to the person involved, declining to answer for another.

To cover up a friend's mistake just helps a friend to avoid his or her own inner enemies. Friends do their best not to create secrets and don't ask others to lie for them.

Self-exploratory Question: How have secrets hurt me in the past?

Affirmation: Today I am neither creating nor keeping secrets.

Principle: Deal honestly with problems within a marriage before romancing another.

Perennial Wisdom Quote: "We are finally being warned that when our hearts are only organs of fire, both our souls and our bodies are likely to get burned." -- Frank Pittman, M.D., author of *Private Lies*

Discussion: The *Harpers Index* in 1991 indicated that 70% of American men earning $70,000 or more said they cheat on their wives. Only 16% of the men earning less than $5000 a year said they cheat on their wives. There might be many reasons for this, but one is certainly that money in America translates into power, and sexual affairs are usually about power, rather than about love.

A sexual affair suggests that one does not feel emotionally connected and empowered in one's marriage. Women, of course, also have sexual affairs. Both women and men in a free society tend to stray outside of their marriages, if they do not feel appreciated and sexually valued within their marriages.

It is only human, however, for both sexes to feel at times sexually attracted outside of marriage. What is the alternative to having a damaging sexual affair? If you feel attracted to someone outside of your marriage, here are some healthy things to do: 1) Ask yourself what aspect of yourself flowers when you are with this person. 2) Avoid the tempting relationship and get busy finding ways to have this aspect of yourself flower on your own. 3) Be honest with your spouse about this aspect of yourself which needs more attention and more appreciation. 4) Collaborate with your spouse about finding ways for this to happen. 5) Seek therapy, if necessary, to achieve successful couple collaboration with making changes within the marriage. 6) If all else fails, get a divorce, and don't start dating anyone else until the divorce is final and settled. Don't date a married person whose divorce isn't final.

Self-exploratory Question: How has my life suffered from sexual infidelity?

Affirmation: I am sexually faithful to my vows, and I do not date married people, other than my own spouse.

June 23
Generosity

Principle: Being generous with one's time, talents and money brings great joy.

Perennial Wisdom Quote: "You may light another's candle at your own without loss." -- Danish saying, "A candle loses nothing by lighting another candle." –James Keller

Discussion: Many Native Americans have "give-away ceremonies" at weddings. This custom involves the young couple giving gifts to all their wedding guests. The gifts traditionally honor special memories of emotional gifts both the bride and the groom have received in the past from family and friends. What do you think of this custom? Do you think it might teach something more important to young couples than the modern Anglo-American custom of wedding guests' giving household gifts to the couple?

The Muslim, Hindu, Buddhist, Jewish and Christian faiths all teach generosity. Proverbs in the *Bible* teaches, "Generosity will be rewarded. Give a cup of water and you will receive a cup of water in return." *The Talmud* teaches, "Living kindness is greater than laws, and the charities of life are more than all ceremonies." "The *Qur'an* teaches, "To be charitable in public is good, but to give alms to the poor in private is better." A Hindu proverb teaches, "He only does not live in vain, who employs his wealth, his thought, his speech to advance the good of others." Buddhism teaches "loving kindness" as one of the greatest virtues.

Generosity opens the heart, connects us with others in need, and dissolves self-pity and self-centeredness. It is powerful medicine.

Self-exploratory Question: Where and how in my life have I been the most generous?

Affirmation: I choose to value generosity more than wealth.

June 24
Hospitality

Principle: Hospitality promotes peace and mutual understanding.

Perennial Wisdom Quote: "Hospitality binds the world together…. Hospitality is the way we come out of ourselves. It is the first step towards dismantling the barriers of the world. Hospitality is the way we turn a prejudiced world around, one heart at a time." -- Joan Chittister

Discussion: Hospitality is defined by Webster as "the act, practice or quality of being hospitable; friendly and solicitous entertainment of guests." It means when someone politely comes to visit our home, we are welcoming, kind and generous. Many residents of rural cultures prided themselves in being hospitable to strangers, because the natural elements were so challenging that strangers had to help one another to survive. Many cultures also based their practices of hospitality on the spiritual belief of the interconnectedness of all life forms. People were encouraged to honor all other life forms as a way of honoring their concept of the Great Spirit, which enlivens all life forms.

Modern secular culture has veered away from some forms of hospitality. A stranger is likely to be greeted at the door with suspicion and, "What do you want?" This is a serious problem because we all <u>do</u> need each other in order to have satisfying lives. Whoever is at the door is more likely to be respectful if we ask, "What can I do for you?" than "What do you want?" We get to choose what foot to start out on in any relationship. All of us may need a good neighbor at any time.

Self-exploratory Question: How do I practice hospitality?

Affirmation: I choose to be hospitable to others, unless they clearly prove themselves unworthy.

June 25
Sacrifice

Principle: When one sacrifices for the benefit of others, one also benefits oneself.

Perennial Wisdom Quote: "Having family responsibilities and concerns just has to make you a more understanding person." -- Sandra Day O'Connor

Discussion: Former U.S. Supreme Court Justice Sandra Day O'Connor has been called the most influential woman in 21st century America. At the same time, she can affirm that her family responsibilities and concerns benefit her by making her more understanding. The sacrifice of time and resources she and others make for their spouses, children, and elderly parents are sources of deepened understanding and personal wisdom. Therefore, they are not a burden, but rather a privilege.

Henry Ward Beecher once said, "No man is more cheated than the selfish man."

He understood the value of sacrifice. Of course, the motivation behind making a sacrifice is also important. The motivation needs to be honest, generous and intended for the benefit of another. If the sacrifice is offered in order to receive personal recognition, the giver receives nothing of significance in return, because the end result is more a manipulation than an honest event. The offering must be unsolicited, un-manipulative, and open-hearted. Then the sacrifice benefits both the giver and the receiver.

Self-exploratory Question: When do I genuinely sacrifice for others?

Affirmation: I grow in understanding when I unselfishly sacrifice for others.

June 26
Praise

Principle: Praise does not involve force and is more enduring than punishment.

Perennial Wisdom Quote: "A little thought and a little kindness are often worth more than a great deal of money." -- John Ruskin

Discussion: Most religions teach the importance of praising God. Most optimists teach the importance of praising life. Most teachers learn the effectiveness of honest, kind praise of effective student effort. Most parents learn the pleasure of genuine praise for their children. Most children learn the pleasure of genuine praise from parents and teachers.

Praise involves honest recognition and the gift of attention given to meritorious behavior and achievement. Praise requires no money and no use of force. Why then is it not more abundant? Perhaps because so many of us struggle with fear and fear tends to block praise. When we are afraid, we tend to use punishment to influence others, rather than praise.

Fearful people look for what others are doing wrong and punish it. Confident, free people look for what others are doing right and praise it. If you experience more punishment than praise in your life, ask yourself what you have done to surround yourself with fearful people. If you experience more praise than punishment in your life, feel good that you have surrounded yourself with confident, free people.

Self-exploratory Question: How can I both offer and receive more praise in my life?

Affirmation: Today I choose to notice others doing things right and praise them for it.

Principle: Appreciation focuses our awareness on the goodness we receive.

Perennial Wisdom Quote: "We measure success by accumulation. The measure is false. The true measure is appreciation. He who loves most has most." -- Henry Van Dyke, "Fisherman's Luck"

Discussion: There is a Creole saying, "Thanks cost nothing." Appreciating others not only costs nothing, but it fills the heart of the giver as well as the receiver. Greeting others with a smile or kind words is also a form of appreciation…. "Namaste" is an Asian Indian greeting meaning "I honor the divine spark within you."

What greeting do you most commonly use? Do you take time to clearly see and quietly appreciate those you greet? Giving ready appreciation also makes it easier to truly receive appreciation. Appreciation needs to be consciously received, as well as consciously given. Appreciation is like rain, and we all need to be like good soil which soaks it up, rather than like rocks, where rain just runs off.

There are also more than human sources of appreciation. Plants and animals offer lots of appreciation, if we are good to them. They appreciate attention, watering, and feeding and welcome us with flowers, tail wags, purrs, or whatever language is in their nature. Loving touch is another way to appreciate others, if we know our touch is welcome. Sometimes our eyes and our hands can communicate even more than our words.

Self-exploratory Question: Whom have I appreciated today?

Affirmation: Today I am taking time to appreciate those around me.

Principle: Talking about people who are not present is rarely helpful.

Perennial Wisdom Quote: "Living kindness is greater than laws, and the charities of life are more than all ceremonies." -- *The Talmud*

Discussion: Gossip is indirect, "triangulated" conversation. This means that one person is talking to another person about someone who is not present. When speaking about someone who is not present, examine your motivation. If it is to inform someone about the need of another, so that the other can receive more assistance, then perhaps the communication is legitimate. But if the words are simply to share information about another, for no purpose other than conversation, it is likely unnecessary gossip.

Most people don't want information shared about them by third parties. They want to be their own information givers. Besides, often "triangulated" conversation contains distorted information, criticism or blame, especially if it has been passed on by a number of people. The Buddhists stress the importance of "Right Speech." Buddhist practitioners are taught to honor silence and to use words thoughtfully only for good purpose. Jesus also taught, "Let he who is without sin throw the first stone." If we are talking about another for no good purpose, it's like throwing a stone.

Words can be even more harmful than stones. Speaking "behind someone's back" usually just ends up in having others "speak behind our own backs." The old advice to not say anything at all, if you can't say something kind, is generally a helpful guideline.

Self-exploratory Question: How can I eliminate gossip from my conversation?

Affirmation: Today I choose not to talk about anyone who is not present.

Principle: Finding fault in others usually just boomerangs back on the fault-finder.

Perennial Wisdom Quote: "Why not look within when things are not going smoothly and see where you are out of tune; never try to blame anyone else for the negative state you are in…. When you realize that you have only yourself to blame when things become difficult and you get out of tune, you will also realize that you are the one to do something about rectifying those wrongs, that you do not have to wait for someone else to change and do something about it. You can start right now doing something about it yourself." -- Eileen Caddy, *Footprints On the Path*

Discussion: Faultfinding is usually a form of unconscious dependency. The person who criticizes others easily is looking outside him or her for approval and happiness, rather than looking inside. Faultfinding spreads negativity and eventually boomerangs.

When others find fault with us, it is helpful to remember that the faultfinder is probably unconsciously blaming others for what he or she feels powerless to change in his or her own situation. We can say something like, "I understand that you think that," or some other neutral way of acknowledging that the complaint was heard, without having to offer agreement, and without trying to change the other's opinion or situation. Of course, all of us need to receive honest, negative feedback at times.

Honest, negative feedback is given respectfully and kindly for the purpose of helpful redirection. Faultfinding is usually delivered disrespectfully, unkindly and simply for the purpose of venting anger and emotionally pushing another away. When we receive this kind of energy, it is best just to give the person space and forget the rude, indirect way it was communicated.

Self-exploratory Question: How can I focus less on finding fault in others?

Affirmation: Today I will not find fault with anyone but myself.

Principle: Scapegoating is hurtful to all parties involved.

Perennial Wisdom Quote: "All our actions take their hue from the complexion of the heart, as landscapes do their variety from light." -- W.T. Bacon

Discussion: Scapegoating involves setting up one person as responsible for the failures of a group. It happens unconsciously, most often within family systems, work groups, and political systems. It usually happens when the family, work group, or political party is invested in avoiding awareness of some reality. For example, a parent might be alcoholic but the whole family is avoiding that reality, so the emotionally weakest child in the family is focused on as causing the family's problems. Or, in a work place, the whole business may be doing very poorly, but that is not being acknowledged; instead one worker is fired and blamed for the business's lack of productivity. Or, in a school system, the whole system might be having problems, but the principal is blamed and fired.

Scapegoating can also happen to a whole culture. The Nazis scapegoated the Jews for Germany's financial problems. Radical religious groups can scapegoat governments or other religious groups for their problems. Radical political groups can scapegoat other political groups or leaders.

To be free of this harmful, avoidant behavior, we have to be able to see reality clearly and point it out. We also need to recognize that at times being rejected by an unhealthy group is actually a release. We may grieve and be sad for the loss of connection, but be better off to leave and find a healthier group to join. If we are materially damaged, of course, it is also important to assert our rights.

Self-exploratory Question: When have I ever been scapegoated or scapegoated another?

Affirmation: I do not allow myself to participate in scapegoating behavior.

Principle: When we give from the heart, we love all to which we have given.

Perennial Wisdom Quote: "Beneficence is a duty; and he who frequently practices it and sees his benevolent intentions realized, at length comes to love him to whom he has done good." -- Kant

Discussion: Learning to understand the natural laws involved in giving and receiving is perhaps more important than anything else in learning how to be happy. Plants give of themselves naturally. The sun and the earth give of themselves naturally. They do not give conditionally, based on what mortals give in return.

There is a natural joy in all life. Life itself wants to continue abundantly. It overflows. This is the same way humans need to give of themselves -- naturally, unconditionally, and without fear. This is the same way we humans need to receive -- naturally, unconditionally, and without fear. This kind of giving and receiving is what literally keeps the whole world alive. It is fear and greed, and the desire to possess property and people, which kill joy.

Study the behavior of raccoons when learning to give. They scout for food in a group and give food to each other. They have a protective lookout when they search for food and always feed him first. They reward those who contribute to the group effort. We have a lot to learn from raccoons.

Self-exploratory Question: Do I know how to take joy in giving?

Affirmation: Today I choose to give of myself and to myself in joyful abundance.

July 2
Creativity

Principle: Creative moments are intrinsically rewarding and revealing.

Perennial Wisdom Quote: "Creativity is not just about what takes place in traditionally recognized creative fields. It's what happens in our small and large moments of empathy and transformation, the moments when we contact our authentically individual and therefore universal experience of truth…. Chaos theory teaches that when our psychological perspective shifts -- through moments of amplification and bifurcation --our degrees of freedom expand and we experience being and truth. We are then creative. And our true self lies there." -- Briggs and Peat, *Seven Life Lessons of Chaos, Timeless Wisdom from the Science of Change*

Discussion: Modern scientists are studying the principles of creation and finding exquisite patterns even in their "chaos." Artists, musicians, dancers, writers, sculptors, gardeners and all persons who joyfully lose themselves and all sense of time while being creative can relate to Briggs' and Peat's words above.

Creative moments are moments in which we are paradoxically both intensely individual and simultaneously very connected to everything around us. Time seems to stand still. Consciousness isn't moving from past to present to future in a progressive line. Consciousness just seems to radiate in a huge circle, centered in the present moment and reaching out in every direction of time and space. Awareness is amplified, and we feel completely free. Differences don't cause conflict; rather they cause connection. We are at peace with what is radiating from inside, and we share our creative impulses without concern as to how they will be received. The expression of these impulses is itself rewarding. There is a childlike purity to these moments which doesn't have to be explained or defended.

Self-exploratory Question: How can I save space in my life for creative moments?

Affirmation: I am joyfully expressing my creativity and connecting to others.

Principle: Expectations ruin the gifts which come from giving.

Perennial Wisdom Quote: "Kindness is greater than law. Act with kindness, but do not exact gratitude." -- Confucius

Discussion: Giving of one's time, energy and thoughts, as well as one's material resources, opens the heart and is very satisfying. But, if we expect gratitude or returned service from those we serve, we short-circuit the creative circle of energy, and our generosity reaps little reward. People who give with expectations for rewards are really just setting up a contract: "I'll do something for you if you do something for me." This isn't love. This is business. It's subtle power-playing. Of course, we have to be sure that we are giving attention, rest, love, food and exercise enough first to ourselves so as to have resources enough to share with others.

Over-giving often stems from subtle power-plays. We want to receive, so we give until we drop, expecting to be rewarded. Our emotionally flattened self can barely get up, much less be genuinely open to receiving life's blessings from wherever it is overflowing. Mental expectations kill creative moments, in one self as well as in others. Dropping these mental expectations opens us up to gratefully receive whatever life is offering us, even if it is painful and not what we desire.

Religious people say this is how "grace" and "blessings" happen. We open ourselves up to receive, without placing preconceived limitations on life. We trust life to give us what we need, even if it isn't what we've asked for.

Self-exploratory Question: Where do I most tend to give with expectations?

Affirmation: When I give, I give without expectations.

Principle: In loving relationships, reciprocity cannot be measured or timed.

Perennial Wisdom Quote: "The only thing that counts in life is love - not just how much love we can give, but we must learn to receive it, because we can give only as much as we allow ourselves to receive. Everything has to be in balance." -- Elizabeth Kubler-Ross, M.D. in an interview with William Elliott

Discussion: We all need a tribe, a family, some sort of supportive network which is committed to principles of reciprocity and loving community. The network doesn't have to have defined edges and identifiers for membership. It can be a loose knit community in which not everyone knows each other. But the community members need to have some commitment to sharing with each other, in difficult times as well as good times. The community needs to function on general guidelines of reciprocity. People need to be committed to giving as well as to receiving. For example, in the Wise Ways Happiness Program and other 12 Step programs, newcomers receive lots of welcoming. After they mature in the Program, they learn that offering this welcoming to other newcomers is how they themselves can grow. We learn best what we share with others.

The giving and receiving are all voluntary. There are no individual expectations placed on anyone. There is no pressure to begin offering service. There is simply encouragement, opportunity, and the example of others who themselves experience service as a great source of personal growth.

Self-exploratory Question: How can I practice reciprocal giving in my support networks, without laying expectations on myself or others?

Affirmation: As I receive, so do I give, freely and not necessarily directly.

Principle: The foundation of personal power is kindness and creativity.

Perennial Wisdom Quote: "Example is not the main thing in influencing others. It's the only thing." -- Albert Schweitzer

Discussion: There are four kinds of power: physical strength, political and economic power, the power of knowledge, and what might be called "personal power." Personal power is the power to influence others through example and through wisdom. More than anything else, this kind of power is built on kindness and creativity. Patricia Evans, Ph.D., in *The Verbally Abusive Relationship,* makes a distinction between "Power Over" and "Personal Power." Power Over she defines as "control and dominance which kills the spirit." "Personal Power" she sees as manifesting in "mutuality and co-creation" and lifting the spirit. She defines it as "the ability to know, to choose and to create from the ground of one's being -- from where one's feelings originate."

Paul Tillich, a famous Christian theologian, defined God as "The Ground of All Being." It might be said that personal power is also spiritual power, power stemming from conscious contact with one's Higher Power. It is an energy which flows from the heart, through the mind, and connecting to the hearts and minds of others. It isn't energy which originates in the ego-mind purely from will. Do you know anyone with this kind of Personal Power? How would you describe him or her? Are you attracted to his or her example? Why? How does this kind of power bring happiness into your life?

Self-exploratory Question: How can I grow stronger in "personal power"?

Affirmation: Today I am growing in kindness, creativity and personal power.

July 6   **Healthy**
Sexuality

Principle: Healthy sexuality is based on honest, mutual, adult consent, reciprocity, emotional intimacy, and loving commitment.

Perennial Wisdom Quote: "What is most important is that sex reflects each individual's warmth and care for the other. It affirms, but is not relied on to create their bond. It is a way to feel close and express care for each other. It is not used as a substitute for solving problems or as a way to create closeness that is otherwise lacking." -- Charlotte Davis Kasl, Ph.D., *Women, Sex and Addiction*

Discussion: Nathaniel Branden, author of *A Psychology of Self Esteem,* asserts that sexual self-esteem is based on 1) a person's ability to choose a partner who is admired and who is a spiritual equal, capable of loving and being loved, and 2) a person's ability to find loving meaning in the sexual act. He says that if a person is sexually motivated just by the sensation of the moment, or the desire to feed one's own pride, admiration or power, sexuality just furthers mental illness.

Sexual intercourse increases hormones related to emotional attachment. Therefore, it is unwise to have sex with someone with whom you do not wish to be emotionally involved. Oscar Wilde offered this humorous sexual advice: "Don't ever go to bed with someone more disturbed than you are." Sexuality can become addictive, meaning compulsive and obsessive and dangerous. This happens when sex is illicit, exploitive, and seductive and draws on fear for excitement, uses conquest as power, and serves to medicate and avoid emotional pain.

Healthy sex is honest, safe, cultivates a sense of being adult and valued, is mutual and intimate, adds to self-esteem, has no victims, is fun and playful, and takes responsibility for needs.

Self-exploratory Question: What are my personal, sexual ethics?

Affirmation: I always make ethical, healthy, sexual choices.

Principle: Healthy adult touch is based on mutual consent and reciprocal caring.

Perennial Wisdom Quote: "Children want to touch everything, to smell the flowers, taste the leaves, dangle their feet in the water, pick apart the scat, carry home the bones. Sometimes I am impatient about this desire for direct contact. 'Have respect!' I want to say. But in the end, I hold my tongue, knowing they pay their respects by making sensual contact with the world. 'The opposite of love,' a friend reminds me, 'is not hatred, but indifference.'" -- Paul Gruchow, *Grass Roots: The University of Home*

Discussion: Children want to touch everything and, in order to help them thrive adults teach them that some touch is not safe. Touching sharp things, hot things, electrical outlets, unknown animals or other's "private parts" can be unsafe. When children are learning about safe and unsafe touch, it is always important to be kind and clear in sharing information. Sometimes adult instruction is harsh and shaming and not accurate. Sometimes adult example is contradictory. Children get confused.

Being clear oneself, as an adult, as to what is safe and unsafe touch is very important, especially when interacting with children. If we don't know, we need to inquire from experts. In emergencies, touch might be hurried and harsh, but the intent is always to be protective and helpful. In general, safe touch between humans is kind, respectful, mutually welcoming, usually gentle and loving. Safe self-pleasuring needs to have similar qualities and to be done in private.

Self-exploratory Question: How do I distinguish between safe and unsafe touch?

Affirmation: I only engage in healthy, safe touching.

July 8   Wise Ways Happiness Step Seven: Emotional Connection

Principle: The Wise Ways Happiness Step 7 reads, "We humbly let go of pride and reach out of our emotional isolation to lovingly connect to others."

Perennial Wisdom Quote: "If you give your life as a wholehearted response to love, then love will wholeheartedly respond to you." -- Marianne Williamson

Discussion: Shame and fear lead to isolation. Some people have grown up in families and communities in which they experienced shame and fear. This usually results in a pattern of isolation, and often addiction. The Wise Ways Happiness Program encourages participants to emotionally connect to others in safe and loving ways. It establishes safe communication guidelines for group gatherings and "dialogues." Its Big Book focuses on ways to emotionally protect one's self while still participating in community. Emotional "boundaries" are discussed, as are the differences between "safe and unsafe" relationships.

New participants in Wise Ways Happiness Support Groups are welcomed, but not pressured in any way to talk or make commitments to the group. They are invited to share, and invited to attend group meetings, but they are not pressured to do so. Only first names are used and discussion of members' social or economic roles outside of the meetings is discouraged, in order to avoid issues of prestige and influence. All participants are equals and are treated with equal respect. This makes emotional connection safe and less threatening than in many group situations.

Self-exploratory Question: How can I be more emotionally connected to others?

Affirmation: I am deepening my safe, emotional connections to others.

Principle: Sexuality can become addictive and damaging.

Perennial Wisdom Quote: "When sex isn't hot, addictive couples view it as a sexual problem. When sex isn't going well, successful couples believe that the problem lies in the climate of the relationship. [They ask] 'What is our problem?' not, 'What's wrong with you?'" -- Charlotte Davis Kasl, *Women Sex and Addiction*

Discussion: Dr. Patrick Carnes, Ph.D., an American psychologist now with The Meadows Treatment Center in Arizona, has dedicated his life to writing about and helping others to heal addictive sexuality. He defines three levels of sex addiction:

1) Compulsive masturbation, pornography, prostitution; 2) exhibitionism, voyeurism, indecent phone calls, and indecent liberties;3) child molestation, incest and rape.

Sex addicts confuse sex with nurturance or power. Sex addicts have mentally and compulsively focused on sex as a means of gratification, rather than experiencing sex as an avenue to adult/adult, loving bonding. Sex addicts are usually starved for attention and touch and are ignorant about the damage done to their victims.

Recovery from sexual addiction usually involves a period of abstinence from all sexual contact with others, while at the same time learning the principles of satisfying love. In some ways recovery from sexual addiction is similar to recovery from food addiction because the individual has to learn first how to abstain from past hurtful behavior, and then how to engage in non-hurtful behavior. Unlike recovery from alcoholism and drug addiction which involves day-by-day total abstinence from the addictive substance, food and sex addicts need to learn abstinence from addictive eating and addictive sex, while also learning how to engage in healthy eating and healthy sexuality.

Self-exploratory Question: How can I protect myself from sex addiction?

Affirmation: I engage in sex only as a healthy, consensual expression of love.

Principle: Being ethical in one's sexual practices is vital to a loving relationship.

Perennial Wisdom Quote: "We can become so emotionally charged by a person that we allow ourselves to be intimate before we know who the person really is. When we give our bodies to another being, we are giving them a piece of our souls. We might want to take the time to find out if they deserve it." -- Iyanla Vanzant, *Acts of Faith*

Discussion: Donald J. Holmes wrote an article called "Sexuality in Medicine, Psychiatry and Law" for the 1972 text called *Psychotherapy*. In it he described sexually "immoral" behaviors as: knowingly and willfully spreading disease, failing to practice contraception control, failing to plan realistically for the care of any resulting child, relying on physical force or threats, capitalizing upon the vulnerability of another, failing to accept another person's right to select and direct his or her own relationship, using any sexual relationship for self-aggrandizement, insulting another with demeaning names, using unnecessary provocation of guilt and the deliberate teaching of untrue things to influence another's choices, being dishonest about intentions or other sexual relationships, and disrespecting another's right to live life as he or she wishes, in so far as it is done with a reciprocal respect for the rights of others.

Would you agree with Dr. Holmes? Would you add or subtract anything from his list? Can you take this list of unethical sexual behaviors and write up your own guidelines for ethical, sexual behavior?

Self-exploratory Question: How would you express your own guidelines for ethical sexual behavior?

Affirmation: I can trust my own sexual ethics to safely guide all my sexual choices.

196

July 11:   Wise Ways Happiness Support Group Tradition 7: Group Self-support

Principle: The Wise Ways Happiness Support Group Tradition Seven reads, "Wise Ways Happiness Support Groups are always self-supporting."

Perennial Wisdom Quote: "Commitment to process can be controlled. Commitment to outcome can not." -- Gay Hendricks, Ph.D., *Conscious Loving*

Discussion: The primary purpose of Wise Ways Happiness Support Group meetings is individual, personal growth. The best way to ensure that this primary purpose is fulfilled is to provide for autonomous, confidential, self-support in each group. Most groups are started up by volunteers.

When a Wise Ways Happiness Support Group is starting up by a professional therapist within an agency, the therapist makes sure Wise Ways Happiness books are available to all members. The therapist explains the meeting guidelines by reading them from the book. The professional does not dominate the group but encourages volunteer chairpersons. If the group is a teen group, the therapist, ideally, purchases the Wise Ways for Teens book available from Deborah Stamm, M.S.

Because Wise Ways Happiness Support Groups are not affiliated with any other organizations, only Wise Ways Happiness literature is read in meetings. If snacks or books are provided at meetings, they are paid for by money contributed by members.

Self-exploratory Question: How do I contribute to my group's self-support?

Affirmation: I am committed to supporting my group's needs, to the best of my ability.

July 12
Solving   **Win/Win Problem**

Principle: Each person in a Win/Win problem solving situation makes sure the other wins, too.

Perennial Wisdom Quote: "With a Win/Win solution, all parties feel good about the decision and feel committed to the action plan." -- Stephen Covey, *Seven Habits of Highly Effective People*

Discussion: The Win/Win conflict-resolution style is positive, specific and prompt. It is the only productive, problem-solving style. A Win/Lose conflict-resolution style is negative, focuses on the past, and presents generalizations. In the Win/Lose style each person is committed to winning, but at the expense of the other. A Lose/Lose conflict resolution style is negative, counter-dependent and future oriented. In this style both people have given up and are trying to take the other down with them.

Gini Graham Scott, Ph.D., in *Resolving Conflict,* describes these six steps for Win/Win problem solving: 1) get emotions under control, 2) set ground rules, 3) clarify positions, 4) explore underlying needs and interests, 5) generate alternatives, 6) agree on the best Win/Win option.

If a person is not practiced in these problem-solving steps, it is helpful to designate specific, weekly, problem-solving sessions with his or her family or roommates. Dr. Scott's book can be purchased, and these six steps can be posted and discussed. Plenty of time for discussion should be provided so that everyone understands the steps and commits to following them. It's helpful to have a volunteer "Process Facilitator" for every session. Ideally this facilitator is a different member of the group each time, so everyone gets to learn how to respectfully keep the group following these steps.

Self-exploratory Question: How can I improve my Win/Win problem-solving skills?

Affirmation: I maintain a Win/Win problem-solving style in all my work and living situations.

Principle: Win/Lose arguments are a waste of time.

Perennial Wisdom Quote: "If we can really understand the problem, the answer will come out of it, because the answer is not separate from the problem." -- Jiddu Krishnamurti, *The Penguin Krishnamurti Reader*

Discussion: In order to be free from Win/Lose arguments, two people must establish these prerequisites: 1) Respect for each other and a desire for Win/Win outcomes, 2) agreement on the steps in a Win/Win problem solving procedure, 3) effective listening skills, 4) effective assertion skills, and 5) effective appreciation skills. These skills need to be practiced by both parties.

Most Win/Lose arguments start up because the intention on at least one person's part is to persuade and/or dominate the other, rather than simply to grow in understanding of the other and of the problem to be solved. Win/Win agreements cannot be reached when one or both parties are not motivated to understand the other's experience, feelings, opinions, and preferences. Understanding takes time and energy. In order for two people to commit this kind of time and energy. Both people need to genuinely appreciate each other as individuals and as a problem-solving team. They need to be able to express this appreciation and reward themselves personally and as a team for making Win/Win problem-solving efforts. It's worth the effort, especially for teams who live or work together on a regular basis.

Self-exploratory Question: Have I established these five "prerequisites" in my most significant relationships?

Affirmation: I choose to stay out of Win/Lose arguments.

July 14
Collaboration

Principle: Collaboration skills are important to any relationship between equals.

Perennial Wisdom Quote: "Kindness in ourselves is the honey that blunts the sting of unkindness in another." -- Letitia Elizabeth Landor

Discussion: When a person feels insecure, usually his or her problem-solving skills deteriorate. Love and respect for the other person in the relationship may be real, but they may be temporarily overwhelmed by feelings of insecurity. This is why kindness is so important when attempting Win/Win problem solving. If one's living or working partner seems to be straying from good problem-solving process, the effective response is to kindly restate one's intention to collaborate as equals on finding a solution to the problem and asking the other whether he or she feels up to a collaborative process at the moment.

When two people collaborate, they respect what each has to offer to the partnership, and they work together as equals on a common problem or project. If this perspective is being lost because someone is feeling insecure, it is best to postpone the problem-solving process until both can feel secure. Sometimes it's possible to simply ask the insecure person, "What can I do to assure you that I respect you as an equal and value your opinions and preferences?" If he or she can respond specifically and positively to this question, then the collaborative, problem-solving process can continue.

Self-exploratory Question: How can I be kinder and more collaborative with others?

Affirmation: I choose to be collaborative and kind with significant others, even if it means postponing a decision.

Principle: Making amends for our own wrongs is necessary to heal ourselves.

Perennial Wisdom Quote: "Complete possession is proved only by giving. All you are unable to give possesses you." -- Andre Gide

Discussion: When we can't make amends to others for wrongs we have done them, we become burdened ourselves by these wrongs. We have to give this burden away to be free of guilt, denial and ignorance. Making amends for a wrongdoing is something we need to do for ourselves. Whatever benefit accrues to the victim of our wrongdoing is secondary to our need to heal ourselves.

Sometimes we can make actual financial or physical restitution for a wrong. Sometimes that is impossible, and all we can do is share a verbal amend, or perhaps offer some labor or service to attempt to rebuild goodwill. This is especially true when our wrong has been accidental. When our wrong has been intentional, we need to dig deep down into ourselves to discover the source of personal ignorance which allowed us to do intentional harm to another.

People who intend harm to others are emotionally and spiritually ignorant. They are usually suffering from old losses which they have not been able to put into a larger context to find some way to remedy without hurting others. They actually believe that revenge will fix their pain. Taking revenge never works. It just makes us angrier and creates more anger and desire to harm in others.

When we have been harmed ourselves, we deserve an amend from the perpetrator, but we can't force the amend. We can confront the perpetrator and demand social justice, if a law has been broken. But this is not revenge. This is simply attempting to assure that the perpetrator doesn't harm anyone else and the ignorance is corrected. (Also see Sept. 6 Reading & Step 9 discussion in Appendix 4.)

Self-exploratory Question: Are there any amends I have neglected to make?

Affirmation: When I have made a mistake, I make amends for it as soon as possible.

Principle: Self-justifications usually just bolster pride and avoidance, not problem solving.

Perennial Wisdom Quote: "Fanaticism consists in redoubling your efforts when you have forgotten your aim." -- George Santayana, *The Life of Reason*

Discussion: Human psyches are not courtrooms. There are no external judges or juries determining percentages of responsibility or blame for an offense. Human psyches are more like coconuts than court rooms. They have light at their core and ever denser defenses at their peripheries. When we try to "present ourselves in the best light" for others, we often neglect really experiencing and expressing our own feelings and preferences in an effective manner.

Determining degrees of fault or blame for the history of a problem usually just sidetracks the problem-solving process. It's most often best to just say something like, "Likely we both contributed to the creation of this problem; now how can we go on and cooperatively solve it together?" When a person isn't able to do this, likely there are deeper relationship issues which need to be addressed before the current topic can be solved. For example, perhaps one person doesn't feel respected or appreciated, so is unconsciously sabotaging the problem-solving, because he or she is losing hope for establishing respect and appreciation in the relationship. When something like this develops, often a professional therapist is needed to help solve the buried issues, so those involved can go on effectively with the immediate issues.

Self-exploratory Question: When am I most apt to defend myself with self-justifications?

Affirmation: I choose to avoid self-justifications and to problem-solve effectively.

Principle: Responsible employment is sustaining, satisfying, and harmful to no one.

Perennial Wisdom Quote: "Wholesome *internal* choices--healthy attitudes about one's work--also contribute to mental happiness and peace of mind. Everyone's livelihood is an opportunity for self-esteem." -- Sylvia Boorstein, Ph.D., *It's Easier Than You Think*

Discussion: Responsible employment means work which is sustaining of one's self and one's dependents and is not abusive or exploitive of anyone. It is also employment which one can engage in with a sense of satisfaction and self-recognition. It is employment which enhances self-esteem and necessitates no self-justification.

Modern society rewards financial success so much that some people rationalize employment that is hurtful to themselves or others just because it is financially rewarding. This is unethical and very unsatisfying because the most important things in life, such as love and self-respect, cannot be purchased with money.

If your present employment is not hurtful to anyone else, but not helpful either, and not satisfying to you, it's important to do all that you can to secure different employment. Time is very precious and not to be wasted on unsatisfying employment any longer than is absolutely necessary for survival.

When we find work that is both satisfying and helpful to others, the blessings multiply. We become more skillful at it, and others benefit more and more, and it takes less and less effort to accomplish. These are all signs of responsible employment.

Self-exploratory Question: Am I responsibly employed?

Affirmation: I choose to be responsibly employed.

Principle: Psychological education and psychotherapy can transform ineffective problem-solving skills.

Perennial Wisdom Quote: "Trouble is a part of life, and if you don't share it, you don't give others the chance to love you enough." -- Dinah Shore

Discussion: Psychotherapy with a licensed, well trained, skillful therapist can transform ineffective problem-solving skills. It is like being tutored in what might be called "emotional hygiene." Most of us get good education in school regarding "physical hygiene," but unfortunately an "emotional hygiene" curriculum is not well developed, at least in many public schools in the United States. As more research is completed regarding the functioning of the brain and the principles of what is now being called "positive psychology," hopefully this will change.

The Wise Ways Happiness Program in this book is offering a curriculum which is founded in research and acceptable to individuals of all religious and non-religious orientations. It is not psychotherapy, because it is usually not facilitated by licensed professionals. It is rather a program of psychological education which can be helpful to anyone.

People who choose to supplement self-help with psychotherapy are similar to students of ancient Socrates. They submit themselves to therapists who ask crucial questions and emotionally support their clients, as the clients learn to effectively answer the questions for themselves. Before entering into psychotherapy, be sure to check out the training and licensing of your therapist and also her or his reputation and confidentiality protection under the laws of your state.

Self-exploratory Question: How could I benefit from more psychological education, and possibly some psychotherapy?

Affirmation: I choose to engage in psychological education. I choose psychotherapy with qualified professionals, if my progress through self-help seems insufficient.

Principle: Effective couple therapy can help to heal couple conflict.

Perennial Wisdom Quote: "It is better to get rid of the problem and keep the person than to get rid of the person and keep the problem." -- Harville Hendrix, Ph.D.

Discussion: Harville Hendrix, Ph.D., conducts couple therapy workshops in which he advises couple education rather than divorce. John Gottman, Ph.D., is another psychologist who has specialized in researching what makes marital relationships work in the United States. Both psychologists have written several excellent books. David Luecke, founder of the Relationship Institute in Virginia, has also written a book called *The Relationship Manual.* It is an excellent relationship workbook with simple summaries of fundamental relationship skills, followed by challenging communication exercises for couples to follow.

Of course, some couples have already gotten into such a crisis in their relationships that professional couple therapy is necessary, in addition to self-help reading and self-examination. Sometimes a person's defenses and fears are so stimulated that a skillful and kind third party is needed to mediate the healing process. When a couple too quickly chooses divorce before doing couple therapy, all too often they simply repeat their mistakes later in a second or third marriage.

Without both partners having certain basic relationship skills, democratic American marriages are very difficult. In a nation in which a person unhappy in marriage can easily file for a divorce, it is unwise to marry in the first place without having some of these skills. Especially if you married young, some professional couple therapy can be very helpful.

Self-exploratory Question: How could my marriage possibly benefit from therapy?

Affirmation: If my spouse and I are unable to solve our problems, we enter therapy.

Principle: Therapeutic couple separation with effective couple therapy can transform marital conflict and sometimes prevent divorce.

Perennial Wisdom Quote: "And I quickly saw that letting go of preconceived ideas about how relationships and life in general 'should be' was an important basic prescription for a good life and a sense of well-being…A 'perfect' marriage is not a marriage without challenges, but a marriage that has the strength to manage the challenges that arise." -- Susan Page, *The Eight Essential Traits of Couples Who Thrive*

Discussion: Many couples in crisis do not consider a "therapeutic couple separation with couple therapy" as a means to repairing seriously damaged relationships. There is a common fear that a separation is just the beginning of a divorce. When a separation is structured effectively by two motivated spouses, and when both spouses agree on seeing a skillful couple therapist during the time-limited separation, huge transformations can happen. The therapist can help each spouse to see his and her own contributions to the marital problems, and can also facilitate problem-solving skills which potentially can resolve the crisis. The couple needs to agree on jointly paying the bills for temporary, separate residences and for time-limited, couple therapy. They need to agree on the length of the structured, trial separation, suitable care for any children, guidelines for each of their social and sexual contacts, and frequency of contact with each other. Ideally, they get together for pleasure at least once a week, have therapy together once a week. Evidence suggests that at least 50% of couples who do this can save their marriages.

Self-exploratory Question: How might a structured separation improve a relationship?

Affirmation: Before considering a divorce, I will consider a therapeutic separation.

Principle: The best protection against divorce is careful choice and good conflict-resolution skills.

Perennial Wisdom Quote: The 1991 *Harper's Index* in the United States cited these statistics: "Estimated chances that an American couple married in 1991 would get divorced: 3 in 5; average duration of an American marriage before divorce: 9.6 years; ratio of number of divorce suits filed by women to number filed by men: 2:1; percent of women who say they are happier since divorce: 85%; percent of men who say they are happier since divorce: 58%."

Discussion: Conflict is a normal part of any close relationship. Whether the conflict destroys the relationship is dependent on the commitment and conflict-resolution skills of both parties. The 1991 *Harper's Index* suggests that women in the United States tend to be more dissatisfied with marriage than men. What is this about? Do you think it relates to how women in the United States prior to about a hundred years ago were considered possessions and could not vote or own property in their own names? Even though the rights of women in the U.S. have dramatically changed since those days, perhaps the culture's skills in teaching adults how to treat each other fairly and kindly has not changed as fast.

There is no required skill test for getting a marriage license, even though wrecking a marriage can cause even more pain and suffering than wrecking a car. Since the basic skills necessary for a successful marriage are now known, perhaps soon a "Marriage License Test" will be required before marriage. Effective conflict-resolution skills would certainly be part of the Test.

Self-exploratory Question: Could I likely pass a "Marriage License Test?"

Affirmation: I practice effective conflict-resolution skills in my marriage.

Principle: Divorce is less painful with effective mediation.

Perennial Wisdom Quote: "Victory breeds hatred, for the conquered is unhappy. He who has given up both victory and defeat, he, the contented, is happy." -- *The Dhammapada*

Discussion: If a divorce cannot be avoided, at least it can be pursued with a Win/Win outcome in mind. This is the only kind of divorce which is stable and less harmful to children. Fortunately, there are now professional divorce "mediators" in most United States cities. These are people who have been trained in conflict-resolution skills, as well as in the divorce laws of their states. If a couple agrees to hire such a professional, prior to securing divorce attorneys, usually the divorce settlement is more just and the post-divorce relationship less damaged.

      If the couple cannot come into agreement on the terms of a divorce with the help of a mediator, it is then still possible for them to secure their own attorneys. But a mediation settlement is always less costly and usually more just. When the judge has to make a decision in the midst of a contested divorce, both spouses often feel un-vindicated anyway and less satisfied with the justice of the outcome. When they can both choose to sacrifice some in order to come into agreement, they can both feel like they have contributed to a positive outcome.

Self-exploratory Question: How can I learn more about mediation?

Affirmation: Should I ever decide on a divorce, I will choose professional mediation.

Principle: Effective mediation can transform hostile divorce and facilitate healthy co-parenting.

Perennial Wisdom Quote: "Quarrels would never last long if the fault was only on one side." -- La Rochefoucauld

Discussion: Ending an unhealthy marriage is sometimes the best solution. If this choice has already been made, the next question is how to leave it in the best possible way, with the least possible hurt to everyone. Usually consulting with a Divorce Mediator is a good place to start. What is different about mediators from traditional divorce attorneys is that they meet with both spouses simultaneously, and cooperatively help them to address all the legal, financial, and child care matters involved with a divorce. Divorce attorneys who have not had training in mediation usually do not do this. Divorce attorneys can only represent one spouse in a divorce action, necessitating both spouses to secure attorneys who then enter into an adversarial win/lose legal struggle, with the outcome determined by a judge who is a stranger to both spouses. This latter divorce process usually leaves both spouses somewhat unhappy with the process and the outcome.

Successful mediation usually leaves both spouses satisfied with the outcome, congratulating themselves for their own successful participation in it, with more money in their pockets, and more able to successfully co-parent children.

Self-exploratory Question: Am I willing to use mediation should I decide on a divorce?

Affirmation: Should I need a divorce, I am capable of creatively participating in mediation.

Principle: All primary care-givers of a child need to creatively cooperate for the well-being of the child.

Perennial Wisdom Quote: "He who establishes his argument by noise and command, shows that his reason is weak." -- Michel de Montaigne

Discussion: Children learn what they see and hear, especially in the early years, and when their caregivers argue over what is best for the child, in front of the child, it is very confusing to the child. Children need to witness significant adults modeling healthy collaboration skills. Some disagreement between caregivers is unavoidable at times, and when it comes up regarding young children, the caregivers need to work out the child care disagreements apart from the children. Children can benefit from seeing adults model healthy conflict-resolution principles, but the content of the modeling should be about issues other than parenting. If parenting is the issue, the parents should seek privacy before working on their parenting conflicts.

Consistent boundaries and limits for the children need to be agreed upon by both parents and applied by both parents. If the parents are divorced and have separate homes, some rules can be different in each home, but ideally the basic values and principles underlying both sets of rules will be compatible. Children need to hear all their caregivers spoken of respectfully. The primary exception to this guideline would be if the child himself or herself is reporting abuse on the part of a caregiver. In such a situation, the adult needs to believe the child, clarify that the reported behavior is abusive, and then search out corroborating information to determine the reality of the situation, before taking action.

Self-exploratory Question: How can I improve my co-parenting skills?

Affirmation: I do my best to collaborate and cooperate with my child's caregivers.

Principle: Responsible interpersonal dynamics transform self-centered, victim-abuser-rescuer "drama triangles."

Perennial Wisdom Quote: "Happy families are all alike; every unhappy family is unhappy in its own way." -- Leo Tolstoy, *Anna Karenina*

Discussion: Basic, healthy conflict-resolution skills are quite similar in most happy families. Dysfunctional dynamics in unhappy families can have many different varieties. However, there is one general way to describe many of these dynamics. It's called "the drama triangle." It involves three or more people, and it is fear-based, controlling, reactive, and shame-based. At least three people distort reality with different types of projection. The result is Lose/Lose for everyone.

One type of distortion is called playing the "victim." This involves seeing one's self as disempowered in the relationship and abused by another. A second type of distortion is called the "abuser" distortion. This comes from the belief that dominance, force, and blame is the only way to resolve conflicts, and the other person is "wrong" and must be made to see it. The third type of distortion is called the "rescuer" distortion. In this distorted perception of reality, the third party agrees that only one of the two others is responsible for the conflict and that the "victim" needs protection.

Dysfunctional people tend to gravitate to one type of distortion, but they also tend to chaotically resort to all of the types. The way out of these unhappy dynamics is for each person to take responsibility for making personal changes, and to respect the equal power and responsibility of all the other adults.

Self-exploratory Question: When am I most likely to participate in a drama triangle?

Affirmation: I am alert to the dangers of drama triangles in my life and avoid them.

Principle: Sometimes we can't control events, but we can always control the way we respond to them.

Perennial Wisdom Quote: "If you are on a road to nowhere, find another road." -- Ashanti proverb

Discussion: People who get stuck in "victim" perceptual distortions are usually people who have been unjustly treated at some time and who have responded with hopelessness and/or dependent behaviors. As children they may have seen adults model only aggressive or non-assertive behaviors, and they may not have learned how to be assertive, nor how to take effective Adult Time Out. (See January 19 Reading.)

"Victims" usually have low self-worth and project their personal power onto someone else. Even if we have been unjustly imprisoned, like Mandella in South Africa, we can still choose honest, assertive and just responses to our jailers and find meaning and personal power in our lives. In domestic situations "victim" behavior often involves over-responsibility, overly empathic responses to others, an over-capacity to tolerate emotional pain, a tendency to personalize other's behaviors, and a tendency to lose oneself within relationship.

Some spouses, of course, are truly abusive. If that is the case, the healthy choice is to separate from that spouse and require intensive psychotherapy for that spouse before considering any private reunions. Abusers have their own problems which are best solved with the help of non-involved professionals.

Self-exploratory Question: When am I most apt to fall into "victim" behaviors?

Affirmation: I am assertive and protect myself from real victimization.

Principle: When angry take Adult Time Out and consult elders before taking action.

Perennial Wisdom Quote: "Those who do not seek the wisdom of their elders are blinded by stubbornness, self-importance and their own folly. Humans can mask their insecurity in many ways. The sure signs are self-importance, addictions, stubbornness, the need to be right, and the refusal to ask for help or advice. Human beings cannot see all of the potential solutions or the possible results of their actions when they are angry, confused or in pain." -- Jamie Sams and David Carson, *Earth Medicine*

Discussion: When people fall into the "abuser" part of the "drama triangle", they are usually still damaged from past experiences and are blaming others for their emotional limitations. They want to punish and prove that someone else is not OK. People in Abuser dynamics resist being told anything. They don't listen. Emotional pain and requests for behavioral change make them anxious, and they cannot engage in Win/Win problem solving when they are so agitated. They temporarily have little capacity for empathy and little impulse control. They do not know how to soothe themselves and restore their brains to effective functioning. Instead they try to control others with domination, distance and fear. When confronted with a person in this state, it is necessary to keep one's self safe by taking "Adult Time Out" and by not returning the aggression.

If you care about the person who is acting aggressively and want to heal the relationship, you can give the person time and space to rest, eat, regain perspective and impulse control, and to regain awareness of his or her own feelings and effective brain functioning. If the behavior includes physical aggression, the abuser needs to seek professional assistance before risking contact again with the abused person.

Self-exploratory Question: How can I best avoid aggressive behavior?

Affirmation: I do not engage in, nor accept, aggressive behavior.

July 28   **Freedom from Unhealthy, Rescuing Behaviors**

Principle: Assuming responsibility for others' problems is disrespectful and damaging.

Perennial Wisdom Quote: "An old error has more friends than a new truth." -- Danish proverb

Discussion: People who tend to fall into the "rescuer" role in "drama triangles" tend to be people who have a strong need to feel needed. They tend to lift responsibility off of "victims'" shoulders, attempting to "fix things." Their intentions are usually good, but they distort reality by projecting their own vulnerability onto a "victim" and their own strength onto an "abuser." Rescuers tend to bind others to them out of need. Friends, family members, therapists, teachers, court systems, and correctional systems are all vulnerable to being drawn into destructive "rescuer" dynamics.

       Rescuers also tend to take on other people's negative moods. Detaching with love is the best way to keep one's serenity when around someone in a bad mood. Detachment does not mean disconnection, rejection or criticism. A loving connection remains when we detach. Self-protective space is simply taken to allow the other person to take responsibility for his or her moods and actions. Remembering that we do not need others' approval is another way to stay free of rescuing actions. We help others the most when we can see their strengths and can encourage them to use their strengths on their own behalf.

Self-exploratory Question: How can I be empathic without rescuing others?

Affirmation: I can care about others without accepting responsibility for fixing their problems.

Principle: In our most important adult relationships respect has to be earned.

Perennial Wisdom Quote: "He that respects himself is safe from others; he wears a coat of mail that no one can pierce." -- Henry Wadsworth Longfellow

Discussion: When we respect ourselves, we have also learned to follow behavioral guidelines which usually earn the respect of others. Such behavioral guidelines include 1) being respectful towards others even when they make mistakes; 2) being assertive, not aggressive; 3) being kind and cooperative; 4) examining our own behavior carefully and readily admitting our mistakes; 5) making amends to others whom we have thoughtlessly hurt or damaged; 6) doing our share of the community work; 7) being of service to needy others; 8) maintaining honest and clear speech; 9) sharing appropriate information with others;10) respecting others' privacy and emotional boundaries; 11) living within our independent means; and 12) maintaining honest employment which damages no one.

Of course, some people will be disrespectful toward us even when we do all of the above things. We can respect ourselves the most when we don't personalize such persons' aggressive behaviors, and when we simply detach from them. Arguing and fighting with disrespectful people just lowers our own standards and makes us reactive and discontented. We can't change others, but we can change ourselves.

Self-exploratory Question: How can I more consistently earn the respect of others?

Affirmation: I respect myself and what I do to earn the respect of others.

Principle: Rewarding children for fulfilling responsibilities appropriate for their age builds character.

Perennial Wisdom Quote: "You don't just luck into things; you build step by step, whether it's friendships or opportunities." -- Barbara Bush

Discussion: Teaching responsibility needs to start early both at home and at school. Parents in the United States are constantly bombarded with advertising about material things which they can give to their children, but parents have little encouragement and help for teaching their children, in step by step ways, to do what they can for themselves and for others.

Busy parents too often find it easier to do FOR their children than to teach children to do for themselves. Parents working long hours outside the home also have little time to teach their children appropriate social skills, such as expressing gratitude, appropriately expressing feelings, and offering appropriate behavioral assistance to others.

Many children in the United States tend to be passive recipients of information via TV, video, internet, teachers and parents, rather than active contributors to their community. Parents, teachers and community members can change this in their homes, schools & community events. They can support such efforts as the Earth Conservation Corps for youth. This non-profit organization's successes in poverty- stricken areas of Washington D.C. have been inspirational. Whole communities need to support parents' efforts to rear responsible children.

Self-exploratory Question: How do I help to raise responsible children in my community?

Affirmation: I do my best to teach children responsibility in and outside of my home.

Principle: Children need healthy mentoring and attention from more than one adult.

Perennial Wisdom Quote: "An effort made for the happiness of others lifts us above ourselves." -- Lydia M. Child

Discussion: Benjamin Franklin once wrote, "What maintains one vice would bring up two children." If adults added up what they spent on mood-altering substances such as tobacco, alcohol and sugar and figured out how that money would benefit children in their family or neighborhood, possibly schools and child welfare organizations might receive more of what is needed to rear healthy, responsible children. If all adults took some community responsibility for the welfare of all the children in their neighborhood, likely children would feel safer and have more resources.

Individuality overshadows civic responsibility in many peoples' value systems. As a result, the American culture and its children are suffering. Freedom is important, but not at the expense of neglecting a nation's children. Also, giving to children creates great happiness in the hearts of the givers, especially elder givers. Somehow the isolation that many American children feel in their small, nuclear families, needs to be overcome by extended family members and community members taking personal interest in helping specific children.

If "no child is to be left behind," we need to be doing more in the United States than increasing academic testing. Each of us needs to be part of the solution to these problems; otherwise we are part of the problem.

Self-exploratory Question: How can I contribute more to the children of my neighborhood and my world?

Affirmation: I do what I can, where I can, to help children.

Principle: Each of us is personally responsible for growing up emotionally.

Perennial Wisdom Quote: "Regret is an appalling waste of energy; you can't build on it; it's only good for wallowing in." -- Katherine Mansfield

Discussion: When we didn't have our emotional needs met well as children, sometimes we carry these wounds on into adulthood, regretting our past but not taking enough responsibility for healing ourselves in the present. Others often then see our wounds simply as emotional immaturity or "victim consciousness." We whine or complain or want to be rescued from our emotional conflicts about which we are simply unaware. We can't see how we are actually giving personal power away to others with our negative, blaming or accusing behavior. We look for rescue from family or friends. Yet, if a friend or family member tries to re-parent us, we just resent it because we really want to be treated as adults, even though we are acting childishly.

Often what we really need is a professional therapist to help us see and take responsibility for our own emotional confusion. Sometimes a self-help group can help, providing modeling of others identifying inner conflicts and responsibly working through them. Sometimes we are handicapped by brain malfunctioning's or chemical imbalances. Fortunately, often our brains can repair themselves with the help of corrective medications, psychotherapy and/or biofeedback. But first we have to get the right diagnosis, then commit ourselves to corrective treatment and follow through. There are no short cuts to growing up.

Self-exploratory Question: How can I help myself to grow into full emotional maturity?

Affirmation: I take full responsibility for recovering from my own emotional wounds.

Commitment

Principle: Learning how to love can most readily happen within a committed family.

Perennial Wisdom Quote: "Real generosity towards the future consists in giving all to what is present." -- Albert Camus

Discussion: None of us can choose what kind of family we are born into. We can choose what we do with the family we have. If our parents were so wounded themselves that they weren't able to meet our childhood needs and model emotional maturity, we can use adult resources to learn to meet our own adult needs and grow into our own emotional maturity. This may include growing awareness of our parents' emotional limitations and the dysfunctional emotional patterns which existed in our families-of-origin. We can still commit to not carrying these dysfunctions on into the families we create as adults ourselves. We can also commit to treating our parents with respect just for their gift of life to us and for their efforts to care for us as much as they were able. We can also treat our siblings with respect and do our best as adults to work out childhood resentments toward them.

       If a family member continues to treat us negatively as an adult, we can do our best not to personalize his or her behavior and to be available should that family member recover from his or her own emotional immaturity. When we don't accept blame from a loved one, when we honestly can feel compassion for our family member's unresolved emotional issues, we aren't as likely to be drawn into dysfunctional "drama triangle" dynamics. We can love, without being necessarily close.

Self-exploratory Question: How can I love my family more, despite dysfunctions?

Affirmation: I am committed to appreciating my family for whatever gifts I received.

Principle: Healing family relationships brings personal growth.

Perennial Wisdom Quote: "Be not ashamed to confess that you have been in the wrong. It is but owning what you need not be ashamed of -- that you now have more sense than you had before to see your error, more humility to acknowledge it, more grace to correct it." -- Jeremiah Seed

Discussion: Pride often gets in the way of healing family rifts. Within a family system each person is responsible for his or her own part of the family dynamics. Even if another family member is behaving badly, it is helpful to look for one's own contribution to the family problem and make amends for it, even if it seems miniscule in comparison to the contributions of other family members.

Modeling corrective, healing behaviors can be very powerful within a family system. Ties of blood and common history are strong, making the family a potentially powerful healing microcosm. An apology can heal one's own pain, even if others do not respond positively to it. It is within the family that we can most readily learn how to respect others' needs.

A family member may be emotionally hurt by some unconscious behavior of our own. When he or she brings it to our attention, we need to respond with concern and a willingness to collaboratively make changes so that the hurt is soothed. This does not mean that we are accepting blame for the family member's hurt. It simply means that we are taking personal responsibility to do our part to maintain a functional, non-hurtful relationship with a family member.

Self-exploratory Question: How can I be more accepting and compassionate with family members?

Affirmation: I am responsible for contributing in a healthy way to my family.

Principle: Respecting a child's core self (soul) facilitates loving child care.

Perennial Wisdom Quote: "Unless you be like little children, you cannot enter the Kingdom of Heaven." -- Jesus Christ

Discussion: It is an awesome task to care for a small child. Human babies come into the world completely dependent, desirous of and in need of attention, and trusting of what adults offer. It is when they are in pain or deprivation or fear that they react negatively. They have to learn to distrust people. At birth they automatically and trustingly reach for contact with a warm adult body. Human adult brains generally have the capacity to understand and respect this vulnerability. Human hearts generally have the capacity to receive pleasure from the process of caring for a vulnerable child. But this care is demanding, and it becomes more and more challenging as the child grows and learns about emotional and social interactions.

Children have to be shown effective coping behaviors. They need instruction and modeling. Parents and child-care givers need to respect the growing little bodies and brains which are in their care and redirect them when they make mistakes. When child-care givers are emotionally needy themselves and have not learned effective adult coping behaviors, they are responsible for securing therapy and education sufficient to remedy these deficits. Children, like water, air, plants, and soil, are gifts from the Universe. They are to be treasured.

Self-exploratory Question: How can I be more loving and respectful to children?

Affirmation: I treasure the privilege of caring for a child and do it respectfully.

Discipline

Principle: Children need limits and guidance.

Perennial Wisdom Quote: "Youth is quick in feeling, but weak in judgment." -- Homer, *Iliad*

Discussion: In general, most professional counselors tend to agree that "authoritative" versus "authoritarian" or "permissive" parenting is the most effective. James Jakob Liszka in *Moral Competence* describes authoritative parenting as 1) warm and loving, yet insistent that children behave appropriately; 2) using mild punishments paired with temporary withdrawal of affection; 3) encouraging independence within well-defined limits; 4) explaining the reasons for rules; and 5) giving permission for children to appropriately express verbal disagreement.

Effective parents help their children to identify and attend to their feelings and needs, but they do not capitulate to their children's demands. Parents need to be able to detach from their children's anger, while also disciplining them with natural consequences. Parents need to be able to set limits for youth regarding such issues as curfews, drugs and alcohol.

Parents need to be able to express their own feelings honestly without emotionally burdening their children. Effective parenting always requires a certain amount of acceptance of chaos, but this does not mean that a parent gives up authority over a child. Experienced parents usually learn to "flow" with their children's interruptions, teaching courtesy to the children, but also not expecting them to wait until a parent's project is totally finished. Effective parenting takes emotional maturity.

Self-exploratory Question: How can I authoritatively discipline children without being authoritarian or permissive?

Affirmation: I am authoritative, and yet loving and accepting with children.

Principle: Parents make mistakes but still deserve respect, especially when elderly.

Perennial Wisdom Quote: "'Honor thy father and mother' stands written among the three laws of most revered righteousness." -- Aeschylus, *Suppliants*

Discussion: As modern medicine extends life expectancy, the challenges of elder care grow. In the United States many elders live ten to thirty-five years past their retirement. Many require assisted living for five to twenty years, as they are no longer able to cook, grocery shop, and drive for themselves. Providing this care in family homes, or in elder communities close enough to visit regularly is a part of respecting our parents.

Hopefully, the elders have thought ahead and financially provided for themselves, but they still need the loving attention of family, even if they are in professional care facilities. They also may need honest, thoughtful oversight of their finances and nursing care during their last years. Parents provide for the care and financial support of their children for up to eighteen years and frequently longer. Increasingly, elders need a similar period of assistance during the last years of their lives. Providing this kind of assistance, either directly or indirectly, helps adult children to prepare themselves for their own elder years.

Elders who keep themselves mentally alert and physically active, as much as possible, as well as in supportive social contact with other elders, make their children's elder care much more manageable and pleasant.

Self-exploratory Question: How can I both respectfully care for my elders and also thoughtfully prepare for my own elder years?

Affirmation: I appreciate the opportunity to offer back to my elders the same kind of loving attention they gave me as a child.

August 7   **"Re-inspirement"**

Principle: Re-inspiring ourselves during retirement can reduce suffering from old age.

Perennial Wisdom Quote: "As I grow older, part of my emotional survival plan must be to actively seek inspiration instead of passively waiting for it to find me." -- Bebe Moore Campbell

Discussion: "Re-inspirement" would be a better term than "retirement" for the post-employment time for elders in modern, economically advanced countries. Usually this time arrives at somewhere between the ages of fifty-five and seventy-five, and the elder usually still has twenty to forty more years to live. Volunteer work, attention to grandchildren, re-education, travel, hobbies and new part-time employment are just some of the many ways in which elders can re-inspire themselves to happy, productive living.

"Downsizing" homes to simplify finances and maintenance and to provide more finances for travel and charity work can be challenging and also very rewarding. Finding new ways to use one's accumulated knowledge, as well as finding new fields of knowledge to explore, keep the mind alert and creative. Exploring music, drama, art, crafts, photography, sculpture, writing, and sports can help to develop talents formerly neglected.

Grandparents can deepen their relationships with grandchildren by occasionally giving their children respites from child care responsibilities. Volunteer work with children in local schools, or far away missions can be inspiring and lead to shared resources and increased gratitude. "Elderhood" can be a time of new inspiration.

Self-exploratory Question: How can I plan my retirement years to be "re-inspiring"?

Affirmation: I look forward to re-inspirement during my retirement years.

224

August 8
"Elderhood"

Principle: The elder years need to be respectfully graced with a term like "elderhood."

Perennial Wisdom Quote: "The innocence of old age is rich. It is rich from experience; it is rich from failures, from successes; it is rich from right actions, from wrong actions; it is rich from all the failure, from all the successes; it is rich multi-dimensionally. Its innocence cannot be synonymous with ignorance. Its innocence can be synonymous only with wisdom." -- Osho, *Maturity*

Discussion: "Elders" are respected in almost all indigenous cultures. Their wisdom was necessary for the survival of the young people. The speed and scope of modern secular knowledge has tended to dwarf the necessity of turning to elders for advice on solving material young adult problems. But in the emotional, social and spiritual realms elders in modern societies still need to be consulted for young people to make wise decisions.

Elders have experience, love for life and time. This cannot always be found among young adults. "Elderhood" is a word which needs to be introduced into the English language to help give the elder years more status than the term "old age" tends to command. In young, modern nations youth and strength and economic resources tend to be equated with status. Older nations and cultures realize that the status of this kind of strength needs to be balanced with the status of the wisdom, which comes with knowledge combined with experience.

Modern community institutions can do more to give elders opportunities to offer wise consultations and mentoring to youth. Senior centers can work with youth and child care centers to see that this happens. In "re-inspirement" years, elders can offer their wisdom to others.

Self-exploratory Question: How can I utilize the wisdom of my elders more effectively?

Affirmation: I make a point to consult elders when I am making important decisions.

August 9   Wise Ways Happiness Support Group Step Eight: Self - Forgiveness

Principle: The Wise Ways Happiness Step 8 reads, "We learn self-forgiveness and how to make amends to others and to ourselves for our past mistakes."

Perennial Wisdom Quote: [Self-forgiveness is the process of shining] "light on the fears and destructive self-judgments that keep us all captive in the role as our own jailer." -- Robin Casarjian, M.A., *Forgiveness, A Bold Choice of a Peaceful Heart*

Discussion: Self-forgiveness is the foundation of all forgiveness. Usually we have trouble forgiving others, because we do not want to look at or cannot forgive ourselves for our part of the problem. We want to blame the problem all on others. We want to make "evil" others into our "enemies" and sanctify ourselves, seeing no wrong in our own behaviors or those of our associates or communities. Or else we see ourselves as "evil" and our own actions as unforgivable.

Self-forgiveness is based on the awareness that all of us are human and make mistakes. If we have not made a mistake personally, perhaps we have condoned or enabled a mistake to be made by an associate or family member. Self-forgiveness involves staying focused in the present moment, rather than dwelling on regrets over the past. Life moves on rapidly, and we need to allow our minds and bodies to move on with it, or we hold ourselves back and distort our awareness. The universe itself is very forgiving. Look at the way human flesh wounds heal and plants recover from temporary droughts.

When we can catch our mistakes early enough, forgive ourselves, make amends for them, and commit ourselves to not repeating mistakes, others forgive us more readily. Attending 12 Step Happiness Support Group meetings can help in this process, because we can see others who have made mistakes and then turned their lives around in amazing ways.

Self-exploratory Question: How can I completely forgive myself for my mistakes?

Affirmation: Self-forgiveness comes through making amends to myself and others.

August 10:   Wise Ways Support Group Tradition 8: Principles, Not Personalities

Principle: The Wise Ways Support Group Tradition 8 reads, "In Wise Ways Happiness Support Groups, principles are always more important than personalities."

Perennial Wisdom Quote: "Those who try to control, who use force to protect their power, go against the direction of the Tao." -- Lao Tzu, *The Tao Te Ching*

Discussion: The leadership in Wise Ways Happiness Support Groups is always directly responsible to those they serve. Force is never used to establish leadership. Democratic discussion of and resolution of disagreements is always the principle.

If a group's good intentions get side-tracked and corrupted by individual self-interests and the ego dynamics of personalities, members can simply break off from the existing leadership to form a new group. This can be done without resentment and can attract new members and is preferable to allowing a resentment between two people to undermine the primary purpose of the group. If one member disagrees with another member's actions, the disagreement can often be solved through the members returning to a study of the Wise Ways Happiness 12 Steps and 12 Traditions. Following well-thought-out principles can heal many a personality problem.

Self-exploratory Question: How can I be sure I am respecting principles more than personalities?

Affirmation: I commit to respecting principles more than personalities.

Principle: Mindfulness is created by staying present with each moment's experience with an observing mind and without resistance, judgement of another or reaction.

Perennial Wisdom Quote: "Some common mindlessness practices are over-watching television, over-playing computer games, and jogging with headphones. We can cultivate mindlessness through mental activities --obsessing, worrying, spacing out, fantasizing. Similar to small children who cling to a favorite toy or blanket, we often seek security in mindlessness." -- Karen Kissel Wegela, Ph.D., *Modern Psychology and Ancient Wisdom,* Sharon G. Mijares, Ph.D., Ed.

Discussion: When we are passive, reactive, "upset", attempting a "geographical cure" or an alcohol or drug binge in order to escape from our present experience, we are experiencing what is called "mindlessness." This kind of "mindlessness" is common in modern secular culture.

When one is "mindful," one is aware of all one's body's changing sensations and perceptions. At the same time a mindful person is mentally present for each current moment, not holding on to some imagined perfect state. Criticisms of others don't distract the mind. Neither do expectations for the future or regrets over the past.

A mindful person doesn't effort at this kind of consciousness. He or she simply maintains a calm, observing mind -- what the yogis call "witness consciousness." This mental state makes it possible to see how one may be causing pain to one's self or to others. It also builds what Karen Kissel Wegela calls "unconditional confidence" -- the recognition that a person is capable and willing to fully experience every moment, whether it be pleasant or unpleasant.

Self-exploratory Question: How can I experience more mindfulness in my life?

Affirmation: My practice of mindfulness is increasing my unconditional confidence.

Principle: Suffering is created by resisting or hanging on to painful experiences.

Perennial Wisdom Quote: "Suffering is described in varying ways, but the core idea is that we tend to deny, hang on to, or push away whatever is painful in our lives." -- Karen Kissel Wegela, Ph.D. in *Modern Psychology and Ancient Wisdom*

Discussion: We cannot prevent pain in our lives. Birth, accident, illness, natural disaster and death usually bring pain. But we can reduce our suffering by not denying, hanging on to, or pushing away physical or psychological pain. The alternative is to stay mindful of the pain, take responsibility for preventing it to the best of our ability, and accepting and witnessing, moment by moment our own contributions to the pain. For example, if we are in a car accident caused by another driver, we could mindlessly choose to verbally assault and threaten the other driver, complain to the ambulance team, abuse the pain medications administered in the hospital, sue the doctor for not adequately relieving our pain, resist the help of the physical therapist and do our best to get set up on disability benefits for the rest of our lives. All these choices would increase our suffering.

The mindful alternative would be to respectfully ask the other driver for help, cooperate quietly with the ambulance team, use pain medications in the hospital judicially, appreciate the doctor for helping, cooperate actively with the physical therapist and do our best to recover completely from the injuries, while also pursuing reimbursement for losses. All these choices would reduce our suffering.

Self-exploratory Question: How can I reduce my suffering and stay mindful?

Affirmation: I accept painful experiences, without rejecting or hanging on to them.

August 13   **Authentic**
Celebration

Principle: Authentic celebration is natural and joyful, and it spreads contagiously.

Perennial Wisdom Quote: "Each day, each moment is so pregnant with eternity that if we 'tune in' to it, we can hardly contain the joy." -- Gloria Gaither

Discussion: Remember your unselfconscious delight as a child to discover something new, to accomplish something special? Change and creativity are naturally celebrated by healthy children. They delight in the sounds of birds and animals. They find the birth of baby chicks a miracle. They find the lick of a playful puppy something to announce to anyone nearby. Such authentic celebration invites others in for enjoyment, brings out laughter and movement, and even promotes healing to the body.

New brain research also confirms that some music promotes integration and heightened functioning of the brain. Dance and authentic movement have a similar effect on the brain. Communal experiences of music and dance tend to bond people to each other and reduce conflict.

It isn't surprising that most religions have developed forms of sacred music and dance, bringing people together for authentic celebration. Agnostics and atheists can also use music, art and dance as ways to come together in community celebration. The human heart longs for such communal experiences, and, if one doesn't adhere to any particular religion, there are still many ways to find authentic celebration. Avoiding isolation and meaninglessness is of utmost importance. Otherwise the human spirit withers.

Self-exploratory Question: How can I authentically celebrate life more often?

Affirmation: I choose to authentically celebrate my life and the life of others.

August 14   **Healthy**
Rituals

Principle: Healthy rituals can energize, protect and heal us.

Perennial Wisdom Quote: "Rituals are a public affirmation of meaning, value, connection. They tie people to each other, to their ancestors and to their place in the world together." -- David Suzuki, *Sacred Balance*

Discussion: Heart-to-heart rituals have positive effects on human immune systems. Dr. Thomas Boyle, a pediatrician and researcher, defines ritual as "the enactment of the sense that certain central, valued elements of life experience are stable and enduring." (Paul Pearsall, Ph.D., *The Heart Code*) Malidoma Patrice Some, Ph.D., in his book, *Ritual, Power, Healing and Community,* lists these four essential aspects of a healthy ritual: 1) It is invocational, i.e. calls on a universal power for support for a specific purpose; 2) It is dialogical, i.e. involves a solemn dialogue between self and spirit; 3) It is repetitive, i.e. involves actions which are repeated by different individuals within a culture at similar life points; and 4) It contains an opening and a closing to the community participation.

Rituals can be as simple as regular family meals at which members begin the meal with appreciation for the food, visit with each other in a supportive fashion, cooperate in cooking, serving, eating, and cleaning up, and stay at the table until the community ritual is complete for everyone. Ritual celebrations are designed to create synergy. Synergy happens when each member of a group contributes their best for the intention of the group. The energy of the group becomes greater than that of its individual members combined. The individuals co-create something new. This helps to give meaning to everyone's lives.

Self-exploratory Question: In what healthy rituals do I participate?

Affirmation: I love to participate in healthy rituals with my family and community.

August 15   **Inspiring Art, Symbol, Writing, Drama and Music**

Principle: Inspiring art, symbol, writing, drama and music can bring unity and integrity to individuals and their communities.

Perennial Wisdom Quote: "Every art requires the whole person." -- French saying

Discussion: The American author, Alice Walker, spoke eloquently about the power of creative energy: "Helped are those who create anything at all, for they shall relive the thrill of their own conception, and realize a partnership in the creation of the Universe that keeps them responsible and cheerful."

Artists of all kinds speak about this kind of energy and mourn its loss when they have "dry" periods. Art appreciators also tap into this energy when they view, read or listen to an art piece. There is an aliveness about good art which connects people. Artists speak of "having to engage" in their art. It is like the art must flow through them for them to feel completely whole. They frequently also feel their art connecting them to others in mysterious ways. Art, drama, storytelling and music have been a part of human celebratory rituals for millennia.

Before paper, art was painted on rocks or human skin or carved into wood or rock. Before modern instruments, ancient flutes were carved of bamboo and voices gathered together into chants. Modern brain research has shown that these activities often have a positive impact on human brain chemistry. Certain ancient symbols, such as the circle used often in dance, have universal harmonizing meanings. Making time for these creative activities helps to keep us alive and well.

Self-exploratory Question: How can I be more inspired by creative art?

Affirmation: Today I am taking time to create and to appreciate the creations of others.

August 16
Concentration

Principle: Concentration requires a quiet, focused mind and body.

Perennial Wisdom Quote: "Training began with children who were taught to sit still and enjoy it. They were taught to use their organs of smell, to look when there was apparently nothing to see, and to listen intently when all seemingly was quiet. A child that cannot sit still is a half-developed child." -- Chief Luther Standing Bear

Discussion: Concentration involves the ability to focus one's attention on one single thing. Concentration practice may be done silently alone or while in a group. The object of concentration can be an art piece, a musical score, a prayer, a yoga stretch, a sports move, woodwork, needlework, whatever. The object doesn't matter so much as the intent of the practice.

When we concentrate our minds, we can both strengthen them and relax them. When beginning concentration training, taking a meditative, silent walk with a mentor or a group can be helpful. The instructions can be simply to concentrate on one's footsteps and breathing pattern, or perhaps to observe in detail sights on the nature trail. What is important is that the practice is supportive and non-judgmental.

Concentration promotes "mindfulness." Mindfulness involves staying calm, alert, and perceptive, not doing anything to change one's experience, rather just accepting it moment by moment.

If concentration is very difficult, it is important to get a medical evaluation. Attention Deficit Disorder is a medical condition in which, when a person attempts to concentrate, there is decreased activity in the prefrontal cortex, rather than the normal increased activity. Medication can help this condition. (See Appendix 1.)

Self-exploratory Question: How can I improve my ability to concentrate?

Affirmation: I am able to concentrate on what I choose and stay focused.

Principle: Accepting emotional pain, when we cannot change a situation, reduces the suffering.

Perennial Wisdom Quote: "[Suffering is] what happens when we struggle with our experience because of our inability to accept it…. [Suffering] is optional." -- Sylvia Boorstein, Ph.D.

Discussion: When we accept our moment-by-moment experiences, even if they are emotionally painful, we don't cling to our desires and preferences. Therefore, we don't create fear for ourselves. Fear is usually a projected loss or pain. If we trust our own ability to manage pain, we don't have to be afraid of fear. It is the fear of fear, or the lack of acceptance of pain, which makes it so unmanageable.

Fear itself can be a passing thought and emotion, if we don't cling to it and make it into worry or even paranoia. Remembering that nothing is permanent is a big help in managing pain and fear. Only taking responsibility for our own thoughts and behaviors, not everything going on around us, is another big help. Sometimes bad things happen to innocent, good people.

Resilient, emotionally healthy people accept this and quickly begin to problem- solve to make the best out of a bad situation. They do this rather than blame others or hang on to self-pity. Blame and self-pity just aggravate bad situations and diminish any likelihood of getting cooperation from others.

Self-exploratory Question: How can I be more accepting of unavoidable emotional pain?

Affirmation: I choose to do my best with difficult emotions and situations.

Principle: Dance can inspire and unify people, as well as be entertaining.

Perennial Wisdom Quote: "Dance is the loftiest, the most moving, the most beautiful of the arts because it is no mere translation or abstraction from life; it is life itself." -- Havelock Ellis, *The Dance of Life*

Discussion: Dance has been held sacred for millennia. Repetitive dance movements can be hypnotic and trance-inducing. Twirling dervishes in the Muslim, mystical Sufi tradition have taught circular dances to induce meditation and also to create community and peace. Dances have been used by aboriginal peoples, accompanied by drums and flutes, for all sorts of ceremonial purposes. As a way to calm the spirit and meditate, yogis have for centuries taught slow-motion hand movements, with the eyes following the movement of the hands. They have also taught slow-motion stretching movements, accompanied by concentration on the breath as a means to enhanced brain functioning.

In more modern times, Western traditions have relegated dance primarily to entertainment, but ancient forms of inspirational and sacred dance are being rediscovered and studied by scientists who are researching the effects of these behaviors on the brain. Likely doctors will someday be recommending certain types of dance as forms of healing, and politicians will someday be joining in dances for community building. We moderns still have much to learn from ancient practices.

Self-exploratory Question: How can I experience dance as a form of inspiration, as well as entertainment?

Affirmation: Moving my body in dance inspires and energizes me.

Principle: Inspiring stories are "chicken soup for the soul."

Perennial Wisdom Quote: "Stories are passed from generation to generation and help to keep the human soul alive." -- Daniel J. Siegel, Ph.D.,*The Developing Mind, How Relationships and The Brain Interact To Shape Who We Are*

Discussion: Stories told about our own lives and about our family members' lives and about notable lives in our culture create the fabric of society. When our parents can tell inspiring stories about their parents' lives and their extended relatives' lives, we grow up placing ourselves in a meaningful and hopeful tapestry of continuity. When we are allowed to be ourselves, with our own uniqueness, and yet accepted into the unique histories of our families, we feel connected and challenged to mature to our fullest.

Dr. Siegel's research has shown how children thrive with parents who have deep self-understanding and have healed from any past losses or traumas. (See his book, *Parenting From the Inside Out.)* Inspiring stories from scriptures, poetry, drama, and history (political, economic, social and artistic) also allow us to benefit from other peoples' experience.

All healthy spiritual groups value these stories and pass them on to future generations. Recently "the storyteller" and storytelling skills are again becoming valued in the United States, especially in their ability to teach cultural and spiritual values. Classes and workshops demonstrate and teach these storytelling skills and inspire budding "storytellers." Whether we attend such classes or simply take pleasure in reading stories and passing on family stories to our children, our efforts are worthwhile. Our children need this sense of cultural and family connection to thrive.

Self-exploration Question: How can I appreciate creative storytelling more?

Affirmation: I value my family's and culture's creative stories and pass them on.

Principle: We can learn from great teachers how to create a meaningful life.

Perennial Wisdom Quote: "The unexamined life is not worth living." -- Socrates

Discussion: Ronald Gross, author of *Peak Learning* and *Socrates' Way, Seven Master Keys to Using Your Mind to the Utmost,* suggests these six ways to create a meaningful life: 1) persistently raise significant questions; 2) involve people in dialogue about their basic values; 3) learn from those with authentic expertise; 4) think productively with friends and colleagues; 5) work together toward the truth; and 6) do the right thing.

Notice how these guidelines would enrich the meaningfulness of a life in any culture and any religion. Notice how Socrates emphasized the importance of learning from experts and connecting in a deep and meaningful way with others. In modern times this also means increasing cross-cultural and cross-religious dialogues to find common guidelines for living peaceful, meaningful lives. We can be Christians, Muslims, Buddhists, Hindus, Native American teachers, agnostics, atheists, whatever, and still follow Socrates' effective guidelines for using our minds in optimal ways to find more meaning in our lives.

Doris Lessing put Socrates' message in simple, modern terms, "What matters most is that we learn from living."

Self-exploratory Question: How can I better follow these Socratic guidelines in my life?

Affirmation: Today I am questioning myself and others about how to lead a more meaningful life.

Principle: For democracy to work, everyone needs to participate in some community effort and thoughtfully vote for the community's leadership.

Perennial Wisdom Quote: "The man's true wealth is the good he does in the world." – Muhammad

Discussion: Democratic decision-making takes more time than autocratic decision-making, but it is inherently more stable. For democracy to continue to thrive, every adult citizen must take his and her voting responsibility seriously. He and she must be active in following national, state and local community issues, in order to give helpful input whenever possible. He and she need to contribute to political campaigns to the best of their financial ability and be active in determining that rich, special interests do not control leaders' votes. As parents, participating on a school board or in PTA's can be rewarding. Attending community council meetings and political party caucuses, answering voters' surveys and sending messages to local, state and national representatives is an important part of keeping a democracy alive.

As the planet becomes more and more economically and politically interconnected, it is also important to be supportive of international, democratically-organized institutions such as the World Court, the World Bank, and the United Nations. Just as individuals cannot live on an island, nations can no longer live isolated from one another.

Democratic institutions grow from the bottom up, rather from than the top down. Chaos often precedes stable democratic leadership, as it takes a while for people to learn how to peacefully promote personal rights and interests. The effort is worthwhile and necessary.

Self-exploratory Question: How can I participate more fully in democratic processes?

Affirmation: I am committed to supporting democratic processes in my community.

August 22
Leadership

Principle: The best leaders are those who can lead selflessly, honestly, democratically, peacefully and joyfully.

Perennial Wisdom Quote: "If we honor ourselves, our roles, our abilities and our talents, we must see those things as sacred. When we choose to share those sacred gifts with others, we can honor ourselves and those we serve only if we do so without looking for reward, accomplishing each deed with a happy heart. Our reward is the joy we find in giving to those we choose to serve." -- Jamie Sams and David Carson, *Earth Medicine*

Discussion: Everyone has some gift to give to others. In the process of giving this talent, this gift, leadership is created. Our gifts might be small and only recognized by one or two other people whom we serve. Or they may be large and recognized in a public way. What is more important than the size of our offered gift of leadership is how we offer the gift. If we lead as a means to promote our own power, prestige, or wealth, we are only engaging in dominant enterprise, not true leadership. This is true even if our leadership is rationalized as promoting the power, prestige and wealth of a group of people.

As human beings develop a richer and richer store of knowledge, the whole world increasingly becomes one family. As the Adam and Eve story in the Bible allegorically tells, human beings all really descended from one set of human parents. As our brains and our technology evolve to allow us more understanding, our leadership needs to focus on service which harms no one, even across national boundaries.

Self-exploratory Question: How can I offer more leadership to my community?

Affirmation: I offer my leadership skills in any area in which I have a special talent.

August 23
Service

Principle: Selfless service is the mark of great leadership.

Perennial Wisdom Quote: "I sought soul and could not see.

I sought God and he eluded me.

I sought my brother and found all three." -- William Blake

Discussion: All the great spiritual teachers have taught the value of selfless service. Buddhists, Muslims, Hindus, Christians, and Native elders from indigenous communities all teach the value of community and selfless service. The United States' culture has emphasized the importance of individuality and personal rights so much recently that the importance of community service has increasingly been overlooked. Somehow this needs to be taught in a "secular" society, or else eventually the foundation of democracy will be undermined by special interests.

For service to be sustainable it needs to be selfless, otherwise resentments find fertile ground. When we offer our service only when we know we will be compensated in some way, we are really just offering a contract, not real service. Of course, some services need to be contracted, and everyone needs to make a living. But when no service is rendered unless a payment is promised, people are only related through business, not through real community. Love is lost, and conflicts grow in such an atmosphere.

Self-exploratory Question: Where in my life do I offer selfless service?

Affirmation: I choose to sometimes volunteer my time and my resources for no reward.

Principle: Do not let resentments get in the way of cooperating with others.

Perennial Wisdom Quote: "Resentment is like holding on to burning wood with the intention of throwing it at another, all the while burning yourself." -- Robin Casarjian, M.A., *Houses of Healing*

Discussion: Resentments get in the way of cooperation. Resentful people choose to use distance and blame to attempt to protect themselves from pain, but it always backfires. They haven't yet learned how to set appropriate emotional boundaries for themselves. They are blocked at looking at their own part in a conflict, as small as their part might be. They simply refuse to contact and cooperate with whomever they judge to be unworthy of them. It is a prideful and controlling defense system which shuts out emotional intimacy.

It is impossible to like everyone all of the time. But we can learn to be cooperative. People are very diverse, and any individual's perspective is always limited. Yet everyone is human and deserving of some respect and some cooperation. Cooperation needs to start with family members, friends and community members, and then spread out to fellow citizens and fellow planet-dwellers.

If we can't respect others' emotional boundaries, even when we don't like the requested boundaries, cooperation breaks down. Soon alienation and misunderstanding result. Families and communities are broken, and everyone suffers more loneliness and isolation. Individuality needs to be balanced with respect for others' emotional, physical, mental and spiritual needs, or else democratic relationships break down into competitive, violent chaos.

Self-exploratory Question: How can I cooperate more with those I care about the most and even with those who are hard to like?

Affirmation: I value cooperative efforts with others, while also keeping my boundaries.

Principle: Polite verbal acknowledgments of contact and withdrawal facilitate respect.

Perennial Wisdom Quote: "The beginnings of all things are small." -- Cicero

Discussion: Human beings are by nature social and verbal beings. As a result, most human cultures have developed rituals of human contact and withdrawal which facilitate cooperative and peaceful co-existence with one another. In English these patterns are often referred to as "common courtesy" guidelines. For example, greeting a person when newly having contact with him or her, especially if both persons are alone in a common space, is considered making appropriate contact. This contact can be made verbally with a "Good morning" or non-verbally with a smile and a nod of the head if passing on the street. If it is with a loved one in the home, it might be an affectionate hug, and a "Hi, Honey" or some other form of endearment.

       To make human contact with another without some sort of respectful acknowledgement in most cultures is considered rude and disrespectful. Similarly, when withdrawing from human contact, some sort of acknowledgement of departure is important. It is considered rude to forget to offer a verbal "Goodbye" or "Goodnight" when leaving a host or hostess at a party. Respectful family members verbally signal other family members when departing to go to bed or to leave the house. Forgetting such courtesies strains relationships and is emotionally isolating.

Self-exploratory Question: How can I be more respectful when contacting or withdrawing from others?

Affirmation: I respect my own and others' emotional needs for contact and space.

242

Principle: Trusting a bigger, meaningful context for our lives reduces suffering.

Perennial Wisdom Quote: "God speaks wherever he finds a humble, listening ear. And the language he uses is kindness." -- Lena Horne

Discussion: When we struggle with life, it is usually because we are taking our own life story too personally and not seeing it as a small part of a great, unfolding cosmic drama over which there is a Higher Power. When we can see suffering that way, it becomes manageable. Whether we are Buddhists, Christians, Muslims, agnostics or whatever, if we can see our lives within a bigger context and trust that bigger context, the suffering becomes meaningful.

Every life exists within a bigger context. Some people just don't take time to discover that context. Instead they resist their painful experiences and forget to look for personal meaning and instruction in them. For example, a person might be incarcerated after committing a very serious crime. He or she might be struggling and suffering a great deal due to the incarceration. He or she might focus only on blaming and shaming the police and legal system which enforced the incarceration. Or this person might take time to find personal meaning in the suffering. This might totally change his or her experience. The larger context for the suffering might be learning how to avoid acting out in anger again. Or the larger context might be learning how to be kind to others in a way which brings happiness to the self, even while serving a life in prison.

Suffering may be reduced by overcoming self-pity, by contributing to the well-being of others and by finding a way to learn from one's losses.

Self-exploratory Question: How can I find meaning in my life in order to reduce my suffering?

Affirmation: I see my life within a large context which reduces my suffering.

Principle: Warfare dehumanizes others and causes unnecessary losses.

Perennial Wisdom Quote: "There never was a war that was not inward. I must fight till I have conquered in myself what causes war." -- Marianne Moore

Discussion: Psychology makes a distinction between "necessary losses" and "unnecessary losses." "Unnecessary losses" cause more suffering. This is because they are preventable. "Necessary losses" such as those due to illness or death from unpreventable disease or natural disasters are painful, but they are somehow easier to accept.

Warfare is the end result of the dehumanization of others. The drive for more power and wealth or the perceived need to protect existing wealth and power or to overthrow existing power is usually the tap-root of warfare. In order for leaders to justify killing other human beings, they have to dehumanize them into "the enemy." They have to believe that they themselves have been so dehumanized that it is legitimate to dehumanize the perpetrators of the first dehumanization.

Violence has a way of spreading, and innocent men, women and children tend to get caught up in the violence, without themselves perpetrating any wrongs. This is why many of the great religious teachers of the world, including Jesus Christ and Buddha, taught non-violence, even in the face of injustice. Some religious leaders have taught that warfare is acceptable in the face of injustice, that war should be fought to reduce the suffering of innocents. Whatever one's personal belief system, it is important to focus on not dehumanizing anyone, including an "enemy." This practice only perpetuates warfare and unjustly rationalizes the eventual killing of innocents.

Self-exploratory Question: How can I avoid dehumanizing anyone?

Affirmation: All human beings deserve respectful treatment, even when, in ignorance and fear, they have been unjust to others.

Principle: When religious people become intolerant, their actions can become evil.

Perennial Wisdom Quote: "Security comes not from having or assuming we have all the answers; it comes from knowing which direction we are going and being able to respond to confusion, crisis, and even calamity on the basis of time-tested principles. The diversity we experience -- in relation to those nearby as well as those who are far away -- need not be seen as a threat; it can become part of the rich texture of life on the journey…. A spiritual compass can help us see religious, ethnic, and national diversity -- in our neighborhoods, country, and world -- as enriching rather than threatening." -- Charles Kimball, Th.D., in *When Religion Becomes Evil*

Discussion: Christian, Jewish, and Islamic traditions all trace their roots to Abraham and all worship the same God. Buddhist, Hindu and Jewish religions have historically been inclusive in their faiths. The Roman Catholic Second Vatican Council's "Light to the Gentiles" embraces the view that salvation is possible for people outside of the Christian church. And yet historically Christianity and Islam have been exclusive in their faith beliefs, claiming heaven only for their own believers. Charles Kimball, an American Baptist, argues persuasively for "an inclusive faith rooted in a tradition." The Dalai Lama says, "My religion is kindness."

Self-exploratory Question: How tolerant and inclusive is my religious faith?

Affirmation: Today I choose to honor the core truths in all the world's major religions

Principle: Avoid addictive and obsessive religious practices to maintain health.

Perennial Wisdom Quote: "We need to be able to perceive others and ourselves as imperfect and still open our hearts." -- Jeremiah Abrams

Discussion: Father Leo Booth in his book *Breaking The Chains* outlines some characteristics of what he calls "religious addiction": negative judgments of others based on their lack of similar beliefs, isolation from others with different beliefs, shaming and blaming others when certain religious practice is not followed, engaging in a religious practice to the point of damaging physical or emotional health, isolation from biological family unless they share similar beliefs, disallowing or shaming the psychological processing of past losses and wounds, keeping secrets, judging and repressing feelings, repressing the free expression of other's feelings, promoting the unquestioning obedience to a religious leader, dishonesty and indirectness in communication.

     Authentic religion always teaches compassion and kindness toward others. When unkindness and rejection are rationalized in the name of religion, the religion has become polluted and addictive. Striving toward human perfection and believing in one's own definitions of perfection to the exclusion of others' definitions is obsessive and dangerous. Doing this with the support of a group is even more dangerous. Many crimes have been committed in the name of divine guidance.

Self-exploratory Question: How am I most likely to become addictive in my religious practices or my humanistic beliefs?

Affirmation: Today I am avoiding addictiveness in the practice of my religion or my humanistic beliefs.

Principle: Healthy spirituality is grounded in compassion and kindness.

Perennial Wisdom Quote: "…all the religions of the world are called upon in these times to re-invite their global citizens to ways of living that are Spirit-filled in their devotion to celebration and the sharing of celebration by way of justice. That is, filled with compassion." -- Mathew Fox, Ph.D., *A Spirituality Named Compassion*

Discussion: Genuine spirituality in any religion includes compassion, kindness, trust, gratitude, acceptance, honesty, lack of criticism and negative judgments of others, relatedness, joy, possible involvement or non-involvement in religious organizations, little focus on property or money other than to serve others, and lack of threat from the separation of church and state.

Religious organizations which have not become corrupted do not ask for blind obedience; they do not make absolute truth claims; they do not justify violent or unethical means to pursue perceived just ends; they do not declare holy war; they do not establish "ideal" times and claim they alone can implement God's vision in the world.

Likely one of the reasons why the various 12 Step self-help programs have been growing in popularity is because their 12 Traditions make the corruption of healthy spirituality within the groups very difficult. The groups do not own any property; they follow principles of attraction more than promotion; they attract new members based on the help and service opportunities they provide. Leaders are "trusted servants," not authority figures.

Healthy spirituality can exist in any religious or 12 Step group if the healthy qualities listed above are prioritized.

Self-exploratory Question: Are all my spiritual practices healthy?

Affirmation: I always determine that a spiritual group is emotionally healthy before I make a commitment to it. I work to help the group stay spiritually healthy.

Principle: Healthy spirituality includes reverence for Nature.

Perennial Wisdom Quote: "The best remedy for those who are afraid, lonely, or unhappy is to go outside, somewhere where they can be quite alone with the heavens, nature, and God. Because only then does one feel that all is as it should be and that God wishes to see people happy amidst the simple beauty of nature." -- Anne Frank

Discussion: Many great religious teachers have emphasized the importance of observing Nature and learning from her. Respect for Nature creates a common ground for all healthy spirituality. It is impossible to walk for long in the woods or on a beach without feeling a Power greater than one's self. The rejuvenating essence of Nature for all humans on the green/blue planet Earth is undeniable.

In most traditions Earth is spoken of in the feminine gender. "Earth Mother" is revered, and her lessons are studied. Native Americans require their youth to go alone into Nature on "vision quests" to discover their own place in the larger scheme of things. Christian youth groups go to "camps" and on "nature walks" to learn to pray and meditate and celebrate God's natural gifts. Buddhist monks meditate as they walk on simple trails bordered by trees and as they make patterns in the sand. Muslim holy places are inlaid with patterns of flowers and plants, often done with semi-precious stones.

Nature herself has a way of healing religious addiction and other forms of addiction. Nature knows that there can be beauty even in death, when the dying are very ill or very harmful to others. Nature's laws reinforce healthy growth and punish human ignorance, greed, addiction and hatred. Taking retreats from our busy lives into natural surroundings brings us back to what is important and sustaining. It also reminds us of the importance of protecting Nature on our beautiful planet.

Self-exploratory Question: How can I more often and beneficially take nature retreats?

How can I also do my part to protect Mother Nature from human pollution?

Affirmation: I periodically retreat for healing and the study of the wisdom of Nature.

September 1
Journaling

Principle: Personal journaling can open doors of self-discovery and transformation.

Perennial Wisdom Quote: "When in doubt, make a fool of yourself. There is a microscopically thin line between being brilliantly creative and acting like the most gigantic idiot on earth. So, what the hell, leap!" -- Cynthia Heimel

Discussion: Readers of *Wise Ways Happiness* principles are encouraged to journal our own private thoughts and life stories on a daily basis, or as often as possible. The daily "principles," "perennial wisdom quotes," "discussions," "self-exploratory questions" and "affirmations" in *365 Wise Ways to a Happy Life* are all designed to stimulate self-examination and exploration. They are also designed to stimulate possible discussions with and support from others.

Journaling is a way of honoring our innermost feelings, thoughts and experiences. We need to have the right to keep our journals completely private, or share parts of them if we wish. They are conversations with ourselves and can easily be misunderstood by others, so we need to be cautious if we share them. We can also use them to help ourselves to remember our dreams, thoughts and feelings. We can even use them to launch a writing career. As Cynthia Heimel reminds us, creativity and foolishness are separated by a very thin line. It makes sense to take the chance and express ourselves.

Self-exploratory Question: How can I use a journal to expand my creative awareness?

Affirmation: I journal on a regular basis for my own personal growth and creativity.

September 2   **Regular**
Dialoguing

Principle: Dialoguing is more than just talking. It's listening, accepting and understanding.

Perennial Wisdom Quote: "Listening is an art. And the first tenet of the skill is paying undivided attention to the other person." -- Mary Kay Ash

Discussion: Appendix 7 contains a list of guidelines for effective dialoguing. They are helpful, not only in a group setting, but also when just two people are struggling to understand each other better so as to be able to work through differences. To effectively problem-solve with another, one has to first be clear about one's own needs, priorities and proposals. But often all of us are unclear about our own needs and priorities and do not feel ready to put forth a proposal for solving some conflict. This is a perfect time to focus on simply dialoguing with each other.

The primary purpose of dialoguing is to arrive gradually at more self-understanding and more understanding of another. To be thoughtfully heard -- to have one's feelings and thoughts accepted -- greatly facilitates self-understanding. To listen to another thoughtfully and carefully greatly facilitates understanding of another. Both these gifts are available through dialoguing.

If you do not have adequate opportunities to dialogue safely with another, starting or joining a group such as a Wise Ways Happiness Support Group can be helpful.

If you do not experience safe dialoguing in your home, consider introducing your family to the information in Appendix 7 and proposing regular times to simply relax and dialogue with one another. Busy modern lives don't provide much time for dialoguing unless it is planned for and committed to ahead of time.

Self-exploratory Question: How can I take more time for creative dialoguing?

Affirmation: I take time for dialoguing, especially with those closest to me.

Principle: Laughter, music, song and dance are good for the body and mind.

Perennial Wisdom Quote: "One who knows how to sing and laugh never brews mischief." -- Iglulik Eskimo saying in *The Sacred Ways*

Discussion: Some Native American tribes have a tradition of "sacred clowning." Tribal members volunteer to be "sacred clowns" at certain community celebrations. They first have to commit to a demanding program of self-examination and emotional cleansing. At the time of the ceremony they paint their bodies black and white in stripes, and their task is to silently mime all that is happening at the ceremony, making people laugh and also making them look into their unconscious, shadowy selves. The clowns are expected to also mime the tribal leaders, and the leaders are expected to humorously accept the non-verbal feedback.

Modern, non-Native comics and clowns have somewhat of a similar role, but they are not as thoughtfully prepared for their roles, and leaders are less expected to be humorously accepting of their feedback. Music, song and dance are also a part of modern culture, but musicians and dancers are also not required to carefully examine themselves and cleanse their own minds and bodies of impurities before performing for others. Perhaps we moderns have a lot to learn from the ancient Native American traditions of "sacred clowning" and community dancing. Sacred clowning is maintained for the betterment of the whole tribe and is taught and supervised by elders who follow ancient community-building principles.

Self-exploratory Question: Are my forms of entertainment all healthy?

Affirmation: I choose healthy entertainment which also benefits my community.

September 4   **Universal Human Rights**

Principle: Individual and governmental respect for universal human rights help to maintain peace.

Perennial Wisdom Quote: "Today countries are concentrating too much on efforts and means to defend their borders. Yet these countries know so little about the poverty and suffering that makes the human beings who live inside such borders feel so lonely!

If instead they would worry about giving these defenseless beings some food, some shelter, some health care, some clothes, it is undeniable that the world would be a more peaceful and happy place to live." -- Mother Teresa

Discussion: In 1948, the United Nations adopted "A Universal Bill of Rights." Eleanor Roosevelt, former "first lady," worked hard with the committee who wrote the document. Among other things, this document assures every human being the right to "life, liberty and security of person," freedom from torture and arbitrary arrest, equal protection under the law including a fair and public hearing in which one is presumed innocent until proven guilty, equal rights in marriage and to own property, a right to freely chose governmental representation, just work conditions, and an education.

Wouldn't it be wonderful if this document were required reading in every public school of every member of the United Nations? Wouldn't it be wonderful if democratic citizens required their representatives to follow these guidelines? Individual citizens must do our best to hold our own governments accountable for respecting these rights and for passing laws that assure that corporate businesses respect these rights.

Self-exploratory Question: How can I do more to promote universal human rights?

Affirmation: I believe in universal human rights and do my best to protect them.

Principle: Appropriate admonition is timely, truthful, gentle, kind and helpful.

Perennial Wisdom Quote: "Appropriate admonition is timely, truthful, gentle, kind and helpful." -- Sylvia Boorstein, Ph.D., *It's Easier Than YouTthink*

Discussion: There is an important difference between inappropriate judgment of another and appropriate admonition. Judgment may be timely and truthful, but isn't always gentle or kind or helpful. To be helpful, the admonisher needs to communicate caring and specifically describe how the person's behavior is causing suffering for another and what corrective behavior needs to be substituted.

Appropriate admonition is necessary at times, especially for children and adults who have not learned to control harmful behavior or are learning a new skill. It is never blaming or shaming.

Awareness of one's intention is vital in all speech. When admonishing another or asking a question, it is best to take time to reflect on your response, examine your intention and check your tone of speech. This takes just a few seconds to do and helps the other person to know that you are respecting him or her, as well as the question or issue being discussed.

Sylvia Boorstein in the above quote lists the necessary qualities in the Buddhist concept of "Right Speech," which is one aspect of "Right Action." For a behavior to be considered "Right Action" it needs to avoid causing others pain and/or be intended to alleviate another's suffering. Other religious groups and many agnostics and atheists, of course, also teach the merits of these "Right Actions".

Self-exploratory Question: How can I improve my ability to give appropriate admonition when it is required?

Affirmation: My admonition of another's behavior is always gentle, kind and helpful.

September 6   **Wise Ways Happiness Step Nine: Making Amends**

Principle: The Wise Ways Happiness Step Nine reads, "We make direct amends to those we have harmed, except when to do so would further harm others."

Perennial Wisdom Quote: "There is a difference between guilt and remorse. When you feel guilty, you keep repeating yourself. When you feel remorse, you stop. Guilt comes from judgment. Remorse comes from love." -- Nogah Lord, *Truth, Simplicity And Love*

Discussion: Making a direct amend to someone we have harmed is a major step in self-forgiveness and in committing to not repeating the harm to anyone else. An amend is different from an apology. It can be easy to say, "I apologize." Making a direct amend involves initiating the contact with a person one has harmed, understanding what caused one's self to engage in this harmful behavior, understanding the damage which has been done to another, empathizing with the pain of the other, asking for help in righting the wrong and learning not to repeat the wrong, and committing to a just settlement and to not repeating the wrong. In some cases, this cannot be done directly with the harmed person, but it can be done with a family member or with another person who would benefit from help. For example, we might have dumped a big bag of trash in someone else's dumpster, and it might be wiser to not repeat this and also spend a few hours picking up trash in that person's neighborhood, rather than making direct amends to a stranger who might become violent. The intent to, as justly as possible, right some wrong, is the essence of making regular amends. (See also Appendix 4.)

Self-exploratory Question: How can I better practice making regular amends?

Affirmation: I commit to making regular amends for all my mistakes.

September 7 Wise Ways Happiness Support Group Tradition Nine: Group Decisions

Principle: The Wise Ways Happiness Support Group Tradition Nine reads, "Wise Ways Happiness Support Group decisions are made by a "group conscious" meeting, ideally by a consensus of the group at the meeting.

Perennial Wisdom Quote: "Communication leads to community -- that is to understanding, intimacy and mutual valuing." -- Rollo May

Discussion: The 9th Tradition of Wise Ways Happiness Groups assures that leadership is a bottom-up process rather than a top-down process. All members are invited to consider questions which affect the whole group. Everyone's vote is respected. As much as possible group decisions are made by consensus.

This tradition is what has made all the 12 Step programs strong and self-sustaining. Wise Ways Happiness Support Groups depend on principles more than personalities. Therefore, they start out small, yet grow and can be ongoing. Following these principles can help groups to avoid the development of unhealthy characteristics in their leadership, such as pride and domination.

Self-exploratory Question: How can I participate more effectively in the leadership of my support group?

Affirmation: I am committed to shared membership participation in my support group.

Principle: Negative thoughts literally damage the brain.

Perennial Wisdom Quote: "Left unchecked, ANTS [Automatic Negative Thoughts] will cause an infection in your whole bodily system." -- Daniel G. Amen, M.D., *Change Your Brain, Change Your Life*

Discussion: Whenever we have angry, sad, or unkind thoughts, our brains release chemicals which activate the deep limbic systems of the brain. When we have positive, happy thoughts, our deep limbic systems calm down. (See Appendix 1.) Negative thoughts are a sort of brain pollution. Often our automatic thoughts are not telling us the truth, but instead are repeating expectations of past negative experiences. We can talk back to our automatic negative thoughts. We can learn to identify "always/never" over-generalizations, mind-reading, labeling others, personalizing and blaming -- all ways to pollute our brains.

Whenever one has a negative thought it should be questioned. For example, "Do I have proof of this reality? Am I over-generalizing here? Am I personalizing or blaming someone in this situation?" In order to question ourselves in these ways, we need to learn to observe our thoughts and feelings and slow down our actions, so we can actually experience reality instead of our own distorted perceptions. If we cannot learn to do this on our own, joining a support group, initiating psychotherapy, or attending a "mindfulness" training class can all be helpful.

Self-exploratory Question: How can I be more vigilant about letting go of negative thoughts?

Affirmation: I can recognize and correct my over-generalizations, mind-readings, and blaming, personalizing thoughts.

Principle: Learning how to manage stress is necessary for a successful life.

Perennial Wisdom Quote: "Changing behavior can also change brain patterns." -- Daniel Amen, M.D.

Discussion: Stress can come from both external and internal sources. We can often not change the external stressors, but we can always change the internal ones. When we feel stuck in repetitive thoughts or worry, we can always distract ourselves and come back to a problem later, instead of trying to force ourselves to prematurely come to a decision or a solution. We can also make it a habit to think through a situation before we automatically say "no" and cause a reaction. We can say, "I need to think about that. I'll get back to you," or we can simply take a few deep breathes and stay silent for a bit while we consider the whole matter.

When we feel stressed and confused, we can take time to write out various options and solutions and possibly even seek advice from someone else. When especially stressed it is always helpful to use a repetitive prayer such as "The Serenity Prayer" (see Appendix 2.), or calming visualizations.

If we are unable to utilize these techniques, likely medication and psychotherapy are necessary. Perhaps even some basic life-style changing decisions need to be made. These can more easily be considered with the help of a therapist and/or a support group.

Self-exploratory Question: How can I more effectively manage my stress?

Affirmation: Stress management is a high priority for me, involving skills which I practice daily.

September 10   **Moral Development**

Principle: Moral reasoning is a skill which takes a lifetime to develop.

Perennial Wisdom Quote: "A person completely wrapped up in himself makes a small package." -- Denzel Washington

Discussion: The American psychologist most noted for developmental studies of moral reasoning is Lawrence Kohlberg, Ph.D. He defined six stages of moral development (from the least developed to the most developed): 1) "Punishment and Reward Reasoning", in which external rules seem imposed upon the self; 2) "Instrumental Purpose and Exchange Reasoning", in which rules are followed only when they meet one's immediate self-interest; 3) "Interpersonal Cooperation Reasoning", in which one meets the expectations of immediate others; 4) "Social Accord and System Maintenance Reasoning", in which duties and obligations of community and nation are respected; 5) "Social Contracts and Rights Reasoning", in which universal justice and human rights are examined and promoted; and 6) "Universal Ethical Principles Reasoning", in which a person actually models applying principles of universal justice and human rights.

As little children all of us start out in Stage One. With good parenting and adult supervision, as children, we learn Stage Two reasoning. While pursuing an education, usually Stage Three reasoning is developed. Stage Four reasoning can start developing in childhood, but it is essential for successful independent young adulthood. Stage Five reasoning develops for some thoughtful and motivated adults. Stage Six moral reasoning develops for some emotionally, socially and intellectually great leaders and teachers.

Self-exploratory Question: In what "stage" of moral reasoning do I now see myself?

Affirmation: I am continually working on advancing my moral reasoning.

Principle: Maturity develops in stages as a person learns to meet basic and higher levels of physical, emotional, social, intellectual and spiritual needs.

Perennial Wisdom Quote: "Of all knowledge the wise and good seek most to know themselves." -- William Shakespeare

Discussion: "The Three R's of Maturity" of the Wise Ways Happiness Program are 1) Respect for self, 2) Respect for others, and 3) Responsibility for all our own actions. Abraham Maslow, Ph.D., a famous American psychologist, defined six levels of developmental, psychological "needs", from the most elemental to the highest. They are correlated with developmental maturity: 1) "physiological" needs; 2) "safety" needs; 3) "belonging-love" needs; 4) "self-esteem" needs; 5) "self-actualization" needs; and 6) "transcendence" needs.

Whether we had our physiological, safety and belonging-love needs met as children or not, it is our responsibility to find a way to meet these needs as independent, "mature" adults. This involves learning how to support one's self financially, learning how to keep one's self emotionally and physically safe, and learning how to love and respect and to be loved and respected by trustworthy others.

As we increasingly accomplish these tasks, our self-esteem is strengthened, and we learn self-confidence and ways to use our talents in service to others, as well as means of self-support. If we are fortunate and live a healthy enough and long enough life, we might also be able to "transcend" these basic needs and realize our spiritual and interpersonal needs to such a degree as to be a model and teacher for others.

Self-exploratory Question: How can I improve my practice of the "3 R's of Maturity?"

Affirmation: I practice respect for myself and others and responsibility for my actions.

Principle: Stages of maturity are also coordinated with levels of consciousness.

Perennial Wisdom Quote: "Mindfulness, the aware, balanced acceptance of present experience, is at the heart of what the Buddha taught." -- Sylvia Boorstein, Ph.D., *It's Easier Than You Think*

Discussion: Eastern philosophies and religions tend to talk about "levels of consciousness" or "mindfulness." Yogis in India taught about seven "levels of consciousness" and "chakras" or centers in the body (from the most fundamental to the highest): 1)Survival (food, shelter, clothing, health); 2) Passion (emotionality and sexuality); 3) Power (of mind, ego and identity); 4) Heart Connection (and acceptance); 5) Expression (creativity and understanding); 6) Compassion ("the 3rd eye" marked by the spot between the eyebrows); and 7) Unity (universal ethical principles).

Notice the parallels between these "levels of consciousness" and Dr. Maslow's "developmental needs" and Dr. Kohlberg's "stages of moral reasoning." (See the September 10 and 11 readings.) A person can move in and out of these different levels of consciousness, depending on his or her current life experience. As one matures more and more, the level of consciousness which is most prevalent can gradually grow higher.

When a person faces awareness of impending death, often he or she can move upward through these levels of consciousness quite rapidly. Children who die young of unpreventable illness often are observed quickly maturing through these levels. Adults who have matured through a full life, frequently can set aside awareness of physical discomfort in order to focus on heart connection and compassion for loved ones as well as unifying thoughts.

Self-exploratory Question: How can I adequately attend to my higher levels of consciousness, and remain non-addictive in my lower levels?

Affirmation: I am non-addictive in my lower levels of consciousness and active in higher levels of consciousness.

Principle: Stages of faith are correlated with levels of maturity and consciousness.

Perennial Wisdom Quote: "People are like stained-glass windows. They sparkle and shine when the sun is out, but when the darkness sets in, their true beauty is revealed only if there is a light from within." -- Elizabeth Kubler-Ross

Discussion: Process definitions of faith are more helpful than content definitions -- the "how's" of faith, rather than the "what's." (See Feb. 14 reading.) James Fowler wrote a ground-breaking book called *Stages of Faith, The Psychology of Human Development And the Quest For Meaning.* In it he defined six "stages of faith": 1) Intuitive-Projective Faith (fantasy-filled and imaginative, usually present at about ages 2-7); 2) Mythic-Literal Faith (usually present at ages 8-12, but can continue into adulthood); 3) Synthetic-Conventional Faith (as teens and older people begin to look for symbolic meaning in literal stories); 4) Individuative-Reflective ("the emergence of the executive ego" creates distance from one's previous assumptive value system"); 5) Conjunctive Faith (the adult willingness to let reality speak its word, regardless of the impact of that word on others or self-security); and 6) Universalizing Faith (adult devotion to "universalizing compassion," however it appears in any religious group's practice.)

Notice the parallels between these stages and Dr. Kohl berg's "stages of moral reasoning."(Sept.10 reading)

Self-exploratory Question: At what "stage of faith" do I see myself?

Affirmation: I am maturing into higher stages of faith.

September 14   **Growing through Stages of Recovery from**
Addiction

Principle: Recovery from any addiction is slow and progresses through stages.

Perennial Wisdom Quote: "A pessimist is someone who complains about the noise when opportunity knocks." -- Michael Levine

Discussion: Addiction is "the noise" of "opportunity" knocking, a warning signal that something serious is wrong with how a person is approaching life (i.e. trying to just dull pain rather than learn from it). The previous four daily readings have focused on stages of moral reasoning, maturity, consciousness and faith. When one has become heavily addicted to a substance or a destructive process, it is impossible to progress through these stages. As long as the addiction continues, maturity is arrested.

Once abstinence from the addictive substance or process is established, then mature development can continue. Usually, however, it first takes at least a year for an individual to just focus on arresting the addiction, one day at a time. Emotional, social and spiritual development often doesn't advance until after a year of stable abstinence in what might be called "stage one" of recovery.

Once "stage one" is well established, then "stage two", involving healing interpersonal conflicts and growing in interpersonal skills, can continue. Service work in 12 Step programs is very important at this stage. Psychotherapy is also often necessary. Stage Three involves the consolidation of spiritual development and the continuation of emotional, moral, and social development. It takes ongoing abstinence from addictions.

Self-exploratory Question: How do I respond when an addictive "opportunity" knocks?

Affirmation: I abstain from addictions one day at a time and progress with my recovery.

Principle: In order for humans to avoid planetary destruction, we must learn how to reduce our desires, reuse materials, recycle materials, and redesign sources of energy.

Perennial Wisdom Quote: "Freedom is not procured by a full enjoyment of what is desired, but by controlling desires." -- Epictetus

Discussion: Human desires and addictions are rapidly destroying the beauty and abundance of the Earth's natural existence. If our planet is to survive the huge current expansion of the human species, and its dependence on polluting fossil fuels, without unrecoverable losses, a majority of human beings need to diligently recover from their addictions and progress at least to "heart" levels of consciousness" (see Sept. 12 reading) and "Individuative-Reflective" levels of faith. (See Sept. 13 reading.)

   We need to get over our mechanistic, desire-based attitudes towards life, or we will literally kill human life on this planet. The September 2002 Supplement to *The National Geographic Magazine* cited these global statistics: every 20 minutes 80 children die due to lack of clean water or sanitation facilities; every day 9,300 people perish from diarrhea, cholera, schistosomiasis and other diseases spread by contaminated water or the lack of water for adequate hygiene. In the U.S. and nearly 1/3rd of the world, aquifers (primary sources of drinking water which take 1000's of years to recharge) are being poisoned; 70% of major commercial fish stocks are depleted, over fished, or exploited beyond maximum sustainable yield; eroded soil and fertilizers have spawned 50 known ocean dead zones, including a massive one in the Gulf of Mexico; humans are now 6.2 billion on the globe, growing by 80 million a year; and they have planted, grazed, paved or built upon roughly 40% of the Earth's land surface. There is little time to waste to save our sustainable resources.

Self-exploratory Question: How can I reduce my desires and protect my planet?

Affirmation: I am reducing my desires, recycling goods, and protecting my planet.

September 16   **Learning "Planetary Competency"**

Principle: The "4 R's of Planetary Competency" include Reduce, Reuse, Recycle and Redesign. (See also <u>March 17</u> reading.)

Perennial Wisdom Quote: "We didn't own the land. We were caretakers. I'd say we owned the path that we walked." -- Curley Bear Wagner, Blackfoot American Indian, *Words of Power,* Norbert S. Hill, Jr., Editor

Discussion: Bill McKibben, the author of *The End of Nature,* in 1998 wrote an article for the *Atlantic Monthly Magazine* which included this information: the human population has grown more since 1950 than it did during the previous four million years. The U.N. predicts 7.7 - 12 billion human beings by the year 2050. This is the maximum population for which the planet can produce adequate food. The U.N. also has projected that an immediate 60% reduction in fossil fuel consumption was necessary to stabilize climate at its current rate of disruption. The bottom line is that the material "good life" as many modern Westerners have come to experience it is unsustainable.

For democracies to protect the future of their children, they must find some way to appropriately reign in the power and economic control of large corporations, or planetary mass starvation and warfare are the inevitable result. Capitalistic, profit-motivated corporations have little current incentive to consider ethical concerns beyond their own "bottom" economic "lines." They only have loyalty to their shareholders and executives. They pay little attention to the welfare of their employees and non-shareholders. And yet these large corporations wield increasing influence on democratic governments.

Somehow democratic peoples need to regain control of their governments and be concerned about overall planetary sustainability issues, or the future will be bleak.

Self-exploratory Question: Am I exercising "planetary competency?"

Affirmation: I commit to being part of the solution to our planet's problems, rather than being part of the problems.

Principle: We can choose healthy or unhealthy responses to desire, fear, anger, and sadness.

Perennial Wisdom Quote: "Surround yourself with people who provide positive bonding." -- Daniel G. Amen, M.D., *Change Your Brain, Change Your Life*

Discussion: A wide range of emotions are normal, necessary and healthy. However, many people tend to get stuck in certain primary emotions, distort their thinking due to this emotional "stuckness," imbalance their brains due to this "stuckness" and make poor behavioral choices. Emotions ideally flow through us quite rapidly, stimulating the lower parts of our brains, and activating the higher parts of our brains which then engage in observing the emotions and making evaluations as to how best to respond to them. This makes for wise behavioral choices. Some brains are not able to function in these optimal ways. (See Appendix 1.) Therefore, they cause people to form mistaken judgments and make unwise choices, such as surrounding themselves with emotionally unhealthy people.

Modern science has learned much about how to rebalance these brain dysfunctions and guide wiser behavioral choices. If a person feels chronically stuck in desire, fear, anxiety, sadness, depression, and/or anger, there are many avenues out of this "stuckness." Reaching out for informed, professional help is the first step. Committed self-help is the second step. (See Appendix 2.)

Self-exploratory Question: How can I best choose healthy responses to my emotions?

Affirmation: I am able to observe my feelings and choose healthy responses to them.

Principle: Violence both produces and is the result of dysfunctional brain activity.

Perennial Wisdom Quote: "Violence is a complex human behavior. There has long been a passionate debate over whether violent behavior is the result of psychological, social, or biological factors.... The brain of the violent patient is clearly different from that of the nonviolent person." -- Daniel G. Amen, M.D., *Change Your Brain, Change Your Life*

Discussion: Aggressive people tend to misinterpret situations and react in impulsive ways. Their cognitive distortions and neurological deficiencies in impulse control can be corrected with a high enough level of motivation and with proper medical and psychological assistance. Aggressive people tend to have problems in the cingulate, basal ganglia, amygdala, and cortex parts of their brains. (See Appendix 1.) These problems result in aggressive ideation and behavior, and also are reinforced by continuing aggressive behavior. What is vital is that the negative cycle of damaged brain functioning and aggressive behavior stops and a recovery cycle begins.

If you suffer from aggressive thoughts and/or behaviors, and many of the principles and behaviors suggested in this book seem impossible or ridiculous to you, it would be helpful for you to seek professional assistance. This book is designed for self-help by motivated individuals who can relate well to the perennial wisdom and modern brain research which it compiles. If self-help doesn't work well for you, some professional assistance is needed first, possibly including an EEG or a SPECT brain evaluation.

Self-exploratory Question: How can I reduce and manage my aggressive thoughts, words and actions?

Affirmation: Today I choose not to use violence in any form, including verbal, to solve my problems.

Principle: Remembering and understanding our night dreams can help us find happiness.

Perennial Wisdom Quote: "Pay heed to the voices in your dreams." -- Cheyenne proverb

Discussion: Sleep is necessary to maintain healthy functioning of the brain. While we sleep, our dreams also give us insight into our unconscious conflicts and needed corrective measures. (See January 5th reading and Appendix 5.)

Many people, however, have difficulty recalling their night dreams. Here are some suggested dream recall aids: keep a notebook and pen at the side of your bed with a low light; make sure the privacy of your dream notebook is protected; and upon wakening, write down the first thing you can remember about your dream, even if it's just one image or word. Don't get out of bed or turn on bright lights prior to writing down your dream. Prod your curiosity about your dreams by talking to yourself about them just before you go to sleep. When you dream about a familiar person, ask yourself both what the dream tells you about your relationship with that person and what the dream tells you about your relationship with an aspect of yourself, represented by that person. Set your alarm on work days so that you have plenty of time to write down your dream and still get to work on time. Share some of your night dreams with supportive family members who will just listen and share theirs.

Self-exploratory Question: How can I recall my dreams more readily?

Affirmation: I recall my dreams, write them down and understand myself better because of them.

Principle: Happiness is our natural state when we do not allow ourselves to dwell too long in desire, fear, anger, or sadness.

Perennial Wisdom Quote: "…emotional disturbance can be defined in the simplest possible terms -- as a general tendency to lapse too readily, or delve too deeply, or to linger too long, in emotional states of desire, fear, anger, or sadness." --Hunter Lewis, *The Beguiling Serpent, A Re-evaluation of Emotions and Values*

Discussion: Hunter Lewis hypothesizes that there are only five primary emotions: desire, fear, anger, sadness and happiness. He calls happiness the "fifth emotion" and describes it as the natural human state of emotional equilibrium when we choose not to dwell too long in the other four primary emotions: desire (grabbing, demanding, bossing), fear (flight, nervousness, avoidance), anger (fighting, attacking, blaming), and sadness (giving up, passivity, dependence).

He describes happiness as a calm, "live and let live" state of satisfying connectedness to one's self and others. He discusses how emotions give rise to value judgments and behavioral choices, how desire can lead to aggressive demands, how fear can lead to avoidance, how anger can lead to verbal or physical attacks, how sadness can lead to doing nothing, and how happiness leads to inviting others into mutually gratifying contact. The first four primary emotions are natural, and yet when we cling to them, we can get ourselves into trouble. When we allow them to flow through ourselves without clinging, we can make good behavioral choices and return to our natural equilibrium, moving back into happiness.

Self-exploratory Question: How can I calmly "live and let live" more frequently?

Affirmation: My natural state is an attitude of calm acceptance and happy connection.

Principle: Integrated brain functioning leads to happier experiences.

Perennial Wisdom Quote: "Not all individuals are able to find emotional well-being in integrating multiple self-states into a coherent experience of the self." -- Daniel J. Siegel, M.D., *The Developing Mind*

Discussion: Daniel J. Siegel, M.D., and Daniel G. Amen, M.D., perhaps more than any other researchers and authors in the 21st century, have helped average, non-medical readers to understand the functioning of the human brain. (See Appendix 1.) Dr. Siegel, in *The Developing Mind,* discusses how optimal brain functioning involves a balanced amount of activity in all the centers of the brain, how over-activity in the limbic brain system, and under-activity in the cortex can lead to getting stuck in such emotions as desire, fear, anger and sadness.

Imbalance in brain functioning can be due to hereditary factors, past traumas, and drug abuse, among other things. What is most important, and what deserves the most attention, is diagnosing the state of one's own brain functioning and learning what must be done to make this functioning optimal. Dr. Amen points out that there are many solutions involving behavioral changes, cognitive changes, nutritional changes, medications, and social changes.

There are both ancient and modern solutions to unintegrated brain functioning. First one must diagnose the problem, then one must select the best treatments, and then actively pursue them.

Self-exploratory Question: How can I know if my brain is functioning in an optimal, integrated fashion?

Affirmation: I commit to doing everything I can to help my brain function optimally.

Principle: Our moods are our own personal responsibilities.

Perennial Wisdom Quote: "Most powerful is he who has himself in his own power."
– Seneca

Discussion: Robert E. Thayer, Ph.D., in *The Origin of Everyday Moods* lists these mood management strategies, from the most to the least effective: 1) active strategies such as relaxation, exercise, meditation, prayer, yoga, positive affirmations, spiritual readings; 2) distraction and pleasure-seeking strategies such as sports, dancing, creative outlets, hobbies, humor; 3) withdrawal-avoidance strategies such as being alone, avoiding persons or things appearing to cause bad moods; 4) ventilation and social support strategies such as talking to a friend or attending social activities; 5) passive strategies such as watching TV, drinking coffee, eating alone, resting; and 6) direct tension-reduction strategies such as taking drugs, drinking alcohol, and having sex.

Dr. Thayer points out that five to ten minutes of walking can enhance mood levels for an hour or more. Sugar snacking causes more tension than it reduces. Caffeine also makes people tense and jittery. Alcohol with the first drink elevates mood, but with more, it is a depressant and reduces energy. Adequate sleep is necessary for good moods, so are a sufficient amount of active mood management strategies. It's vital to become a good self-observer of one's moods and mood-regulating behaviors.

Self-exploratory Question: How can I improve my mood management strategies?

Affirmation: I use active mood management strategies such as relaxation, exercise, meditation, prayer, yoga, positive affirmations and spiritual readings.

Principle: Becoming adept at observing one's cognitive and emotional choices can greatly enhance one's moods.

Perennial Wisdom Quote: "A tree falls the way it leans." -- Walloon saying

Discussion: Modern culture generally attempts to teach young people to be responsible for their behaviors. It tends, however, to overlook teaching young people to be responsible for their own thoughts, feelings and moods. Although modern research now understands a great deal about how to manage moods and improve brain chemistry and activity, little of this information is a standard part of junior high and high school curricula. Hopefully this will change rapidly.

Hanging on to blaming thoughts tends to promote angry moods. Angry moods are harmful to the heart and the brain, just to mention two vital parts of the body. They also are harmful to relationships. Hanging on to desirous thoughts tends to promote attaching and grasping, which tend to harm relationships and promote dissatisfaction. Hanging on to sad thoughts tends to promote depression. Depressive moods are also harmful to the brain. Hanging on to shaming thoughts tends to promote both anger and depression. Hanging on to fearful thoughts tends to promote anxiety and avoidance.

Hanging on to accepting and loving thoughts tends to promote happiness. We get to choose what thoughts we hang on to and what moods we create. If we cannot control our thoughts and moods, professional therapy, behavioral changes and medication can all help to give us control.

Self-exploratory Question: How can I become more aware of my mental and emotional choices and choose more wisely?

Affirmation: Today I choose to hang on to accepting and loving thoughts and moods.

September 24   **"The Golden Rule" and Mood**
Management

Principle: Practicing the "Golden Rule" helps with mood management.

Perennial Wisdom Quote: "The essence of all growth is a willingness to change for the better and then an unremitting willingness to shoulder whatever responsibility this entails." -- Bill Wilson, *As Bill Sees It*

Discussion: Practicing the Golden Rule (See April 28 reading.) is very beneficial for mood management. Consistently practicing the Golden Rule is not easy; therefore, being consistently responsible for one's own lapses in this practice and learning how to make amends for them is vital to mood management. When we have violated our own ethics and when we have caused harm to others, guilt and shame often follow. This is because it is easy to avoid responsibility for our mistakes and very difficult to experience healthy remorse and make productive amends.

Careful, consistent ethical behavioral practice is, therefore, a vital part of mood management. None of us is behaviorally perfect, but all of us are capable of learning healthier, better thoughts, moods and behaviors and unremittingly taking responsibility for bettering ourselves. Practicing active, "direct" mood management strategies versus passive, "indirect" ones is also essential. (See September 22 reading.)

Self-exploratory Question: How can I improve my practice of the Golden Rule and thereby improve my moods?

Affirmation: Practicing the Golden Rule is one of my vital mood management strategies.

Principle: Healthy moods involve attention to Rights, Respect, and Responsibilities.

Perennial Wisdom Quote: "I long to accomplish a great and noble task, but it is my chief duty to accomplish small tasks as if they were great and noble." -- Helen Keller

Discussion: Helen Keller became blind and deaf at 18 months old, and yet she became a famous inspirational speaker, writer and teacher. She learned how to respect her disabilities and herself by overcoming her disabilities. She learned how to be responsible for her limitations and thereby surpass them. She learned her rights and those of her fellow American citizens, and she advocated for them. She learned how to behave respectfully even to those who were ignorant and disrespectful. She saw each of her tasks as small and accomplished them one at a time, dutifully, thereby becoming great and someone to be quoted and remembered.

There have been many other such great individuals, some remembered and some not. It is more important to daily observe our thoughts, feelings, moods and actions and keep them healthy and respectful to ourselves and others, than it is to be great and remembered. One day at a time, maintaining respectful behavior towards ourselves and others is much more important than material wealth or social and political power.

When our last days come and we look back on our lives, it is unlikely that we will consider how much money or social and political power we once had. Instead, we will want to be thought of by our loved ones as loving, kind, and respectful. We will want them near us as we say goodbye to the world, and we will want them to remember us with open hearts. Only love lasts beyond the grave.

Self-exploratory Question: How can I best maintain respectful behavior at all times?

Affirmation: Maintaining respectful behavior is more important to me than wealth and power.

September 26 **Freedom from Common "Thinking Errors"**

Principle: A common "thinking error" is to believe that others cause our feelings.

Perennial Wisdom Quote: "As long as your happiness is caused or sustained by something or someone outside of you, you are still in the land of the dead. The day you are happy for no reason whatsoever, the day you find yourself taking delight in everything and in nothing, you will know that you have found the land of unending joy called the Kingdom." -- Anthony de Mello, *The Way To Love*

Discussion: Feelings are caused in our own bodies, not in the bodies of others. Others don't "make us" happy or sad. We choose to respond to others with happiness or sadness. There are many different ways to respond to any given external situation. We always have the choice as to how to respond.

We cannot determine what other people say and do, but we can decide how to respond to these actions. For example, if someone says something mean to me, I can choose to see it as a personal slight, reflecting some false judgment of me, and then get angry and resentful. Or I can choose to see the mean individual as uninformed and ignorant and not worthy of my getting upset, allowing me to just ignore him or her. The choice is mine. Nobody "makes me" angry, sad, or happy. I am in charge of my own feelings.

Self-exploratory Question: Am I able to take responsibility for ALL my feelings?

Affirmation: Today I choose to take responsibility for ALL my feelings.

September 27   **Freedom from More Common "Thinking Errors"**

Principle: A common "thinking error" is that anger makes a person more powerful.

Perennial Wisdom Quote: "But in fact, anger and resentment usually mask feelings of fear, helplessness, disappointment, or insecurity. Most often, anger and resentment are used as substitutes for feelings of genuine personal power." -- Robin Casarjian, *Houses of Healing, A Prisoner's Guide to Inner Power and Freedom*

Discussion: Anger is energizing but, when it is not tempered by calm thought, it is actually dis-empowering. Anger is the fiery emotion which wells up inside of us when we feel wronged. It is helpful in that it identifies the wrong, but when anger's energy is not followed by observations of one's own part in a situation, and thoughts about how most effectively and harmlessly to correct the situation, it becomes destructive and usually adds to the problematic situation.

Learning to observe one's anger before making a decision about action is vital. In the reading for July 5, we discussed how personal power is the power to influence others through example and through wisdom. Personal power is not based on one's ability to force an outcome. This is because forced outcomes only last as long as one maintains an ability to dominate and control others. This ability is usually exhausting and short-lived, at least in democratic societies. We need to learn how to channel the energy of our anger into wise words and wise behaviors. This takes a lot of self-observation, as well as observations of others who have learned to do this. (The readings for January 18, June 8 and June10 describe essential anger management skills.)

Self-exploratory Question: How can I observe and use my anger more effectively?

Affirmation: I am making choices which enhance my genuine personal power.

Principle: When we allow others to rob us of our inner peace, we are giving away power.

Perennial Wisdom Quote: "You hold the power for your inner state -- unless you give it away. You give a situation the meaning it has for you." -- Robin Casarjian, *Houses of Healing*

Discussion: Robin Casarjian gives the example of a prisoner who hands over to a correctional officer the power to determine how she feels. She feels insulted by the officer and robbed of her inner peace. By dwelling on her resentments towards the officer, she gives her power away. By seeing the officer simply as an abuser, rather than as a person who is out of contact with her higher Self and lost in her own ignorance, the prisoner cannot emotionally separate herself from the officer and stays emotionally enmeshed with someone whom she doesn't like or respect. The resentments keep the prisoner also out of contact with her higher Self.

Such vicious cycles can go on and on, creating very destructive enmity. History is full of stories of leaders of nations who have gotten caught up in such crazy enmeshed dynamics and led armies into the loss of thousands of lives. The way out of such fruitless behavior is to recognize that we don't have to angrily react to people who insult us or abuse us. We can protect ourselves by walking away and internally acknowledging the ignorance of the other, by reporting the physical or verbal abuse to higher authorities, and emotionally letting go of the put-downs. If we know the accusations are false, there is no need to harbor resentment. If any small part of the accusations is true, we can focus on ways to remedy that wrong. In any case, the emotionally healthy path is to move on and not focus on past slights.

Self-exploratory Question: How do I give my power away to others?

Affirmation: My inner peace is my responsibility, no matter what is happening outside.

Principle: It is a "thinking error" to see all guilt as unhealthy.

Perennial Wisdom Quote: "Healthy guilt is a feeling that arises when we believe we have done something wrong or immoral. It is a matter of responding to our own highest sense of integrity. It relates to behaviors or thoughts that we don't condone, that don't reflect our deepest sense of what is respectful, honest, and just…. Healthy guilt guides our conscience." -- Robin Casarjian, *Houses of Healing, A Prisoner's Guide to Inner Power and Freedom*

Discussion: Unfortunately, in the United States when a person wants to have a fair trial to review his or her inappropriate behavior, he or she has to plead "not guilty." Defense lawyers therefore coach their clients to plead this way, even when they are admitting their guilt to their attorney. This adds to a common perception that guilt means "getting caught," not just committing the crime.

Teachers and counselors in prisons try to teach prisoners how to experience "healthy guilt," but the legal system itself tends to reinforce "beating the rap" rather than being up-front, and with remorse, admitting guilt. But individuals can resist the dysfunctional elements of this system and learn to understand that, if they are to live satisfying lives out of prison, they will first have to develop healthy guilt and strong consciences which guide them away from behavior which is harmful to themselves or others.

Self-exploratory Question: How do I determine the difference between healthy and unhealthy guilt?

Affirmation: Healthy guilt guides my conscience and keeps me from doing wrong.

Principle: Compassion for people who ignorantly make mistakes can replace revenge.

Perennial Wisdom Quote: "Remember, what we are forgiving is not the act --- not the violence, or neglect, or insensitivity -- we are forgiving the people. We are forgiving their ignorance, their suffering, their confusion." -- Robin Casarjian

Discussion: Forgiveness is the path to freedom from revengeful acts and spiraling cycles of violence. As Robin Casarjian says so well in her book, *Houses of Healing,* when we forgive, we are forgiving another's ignorance, suffering and confusion, not another's acts. Violent acts are not to be forgiven. Violent people can be forgiven, especially when they learn to see their own ignorance and change their ways.

The Christian Bible has an excellent story of a violent person who turns his life around. It is the story of Paul, a man who violently persecuted early Christians and then saw his ignorance and became a strong Christian teacher himself. Paul actually wrote many of the books in the New Testament. Much of his theology is now a core part of the Christian religion. And all this came from a man who was violent and angry as a young man.

People can change. If Christians had not forgiven Paul for his earlier behaviors, if they had taken revenge on him because he had been violent towards them, the Christian community would have likely withered and died rather than becoming one of the largest religious communities in the world.

Self-exploratory Question: When I am wronged, how can I forgive the wrong-doer but not the wrongful act?

Affirmation: When I am wronged, I let go of thoughts of revenge.

Principle: Careful conflict-resolution processing improves loving relationships.

Perennial Wisdom Quote: "Loving someone and pleasing someone are two different things." -- Jerry Jampolski, Ph.D.

Discussion: Frequently people make the mistake of thinking that avoiding conflict is the best way to maintain intimate relationships. Actually, a certain amount of conflict and disagreement is natural in any relationship and, when handled appropriately, increases intimacy and affection. Sometimes people become conflict avoidant because of chronic anxiety related to overactive limbic brain systems. (See Appendix 1.) If this is a problem, the person needs to secure appropriate medication and cognitive/behavioral psychotherapy.

If a person is in a relationship with a conflict-avoidant person, it is helpful to attempt to diminish the avoidant person's anxiety before attempting problem- solving. Some measures to do this are as follows: select a regular weekly time when both parties are rested and well-fed; and then sit down and routinely discuss ways to improve the relationship. Families can create weekly "Family Meetings", and adult couples can create weekly "Couple Conferences." Everyone can agree on starting these sessions with words of appreciation for each other, followed by a democratic "agenda setting" process to assure that everyone's issues get addressed.

Everyone can also agree on specific problem-solving steps which will be followed at these meetings. (See Oct. 3 – 5 readings.) Everyone can also agree that if a serious impasse is reached in attempting to solve an important problem, a neutral mediator will be chosen to be "chairperson" at the next problem-solving meeting.

Self-exploratory Question: How can I help my family and workplace to effectively address problems?

Affirmation: I set aside time and energy for problem-solving with others.

Principle: Calm, cooperative attention is needed to solve interpersonal conflicts.

Perennial Wisdom Quote: "HALT when you are Hungry, Angry, Lonely, or Tired." Don't try to problem solve under these conditions. -- Anonymous

Discussion: Healthy people neither avoid nor seek conflict. They deal with conflict in effective ways when it occurs, but do not go out of their way to create it. People with overactive limbic brain systems and underactive prefrontal cortex systems, however, have a tendency to unconsciously seek out conflict. This is because their prefrontal cortexes are craving stimulation. Their brains crave the adrenaline which increases with conflict. This problem can be corrected with medication and appropriate behavioral instruction, but until the corrections are made, people around them need to respond thoughtfully.

Here are some of the most effective responses to others' conflict-seeking behaviors: avoid yelling, lower your own voice as the other's voice rises, take Adult Time Out when needed (possibly just say you need to use the restroom), use humor (not sarcasm or angry humor), be a good listener, and explain that you want to understand and address the problem, but you need to be able to talk about it calmly first.

Self-exploratory Question: How can I personally deal better with conflict-seeking behavior?

Affirmation: I choose neither to seek, nor to avoid conflict; rather I choose to calmly deal with it.

October 3   **Wise Ways Happiness Step Ten: Continual**
Honesty

Principle: The Wise Ways Happiness Step Ten reads, "We continue honest daily self-examination, and when mistakes are found, we promptly admit them."

Perennial Wisdom Quote: "Dishonesty is a forsaking of permanent for temporary advantages." -- Christian Bovee

Discussion: In learning to take honest self-inventories, it is often helpful to have a support group. Otherwise, it is too easy for some to avoid looking at weaknesses and too easy for some to overlook strengths. If we are fortunate, we have loving family and friends who know how to give us honest feedback; but many people are not this fortunate. Many family members and friends fear reprisals or abandonment if they give honest feedback, so they are avoidant. This is why the Wise Ways Happiness Program encourages members to form or join Happiness Support Groups in which honest self-inventories can be taken and healthy support for positive self-improvement is reliable.

Promptly admitting a mistake in a safe setting from which there will be no reprisals is an important goal. If one cannot find a safe group in which to do this, seeking a professional relationship with a therapist, minister, priest, rabbi or other person who has confidentiality privilege under the law is very helpful. When we hide from ourselves and others under cloaks of lies and informational distortions, we end up further hurting ourselves and blocking our self-improvement. When we disavow our strengths and leadership capacities, we cheat ourselves and others. The continual practice of Happiness Step Ten is an important part of the Wise Ways Happiness Program. (See Appendix 4 for more discussion of all 12 Happiness Steps.)

Self-exploratory Question: How can I continually be honest with myself and others?

Affirmation: I am committed to honesty and the prompt admission of my mistakes.

October 4   Wise Ways Support Groups' Tradition Ten: No Other Group Affiliations

Principle: The Wise Ways Happiness Support Group Tradition Ten reads, "Wise Ways Happiness Support Groups have no other affiliation and neither endorse, finance, nor lend their name to any other enterprise, lest problems of money or prestige divert them from their primary purpose. Professionally facilitated Wise Ways Happiness Counseling groups have permission to use the Wise Ways Happiness name as long as they are using this book for their meetings."

Perennial Wisdom Quote: "Love of money is the mother of all evils." -- Diogenes

Discussion: Money, prestige and a desire for personal power can get in the way of a group's original service goals. Alcoholics Anonymous broke away from the Oxford Group, which started out as a very healthy spiritual study network but eventually died as it became too political. Politics, even in democracies, are very influenced by money, property and prestige. It is therefore vital for Wise Ways Happiness groups to always follow Tradition Ten.

The Wise Ways Happiness Support Groups must never endorse other organizations in any direct way or allow themselves to be limited by an endorsement by another organization. Wise Ways Happiness Support Groups need to remain independent and follow the 12 Traditions in order to maintain healthy group process and leadership. Wise Ways Happiness Counseling Groups need to be as low-cost as possible.

Self-exploratory Question: How can I help my Wise Ways Happiness Support Group to keep the Tenth Tradition?

Affirmation: I respect the primary self-help purpose of my Wise Ways Happiness Support Group and do my best not to allow it to become side-tracked into other endeavors.

October 5   **Healthy**
Nutrition

Principle: Healthy nutrition is essential for a healthy brain and a sense of well-being.

Perennial Wisdom Quote: "Low levels of dopamine, serotonin, and norepinephrine have all been implicated in depression and mood disorders. It is essential to eat enough protein in balanced amounts with fats and carbohydrates." -- Daniel G. Amen, M.D., *Change Your Brain, Change Your Life*

Discussion: Lean fish and meat, cheese, beans, and nuts are all rich sources of protein. Whole grain crackers, bread and cereals give essential complex carbohydrates. L-tryptophan is an essential amino acid found in milk, meat and eggs and is necessary for good sleep and healthy moods. Avoiding simple carbohydrates such as white bread, white pasta, cake and candy is also important. Simple sugars in large amounts can promote depression and should be avoided, especially for persons with concentration problems. Eating a healthy breakfast and lunch, rather than having most food intake in the evening is also helpful. Taking herbal and vitamin supplements, with the advice of a doctor or nutritionist is also advisable. Dr. Amen recommends l-tryptophan, tyrosine, dl-phenylalanine, and B vitamins for correcting moodiness and irritability due to imbalances in the limbic brain system. Be sure to consult with a professional to determine proper doses.

Self-exploratory Question: How can I improve my food and supplement intake?

Affirmation: I eat healthy foods, in healthy amounts, at healthy times, and include important supplements.

October 6
Companionship

Healthy Dating and

Principle: Teenagers need to develop social skills with groups of peers of both genders before they begin seriously dating just one person.

Perennial Wisdom Quote: "If you want to marry wisely, marry your equal." -- Spanish saying

Discussion: Many cultures perform "coming into adulthood" rituals before their teenagers are allowed to look for mates. Usually teenagers are encouraged to socialize, talk, dance, sing, play sports, etc., in group settings with adults present for some time before they are allowed to complete the adulthood transition rituals. In some cultures, "vision quests" and other tests of self-sufficiency are also expected and supervised by adults before teenagers are allowed adulthood status. Unfortunately, many "developed" countries no longer have these rituals and many teenagers and parents have little adult community support for handling these difficult transitions.

A good general guideline for parents to follow is that a teenager needs to have learned how to deal with casual acquaintanceship contact and casual companionship contact with a potential romantic interests, before being allowed to date independently. The chronological age when a teen is ready for this will vary with individual teens.

Adults who are newly single after a divorce also need to give themselves plenty of time and opportunity to socialize in casual acquaintanceship and companionship settings before developing a primary friendship with a potential romantic interest. Otherwise sexual feelings can become overwhelming before emotional, social and intellectual compatibility can be determined.

Self-exploratory Question: After becoming a single adult, how can I appropriately and gradually form a companionable friendship with someone prior to becoming romantic?

Affirmation: I am careful to form relationships slowly, especially with a potential mate.

Principle: Building a healthy friendship is much more difficult than just having sex.

Perennial Wisdom Quote: "Love is never lost. If not reciprocated, it will flow back and soften and purify the heart." -- Washington Irving

Discussion: Companionship involving shared interests and activities usually comes before friendship. Healthy individuals usually have a number of companionship relationships. When the personal contact with a companion becomes even more important than a shared activity, then friendship grows. At this stage of relationship people learn to accept each other's weaknesses, and they help each other out when the other is in trouble. They learn that they can disagree about something, and even become angry with one another over an issue, but the friendship is strong enough to lead to forgiveness and acceptance. Because of the trust and compassion which grows, shared activities become even more enjoyable. As friends, histories and personal realities are honestly shared.

   Friends learn about each other's emotional commitments and involvements with other people. They respect these involvements. They don't initiate a sexual relationship unless both parties are independent adults and free of other sexual commitments. They respect marriage vows. They can love each other as friends, even though sexual attraction might not be reciprocal. They can let go of friendship, with love, if it just becomes too painful, due to unreciprocated feelings. Friendship is the foundation of healthy sex. Sex before friendship is dangerous.

Self-exploratory Question: When dating, do I know how to form honest friendships, postponing sexuality?

Affirmation: I choose not to be sexual when it could endanger my emotional health.

Principle: Friendships need to establish trust, respect and independence before sex.

Perennial Wisdom Quote: "True love comes quietly, without banners or flashing lights. If you hear bells, get your ears checked." -- Erich Segal

Discussion: Many cultures and religions advise young people to wait until after marriage before being sexual. This is good advice, but with the advent of birth control, it is often not followed. Often the best a modern young person can do is to wait to be sexual until he or she is 1) living independently from family, 2) capable of financial self-support, 3) capable of socializing happily with peers of both sexes, 4) confident of healthy friendship and companionship with supportive others, and 5) sexually attracted to an emotionally available, healthy friend -- one who is not romantically or sexually involved with anyone else.

For some modern couples even all these criteria seem very hard to meet. But when sexuality is initiated with a partner who does not meet these criteria, or when you yourself do not meet these criteria, usually trouble and heartbreak are the result. The biology and chemistry of sexuality promote emotional attachment. It's risky to become sexual with someone whom you don't consider an equal and whom you do not yet know as a friend. Our bodies and emotions are precious parts of ourselves and need to be protected. Waiting for the right time to be sexual, be it after marriage or after a trustworthy friendship has been established, is well worth the wait.

Self-exploratory Question: How can I determine whether I am ready for sex?

Affirmation: I choose only to be sexual when I know I can trust my partner to be an honest, adult, independent, true friend.

Principle: A love commitment takes time and needs to be respected.

Perennial Wisdom Quote: "Effort matters in everything, love included. Learning to love is purposeful work." -- Michael Levine

Discussion: Goethe years ago wrote about how "the moment one definitely commits oneself, providence moves, too. A whole stream of events issues from the decision, raising in one's favor all manner of unforeseen incidents and meetings and material assistance, which no [one] could have dreamt would come…. Boldness has genius, power, and magic in it."

M. Scott Peck, M.D., more recently became famous for his belief that "love is primarily a matter of decision and action," different from liking or affection, which is "primarily a feeling." Making a commitment to get married, setting a date usually at least three months away, and informing one's friends and family about the decision begins an intimacy-building process which can be turbulent. This turbulence, however, and how one handles the turbulence, is a good practice zone for marriage. If the couple can't manage the turbulence, then likely the marriage wouldn't work out well.

Marital engagements in some cultures have become almost old fashioned. This is sad because they served many purposes: 1) giving the couple time to explore "couplehood" before a legal commitment; 2) giving two families time to get used to joining together as in-laws; 3) giving friends time to make the emotional adjustments; and 4) giving everyone time to plan a meaningful marriage ceremony.

Self-exploratory Question: How can I be sure of compatibility before marriage?

Affirmation: If I make a marriage commitment, I will do it seriously and slow.

October 10   **Seeing the Difference Between Love and Attachment**

Principle: Love often involves some attachment, but attachment does not always involve love.

Perennial Wisdom Quote: "Love is the force that focuses its light on the deepest shadowy parts of ourselves. It brings to the surface the parts of ourselves that we most desperately try to keep hidden." -- Gay and Kathlyn Hendricks, Ph.D., *Conscious Loving*

Discussion: Human babies are born with the ability and even necessity of emotional attachment. But when our childhood attachment needs are not met well by our adult care givers, people sometimes carry their needs for childlike attachment into adulthood. Childlike attachment involves a child placing his or her dependency needs on an adult.

When, as an adult, we place our unmet childhood dependency needs on another adult, we usually establish an attachment, which may be temporarily functional in some ways but which blocks our maturity as individuals. This attachment can include a fear of abandonment on one person's part and a fear of emotional engulfment on another person's part. Such a combination can become problematic.

To form a stable, loving, committed relationship, both persons must take individual responsibility for working through any of their own childhood abandonment or engulfment issues. They need to be able to maturely face the unwanted discoveries about themselves and each other which will be revealed in their intimate relationship. Unless this happens, marriage can become more of a battle than a loving relationship.

Young couples often have some issues from childhood which need to be worked out cooperatively and sometimes with the help of professional therapists. When they commit to doing this, a stable, loving marriage can develop. When there is no commitment to this, divorce is likely.

Self-exploratory Question: How would I define the difference between attachment and adult love?

Affirmation: I am gradually maturing in my capacity for adult, committed love.

Principle: Engagement to marriage is a time in which friendship is strengthened, collaborative planning grows, and two "in-law" families get to know each other.

Perennial Wisdom Quote: "To dare to make and care to keep commitments, this is love." -- Lewis B. Smedes

Discussion: Terry Gorsky, Ph.D., an American psychologist who has written a great deal about freedom from addictive relationships, talks about marriage as actually being "stage five" in the development of a healthy, lasting, intimate relationship. He describes the first four stages as: "casual/superficial acquaintanceship," "companionship," "friendship," and "romantic love/sexy friendship." (See Oct. 6-9 readings.) He stresses that many modern, addictive individuals can rush into sexual relationships and then find themselves emotionally attached, but not well suited for each other. This can lead to "stalking" and "domestic violence."

Individuals who have grown up in dysfunctional families and witnessed their parents being emotionally attached but not loving with one another, are particularly vulnerable to forming these kinds of relationships themselves as adults. The remedy is building relationships slowly and carefully, being sure that adequate time is taken in the acquaintanceship, companionship and friendship stages before sexuality and committed co-residence or marriage.

It is best to postpone sexuality until after marriage, or at least until after friendship and engagement.

Self-exploratory Question: How can I commit to friendship before marriage?

Affirmation: Should I commit to a marriage, I am first committing to a solid friendship.

October 12   **Recognizing Romance: Stage One of Intimate Relationships**

Principle: Stage One of an intimate relationship focuses on pleasurable commonalities.

Perennial Wisdom Quote: "In real love you want the other person's good. In romantic love you want the other person." -- Margaret Anderson

Discussion: Susan Campbell, Ph.D., who wrote *Couple Journey*, was one of the first American psychologists to address the issue of "stages" in the development of intimate relationships. Many other writers, since Dr. Campbell's pioneering book, have addressed this issue. Different authors label the stages somewhat differently, but most of them usually define three to five "stages."

Dr. Campbell calls the first stage the "Romance Stage." In this stage we sense our possibilities as a couple, and we create a shared vision. This is an exciting, hormone-surging stage in which individuals focus on commonalities and the pleasure of shared experiences and learning about each other's histories. In this stage, differences are usually overlooked and not considered important. The main danger in this stage of relationship is idealization of each other and of the possibilities of a couple relationship.

When there is fear that conflict will destroy the couple vision, the foundation of the relationship becomes weak. One or both persons over-compromise themselves and minimize their individual needs, sacrificing their individuality at the altar of the relationship. This leads to trouble later in the relationship.

When the couple faces conflict honestly and begins to see and appreciate individual differences, then a healthy foundation for a Stage Two relationship is built.

Self-exploratory Question: How can I experience romance, even when differences of opinion exist?

Affirmation: I am open to romance and also to the processing of differences of opinion.

October 13   Working Through Power Struggles: Stage 2 of Intimate Relationships

Principle: Stage Two of an intimate relationship involves the exploration of differences.

Perennial Wisdom Quote: "If you would be loved, love and be lovable." – Ben Franklin

Discussion: Stage Two of an intimate relationship is inevitable and can start developing within the first few weeks or the first two years. In this stage the differences between two people begin to surface along with areas of disagreement. In an egalitarian relationship which facilitates emotional intimacy, there is usually some struggle in working out power and security needs. Neither party wants to be dominated, or to give up the relationship.

In this stage of relationship, a sense of humor and respect for differences and the basic adult equality of both members of the relationship is vital. Each person needs to genuinely want to understand the other's feelings and needs. The couple must find solutions which meet both parties' needs. If one or both parties have not witnessed successful conflict-resolution between equal, loving adults, sometimes domination and manipulation techniques begin to undermine trust and respect in the relationship. If this happens, professional couple therapy is needed.

Individuals in this stage of relationship need to 1) learn to ask for what they want, 2) learn to overcome the illusion that one can change another to fit personal expectations, and 3) learn to overcome the need to retaliate when one doesn't get what is wanted.

Self-exploratory Question: How can I more securely let go of any need to dominate or manipulate my intimate other?

Affirmation: I respect conflict as part of any intimate relationship, and I welcome respectful and cooperative discussion of differences and possible solutions.

October 14   **Arriving at Stability: Stage 3 of Intimate Relationships**

Principle: Stage Three of intimate relationships involves increased stability.

Perennial Wisdom Quote: "All the paths of the Lord are steadfast love and faithfulness." -- The Bible, *Psalms* 25:10

Discussion: In the third stage of an intimate relationship each person gradually learns to take responsibility for formerly unconscious processes. Individuals clarify and expand their senses of identity through respectful dialogue with each other. Both parties overcome the illusion that differences will disappear in the relationship. Rather they come to appreciate the differences. They grow in awareness of how accepting differences helps each to better understand the other, and how this promotes couple creativity.

Differences are confronted in a way that builds stability in the relationship rather than challenging it. Each person appreciates more and more how learning from the differences is a benefit rather than a loss. Each person grows to see more clearly the benefits of the partnership and does not want to sacrifice the benefits because of some stubborn need to have one's own way.

If the couple has entered professional couple therapy, the couple sessions become less heated, and the strengths of the partnership become more obvious and appreciated. Therapy often needs to continue for a while, however, so that these strengths can become well-established and so that the couple learns how to successfully work through conflict without the help of a therapist.

Self-exploratory Question: How can I help to recreate stability in my intimate relationship after every episode of struggling over differences?

Affirmation: I value my intimate relationship so much that I do not allow differences of opinion to permanently destabilize it.

October 15   Establishing Deep Commitment: Stage 4 of Intimate Relationships

Principle: Stage Four of an intimate relationship is deep commitment.

Perennial Wisdom Quote: "Care is <u>c</u>ommitment, <u>a</u>ltruism, <u>r</u>espect, and <u>e</u>mpathy, given as a gift…" -- Malcolm L. Smith, *Meditations on the Art of Peaceful Intervention*

Discussion: According to Susan Campbell, Ph.D., in Stage Four of an intimate relationship the couple begins to experience themselves as an interdependent, synergistic "we-system." They learn to live with life's insoluble dilemmas and paradoxes. Differences are accepted and managed with less conflict.

The challenge in this stage of relationship is to avoid complacency. Complacency diminishes liveliness and passion in a relationship and in each individual's life. The couple also needs to avoid becoming too insular and isolated in this stage. Each person needs to have some activities and friendships outside of the marriage, friendships which are respected by each partner.

Each partner needs also to find individual purpose and meaning in life, not just couple meaning and purpose. Otherwise, should there be a death or major illness, individuals can become terribly traumatized and not have enough resilience to cope with the loss.

Self-exploratory Question: How can I learn to be more committed in an intimate relationship?

Affirmation: I am learning deeper and deeper commitment in my intimate relationship.

October 16   **Co-Creation: Stage 5 of Intimate Relationships**

Principle: Stage Five in an intimate relationship involves "co-creation."

Perennial Wisdom Quote: "I think true love is never blind,

But rather brings an added light,

An inner vision quick to find,

The beauties hid from common sight."

Phoebe Cary in *True Love*

Discussion: Susan Campbell, Ph.D., describes how in Stage Five of a committed, intimate relationship, a "co-creative" energy exists. The partnership is involved in creating its own experience, and both persons' lives are increasingly enriched. A spiritual dimension to the relationship grows. Each person experiences himself or herself as interdependent with all of life.

It is still important to pay attention to "the care and feeding of the relationship." However, both people also feel empowered to be more creative in the larger world. Balanced attention is given to the relationship itself and to outer creative efforts.

Sometimes struggle is again inevitable, and it seems that Stage Two of the relationship has reappeared. But the couple has experience working out differences, so there is more confidence that the new challenges will not destroy the relationship. Instead both persons willingly enter into the struggle and stay committed to resolving the new issues in a way which does not destroy the partnership's co-creativity.

Self-exploratory Question: How can I enjoy the co-creative energy of my partnership and also be individually committed to working out new power struggle stages?

Affirmation: I am committed to both enjoying the co-creative energy of my partnership and working through any new power struggle issues.

October 17   **Learning about Stage One of Functional Conflict-Resolution**

Principle: Stage One of functional conflict-resolution involves respectful listening and clarification of the problem.

Perennial Wisdom Quote: "Until one is committed, there is hesitancy, the choice to draw back, always ineffectiveness." -- Goethe

Discussion: Disagreement and conflicts of interests are natural in any relationship. It's important not to be surprised by them. Rather, we need to be thankful that differences of opinion can be honestly and safely expressed. The difference between healthy and unhealthy relationships is how they deal with conflict. In healthy relationships individuals are motivated to understand and accept each other.

Stage One of functional conflict- resolution is carefully listening to each person's feelings and points-of-view, not interrupting and not focusing on pressing one's own point of view. Often people just need to be heard, feel valuable and have their feelings and point-of-view accepted. They need to feel respected.

Many people make the mistake of insecurely pushing too quickly to the latter stages of conflict-resolution, i.e. the discussion and selection of a solution to the problem, before checking to make sure that everyone's point-of-view on the problem is adequately heard. Respectful listening needs to come before the brainstorming of solutions.

Sometimes it's helpful to also have a "chairperson" or mediator for a conflict-resolution session, someone who makes sure interruptions are not tolerated and someone who respectfully summarizes each person's feelings and point-of-view, maybe even writing them down where all can see. Practicing being this "chairperson" who remains neutral and focuses on healthy group process can be a very good exercise for all members of a group. Ideally this role is rotated.

Self-exploratory Question: How can I better practice Stage One of conflict-resolution?

Affirmation: I take time to listen to everyone before proposing solutions to conflicts.

October 18   **Practicing Stage 2 of Functional Conflict-Resolution**

Principle: Stage Two of functional conflict resolution involves respectfully brainstorming solutions to the problem.

Perennial Wisdom Quote: "Love is the child of freedom, never that of domination." -- Erich Fromm, *Escapes From Freedom*

Discussion: Only after every party in a dispute has been respectfully heard is it time to begin brainstorming solutions to the problem. During this stage of conflict-resolution, it is important not to push too quickly to evaluating the proposed solutions. First, each person needs to have his or her proposed solution heard and considered on a par with everyone else's solution. In "family meetings" even little children need to have an opportunity to propose solutions and have them considered respectfully. This teaches them to also respect the solutions of others. If the conflict involves more than two people, it is often helpful to write down the proposals where all can see them. This helps each person making a proposal to carefully state it.

Only after all the proposals are given is it time to evaluate the proposals in terms of their pros and cons. This needs to be done impersonally, with no shaming of the person who might have proposed a solution with many cons and few pros to it. Everyone needs to be given time to brainstorm the pros and cons for each proposed solution. This is a time-consuming process, but it teaches trust, respect and good judgment.

Only after Stage Two is completed is it time to move ahead to actually selecting a solution (Stage Three).

Self-exploratory Question: How can I more effectively participate in brainstorming solutions to relationship problems?

Affirmation: I am committed to respectful brainstorming before selecting a solution to a problem.

Principle: Stage Three of functional conflict-resolution involves actually selecting a solution and agreeing on a re-evaluation time.

Perennial Wisdom Quote: "Hatred does not cease through hatred at any time. Hatred ceases through love; this is an unalterable law." -- Buddha

Discussion: Forced solutions are never stable. They always breed hatred. And when hatred is returned with hatred, no stable solutions are possible. Buddha, Jesus Christ, Confucius and many other great teachers stressed this "unalterable" metaphysical law.

When there is disagreement in a conflict, every party in the conflict needs to respect the needs of every other party, even if one of the parties has made mistakes in the past. The solution needs to be democratically, respectfully reached by at least a majority, after the minority views have also been respectfully heard. Inevitably some compromise is needed and must be reached without resentment, but instead with the recognition that the needs of the whole are greater than the needs of any individual. There is power and creativity in the partnership or group and the needs of the whole are more important than the needs of one individual.

This principle is the first Tradition of all the various 12 Step self-help programs, including the Wise Ways Happiness Program. When a decision is reached by a majority of a group or by the consensus of a group of two, it is also helpful to agree on a time for re-evaluating the success of the selected solution. This provides time for later consensus-building or change, if necessary, in the solution.

Self-exploratory Question: How can I more lovingly cooperate in the final, third stage of conflict-resolution discussions?

Affirmation: I value democratic decision making and cooperative re-evaluation of decisions.

Principle: Alcohol abuse damages the brain.

Perennial Wisdom Quote: "There is a devil in every berry of the grape." -- *The Qu'ran*

Discussion: Small doses of alcohol produce brain activation. However, higher doses result in overall decreased brain activity. Alcohol is actually a central nervous system depressant. SPECT brain studies tend to be abnormal for individuals who have alcohol abuse in their families.

Chronic alcohol abuse decreases thiamine, a B vitamin necessary for cognitive functioning, and puts people at risk for Korsakoff's syndrome (an inability to record new memory). Recently it has also been discovered that the brain damage in newborns thought to be caused by cocaine or other drug abuse, is often actually caused by alcohol use. Amazingly, alcohol use by a pregnant woman is now thought to be more dangerous even than cocaine abuse. Even as little as one or two glasses of beer taken by a pregnant woman can cause a negative effect on her developing fetus.

There is also some evidence to suggest that the earlier you start using alcohol, the more damage the alcohol can cause to the brain. Scientific research supports waiting to drink alcohol until age 21 when the brain in more developed and organized and suffers less damage from alcohol. It's best not to drink alcohol at all if you are underage or could get pregnant, or if you can't stop after one or two drinks.

Self-exploratory Question: How can I protect myself from alcohol abuse?

Affirmation: If I am over 21 and not pregnant, I allow myself one or two beers or glasses of wines a day, or I completely abstain from alcohol. I do not abuse alcohol.

Principle: Illegal drug use damages the brain.

Perennial Wisdom Quote: "Put a rope around your neck and many will be happy to drag you along." -- Egyptian saying

Discussion: A twenty-year heroin addiction can cause a brain to act similarly to that of a senior citizen with dementia. Dr. Amen uses the term "brain melt" to describe the brains of opiate abusers. Alcohol (more than a glass or two of beer or wine), marijuana, heroin, cocaine, methamphetamine (doses which are 10-50 times what doctors prescribe for ADD), LSD, PCP and inhalants all can cause brain damage. When the brains of amphetamine and cocaine abusers are studied with SPECT tests, they look like they have had mini-strokes. Symptoms include deficits in concentration, new learning, visual and verbal memory, visual-motor integration and word production. Crack abuse decreases cerebral blood flow. When combined with cigarette dependency, crack smokers have shown 42 percent decrease in brain blood flow. (See Dr. Amen's book *Change Your Brain, Change Your Life.*)

Marijuana is also not a safe drug to use frequently. Long term, regular use of it has been shown to cause seriously reduced activity in the temporal lobes of the brain, causing memory, learning, and motivation problems.

Self-exploratory Question: How can I protect myself from drug abuse?

Affirmation: Today I am abstaining from all illegal drugs.

October 22   **Brain Recovery from Alcohol and Drug Abuse**

Principle: Brains can recover from alcohol and drug abuse, if treated early enough.

Perennial Wisdom Quote: "Falling is easier than rising." -- Irish saying

Discussion: Dr. Amen's book, *Change Your Brain, Change Your Life*, especially his chapter, "The Impact of Drugs and Alcohol on the Brain," should be required reading for all high school students. It would likely change more teenagers' dangerous behavior than current drug education. This book is both sobering and encouraging. Its case studies suggest, not only the devastating damage which alcohol and drug abuse do to brains, but also how miraculously brains can regenerate if the abuse is caught early enough and if the person in recovery uses good nutrition, good exercise, good psychological principles, and (in some cases) the appropriate medically-prescribed medication.

This does not mean that recovery is easy. It is not. Preventing the abuse from starting in the first place is much easier than recovering after abuse has taken place. Dr. Amen's book clearly shows how Vitamin B supplements, a good diet, good exercise, and good cognitive/behavioral education can help most recovering addicts. Reading his book should also be required for all drug rehabilitation staff members and clients. Revolutionary changes in the social, psychological, and legal treatment of addicts will likely eventually result from more brain testing.

Meanwhile, if you are or if a loved one is an addict, it is important to both read about new brain research and do 12 Step, behavioral recovery work. (See Appendix 1 and 4.)

Self-exploratory Question: How can I help my brain to recover from any toxicity?

Affirmation: I am doing everything I can to heal my brain from past abuses.

Principle: Caffeine and nicotine adversely affect brains and need to be avoided.

Perennial Wisdom Quote: "Destruction never comes with weapon in hand. It comes on tiptoe, seeing good in bad and bad in good." -- *The Mahabharata*

Discussion: Published research indicates that caffeine, even in small does, decreases blood flow in the brain, causing under-activity. Caffeine is found in many cold remedies, coffee, tea, many sodas, and chocolate. In the short run caffeine might help a person to become alert or stop a headache, but in the long run it makes things worse. People begin using more caffeine to correct the under-activity caused by previous caffeine withdrawal. Caffeine addiction sets in, indicated by the presence of headaches during withdrawal.

More than two cups of coffee or tea a day is to be avoided. If you can't stop at two cups, then totally abstain. After a few days of headache withdrawal you'll feel better and can start off your day with a high B Vitamin drink such as Emergen-C and be more alert than when you were using coffee.

The damage that nicotine causes to lungs, and whatever part of the body is most exposed to it, is well documented. The research on secondary nicotine inhalation is causing more governments to ban tobacco from public places. Everyone has a right to ask a smoker to step outside of his or her home to smoke. Actually, stepping outside a home to smoke is a courtesy which should be offered without its even being requested.

As with other drugs, the good news about tobacco is that, if the use is stopped early enough, the body has an amazing capacity to heal itself. If the use lasts too long, however, even this capacity is overwhelmed.

Self-exploratory Question: How can I reduce my use of or abstain from caffeine and nicotine?

Affirmation: I deserve to have a nicotine-free body and mind.

Principle: Exposure to SPECT test pictures and Referenced EEG pictures of drug abused brains can help to reduce potential drug abuse in pre-teens and teens.

Perennial Wisdom Quote: "Normal brain is smooth, symmetrical, and full. The heroin brain shows massive areas of decreased activity throughout. The cocaine and meth brain shows multiple small holes across the cerebral cortex. The alcoholic brain looks shriveled. The marijuana brain looks as though areas are eaten away, especially in the temporal lobe region, the seat of language and learning." -- Daniel G. Amen, M.D., *Change Your Brain, Change Your Life*

Discussion: Wouldn't it be wonderful if "Brain Hygiene" were taught in junior high and high school, just like dental and body hygiene is taught? The research is in. It just is taking a while for the educational curriculum systems to catch up. Meanwhile, parents can buy Dr. Amen's books and show the pictures to their middle school and high school children. Pictures of actual brains, accompanied with the information about what likely caused the brain problems, can speak much louder than general cautionary words.

Children can be bringing home up-to-date health information which perhaps their hardworking parents are too busy to gather. Teenagers can start believing the anti-drug messages they hear in school, because they have actually seen pictures of brains which have been damaged by illegal drugs and alcohol.

Self-exploratory Question: How can I use new brain research more effectively?

Affirmation: I am educating myself and my children about new brain research and drugs and exposing them to Wise Ways Happiness principles.

Principle: As adults we can respect our parents and families-of-origin, and we can also detach from their dysfunctional behaviors and surround ourselves with functional others.

Perennial Wisdom Quote: "You can never get even with someone who has harmed you. Any attempt to do so puts you behind the eight ball, again. Two wrongs never make a right…. The pendulum of life swings both ways and brings rewards at both ends of the spectrum. If you use your mind, time and energy to cause harm to anyone, the pendulum will sooner or later move in your direction." -- Iyanda Vanzant, *Acts of Faith*

Discussion: When people act out their pain and suffering onto others, the pain and suffering eventually come back their way. Injustice exists in the world. Accidents and abusive behavior hurt others. But when we engage in punishment to try to correct another's behavior, it usually backfires onto us.

Of course, society needs to do its best to prevent and contain abusive behavior, but the focus needs to be, not only on protecting the innocent, but on healing the abusers. Dysfunctional families engage in punishing behavior, not just for containment and prevention but for revenge and angry catharsis. Dysfunctional families include adults who escape from their thoughts and feelings through blame, shame, and other forms of behavioral self-abuse and abuse towards others.

To free ourselves from dysfunctional behaviors which have existed in our families, we need to take responsibility for not engaging in dysfunctional behaviors ourselves, no matter what modeling we have received. We need to surround ourselves, to the best of our ability, with functional, emotional healthy friends and "families of choice." We need to be sure our own friendship and support to others is healthy and kind. It is never too late to "grow up", and it's never too late to adopt a healthy "family."

Self-exploratory Question: How can I best recover from family dysfunctions?

Affirmation: I am responsible for my own behaviors, not my family's behaviors.

Principle: Maintaining clear awareness if often painful.

Perennial Wisdom Quote: "There is no birth of consciousness without pain." -- Carl Jung

Discussion: Most often we avoid awareness in order to avoid pain. Consciously or unconsciously we don't want to experience clear awareness of something, so we avoid it. Unfortunately, this is like sweeping dirt under a rug -- the pile just gets deeper and easier to trip over.

The belief that avoidance will make things easier is only true in the short run. In the long run avoidance of awareness always makes things harder, and often it is hurtful to others as well. It's OK to choose not to take action in many situations, but when we do so by blocking out clear awareness of what is happening, we don't take good care of ourselves.

It's important to want to KNOW what is, and be willing to experience some pain in the process of knowing. Ignorance is blinding. George G. N. Byron once said, "A man can see further through a tear than a telescope." Wanting to see clearly needs to be more important than avoiding immediate pain. Trusting in one's self to tolerate and learn from pain is vital to strengthening wisdom. Without this trust we hide in shadows and remain fearful children.

Self-exploratory Question: How can I trust myself to learn more, despite related pain?

Affirmation: I am committed to learning and growing, despite painful new awareness.

Principle: The human mind is very prone to projection, especially when afraid.

Perennial Wisdom Quote: "Speak when you are angry and you will make the best speech you will ever regret." -- Ambrose Bierce, *The Devil's Dictionary*

Discussion: "Projection" is a psychological term meaning seeing outside of one's self the feelings and intentions which exist unconsciously inside of one's self. It involves evaluating present situations on the basis of past experiences, without looking clearly and carefully at both what is outside and inside. When this happens, injustice usually is the result.

Anger is an emotion which is easily projected, causing much unnecessary suffering. We can see others as being angry and therefore threatening, when in actuality we are angry ourselves and fearful of threat, possibly without any external threat existing. This kind of projection destroys real safety.

To be free from projection, we must develop careful, calm, realistic ways of observing our environment, our thoughts and our emotions. If we observe that we are angry, we need to be careful before we assume that those outside of us are dangerous. If we observe that we are afraid, we need to be cautious and take care of ourselves, but not necessarily assume that there is an external threat. External threats may or may not exist. We may just have had many attacks and losses in the past and be projecting threat on to the current situation. We may end up unnecessarily rejecting or harming someone.

One good way to determine whether we are projecting or not, is to check out our perceptions with reliable others. This may take time, but often prevents making mistakes. Usually if others perceive a person or a situation very differently from our own perceptions, our own perceptions need to be corrected. It's possible that our perceptions might be more accurate than everyone else's, but not statistically likely. At least taking time to gather more information about a person or situation is usually wise.

Self-exploratory Question: What strategies do I use to check myself for projections?

Affirmation: I do my very best to check out my perceptions, rather than project assumptions.

Principle: It is best to assume a person is innocent unless proven guilty.

Perennial Wisdom Quote: "I will chide no brother in the world but myself, against whom I know most faults." -- Shakespeare

Discussion: When an optimistic person experiences a negative event or feeling, he or she perceives it as something temporary and to be overcome. There is hope and reinforcement for positive change. When a pessimist experiences a negative event or feeling, he or she perceives it as permanent and related to personal traits, behaviors or inadequacies. This is based on research by Dr. Martin Seligman of the University of Pennsylvania.

Pessimists tend to "personalize" things and to hold grudges. Suspicion thrives in pessimistic minds. Once wronged, a pessimist expects always to be wronged. Negative projection thrives in pessimistic minds. It's important to be realistic and protect ourselves from actual danger, but it is also important not to project trouble which isn't there. These kinds of projections can actually create negative consequences which wouldn't have happened without such projection.

To be free from suspicion, it is best to assume a person innocent unless he or she is proven guilty. The justice system in the U.S. is built on this principle. Collecting objective facts about a situation is necessary before assuming negative intention or damaging behavior.

Self-exploratory Question: How can I become less suspicious?

Affirmation: I focus on the proven present and avoid making assumptions.

Principle: Challenging catastrophic thoughts and being around optimistic people tend to overcome pessimism.

Perennial Wisdom Quote: "Defeat makes optimists try harder. Defeat makes pessimists try less." -- Martin Seligman, Ph.D., lecture

Discussion: Pessimism is a risk factor for depression. Optimism is a protective factor against depression. Optimistic sport teams tend to beat the predicted "point spreads." Optimistic students tend to get better grades than their objective test scores would predict. This is likely because of the "try harder" factor. Optimistic people are not easily defeated. They take defeat as a learning experience, not a closed door or a statement of their inadequacies. They redirect their energies after a defeat and don't give up.

We can train ourselves to recognize pessimistic, catastrophic thoughts and then dispute them in our minds, rather than acting on them. A disappointment can be reframed in one's mind as a temporary, local, external setback, rather than a permanent, pervasive, internal defeat. Surrounding ourselves with optimistic people also helps. Attitudes tend to be contagious.

Finding purpose and meaning in one's life which is greater than just personal pleasures also helps. Pursuing activities which promote this purpose and meaning can bring absorption and interpersonal connection, which is much more satisfying than brief, personal pleasures. This satisfaction can promote hope and social connections, which in turn further optimism. (See Dr. Martin Seligman's writings on "Learned Optimism" and visit www.authentichappiness.org.)

Self-exploratory Question: How can I reframe my catastrophic thoughts and surround myself with optimistic people?

Affirmation: I replace my catastrophic thoughts with optimistic ones.

Principle: When we suppress or repress feelings, they remain locked in our "low brains" and tend to separate us from satisfying experiences and emotional intimacy.

Perennial Wisdom Quote: "Shame is the emotion generated when we really need and want to connect to another and the other can't give us emotional attunement." -- Daniel Siegel M.D., lecture

Discussion: Emotional numbness tends to be the result of internalized toxic shame and suppression of feelings. Daniel Siegel, M.D.'s writings on childhood attachment problems (see *Parenting From The Inside Out*) indicate that children who are not met with congruent, consistent, supportive responses from their primary caregivers tend to push painful experiences away, but then also feel defective themselves. They do not yet see the larger picture of their caregivers' past traumas and limitations, so their young minds assume that they are flawed because they are not able to elicit the supportive responses they need.

To avoid becoming suicidal, painful childhood memories and the beliefs they generated tend to be pushed out of awareness. To heal these memories and the damage past traumas have done to our brains, we need, as adults, to find a supportive person or persons, with whom we can review our memories and childhood conclusions. Thereby, we can correct our inadequacy beliefs and release our toxic shame. We need to do this for ourselves, as well as for our children. If we don't do this, our brains will not function optimally and our lack of deep self-understanding will limit our children's ability to thrive.

Self-exploratory Question: How can I release my emotional numbness?

Affirmation: I am receiving support for releasing my emotional numbness.

October 31
Toughness

Freedom from Emotional

Principle: Emotional toughness is one form of emotional numbness.

Perennial Wisdom Quote: "Love they neighbor as thyself, but choose your neighborhood." -- Louise Beal

Discussion: Emotionally "tough" people tend to have grown up in "tough" neighborhoods, by choice and/or by circumstance. When environments are not physically and/or emotionally safe and nurturing, children and adults protect themselves with a layer of "toughness" -- "I don't care" and "I don't know" and "You can't make me" defensive attitudes.

These attitudes might have been necessary at one time for survival, but when we maintain them as adults our lives are stunted and dissatisfying. Human minds are evolutionarily social. We are designed to connect to each other in mutually satisfying ways and work and play together for joy and community benefit. This is how our brains develop optimally. When we don't know how to do these things, it is important to surround ourselves with people who do know how and who will teach us.

We can learn how to choose "safe friends." (See May 2-4 Readings.) We can join healthy spiritual communities. We can form a Wise Ways Happiness Support Group or join another 12 Step group. We can pursue professional therapy. There are many ways to overcome emotional toughness.

Self-exploratory Question: How can I soften my emotional "toughness"?

Affirmation: I welcome my feelings and surround myself with kind, supportive others.

Principle: Healing our own past traumas and losses and finding satisfaction and meaning in our own lives is a part of healthy parenting.

Perennial Wisdom Quote: "…parental lack of resolution of trauma or loss has been demonstrated by attachment research to be a major factor associated with the most disturbed child form of attachment, disorganization/disoriented." -- Daniel Siegel, M.D., *The Developing Mind.*

Discussion: Good parenting requires attunement to the emotional, intellectual and social needs of our children, and it also requires parents to be mentally healthy themselves. Daniel Siegel, M.D. and other U.S. researchers of childhood attachment issues write in *Healing Trauma* about the importance of parents' taking care of themselves emotionally. If childhood or adult traumas have been simply suppressed with an "I'm OK; I just need to focus on my child" attitude, they can still inhibit healthy parenting.

How we feel and felt toward our own childhood caregivers, and what we experienced in our own childhoods, does influence how we parent our children. Dr. Siegel, a child psychiatrist, in *Parenting From The Inside Out,* discusses how healing one's own traumas and arriving at a deeper self-understanding can help a parent to raise children who thrive. He shows how parental emotional patterns influence the actual brain development of their children. He shows how adults who have not been well-parented themselves need to do remedial work on themselves in order to help their children develop secure emotional attachments and healthy brain functioning.

Self-exploratory Question: Have I sufficiently dealt with my own childhood losses and come to a deep understanding of myself?

Affirmation: I take my own emotional healing seriously, as a part of good parenting.

November 2
Depression

Freedom from

Principle: Depression inhibits interpersonal satisfaction and healthy parenting.

Perennial Wisdom Quote: "Research also suggests that depression is associated with a decreased capacity to perceive the emotional expressions of others." -- Daniel Siegel, M.D., *The Developing Mind*

Discussion: It is no longer necessary to just put up with and suffer from depression. Modern science can now accurately measure malfunctioning of the brain and the treatments necessary to heal them. Depression, like drug and alcohol addiction, is very damaging to family systems, as well. Parents who are depressed and either neglect their children and/or respond to them inappropriately can get professional help themselves, which will also indirectly help their children.

If previous attempts at psychotherapy and/or medication have not been encouraging, modern science has developed new diagnostic tools which can individualize assessments more accurately and also point to individualized treatments. Loving parents who are attempting to do the best they can with parenting, and yet still become frequently reactive, can now get more help and less judgment from informed professionals.

Every parent becomes reactive and un-empathic at times, but when it is a chronic problem, professional help is needed. It is depressing to want to do well in one's primary relationships, and yet do poorly in them. Good people sometimes do bad things due to their own unresolved psychological issues. Help is available.

Self-exploratory Question: How can I better examine myself for hidden depression?

Affirmation: I am using all available resources to have a good life and be a good parent.

Principle: Depending on a person who is himself or herself dependent on addictive substances or processes is not self-responsible.

Perennial Wisdom Quote: "Forgiveness is another word for letting go." -- Matthew Fox

Discussion: Beginning in the 1980's in the U.S., there was a popular movement involving looking at one's current or past family dysfunctional behaviors and recovering from them, using a 12 Step recovery approach. Al-Anon Family Groups for friends and families of alcoholics and drug abusers, and the various Adult Child of Alcoholic groups, were and still can be very helpful to individuals who find themselves loyal to a psychologically dependent adult. These groups, as well as the Wise Ways Happiness Support Groups, can help an individual to discover how to "let go with love" as well as how to do an effective "intervention" on a loved one who is being dangerously self-destructive.

Forgiving a family member and/or loved one for past wrongs and destructive behaviors can also involve letting go of trying to "fix them" or trying to punish them. Instead it involves focusing on one's own recovery from past losses and building on one's own current strengths. Melody Beattie's *Co-dependent No More* is a classic self-help guidebook for individuals caught in emotional attachments to dependent adults.

Self-exploratory Question: How can I remove myself from destructive dependency on a dependent adult?

Affirmation: I am responsible for my own self-care and for preventing my love for others from interfering with my emotional health.

Principle: Drug abuse, violence and prison time tend to go hand in hand.

Perennial Wisdom Quote: "Seek not good from without; seek it within yourselves, or you will never find it." – Epictetus

Discussion: The substances currently most linked with violence are alcohol, cocaine, methamphetamines, phencyclidine, and anabolic steroids. (See Dr. Amen's book, *Change Your Brain, Change Your Life.*) All of these substances cause abnormal flow of fluid in the brain. Nicotine and caffeine may also magnify the negative effects of these three substances. Danger from these substances may be especially pronounced if a person is already genetically predisposed with abnormalities in the prefrontal, cingulate, dominant temporal lobes, and dominant limbic and basal ganglia areas. (See Appendix 1.)

Substance abusers are often trying to ineffectively self-medicate for pre-existing brain abnormalities. The substance abuse then just makes matters much worse. All substance abusers and violent individuals should be screened for underlying psychiatric or neurological conditions, such as ADHD, bipolar disorder, learning disabilities, head traumas, Fetal Alcohol Syndrome or Effect, etc. In severe situations, brain SPECT imaging can be used to 1) uncover past brain trauma, 2) help clinicians choose appropriate medications, 3) allow family members and the legal system to see the medical aspects of a person's problems, and 4) help convince the drug abuser to get treatment in order to abstain from drugs and repair existing brain damage.

Self-exploratory Question: How can I protect myself better from drug abuse and violence?

Affirmation: Today I am protecting myself from drug abuse and violence.

Principle: Prejudice limits our awareness and the potential for national security and world peace.

Perennial Wisdom Quote: "If we are to achieve a richer culture, rich in contrasting values, we must recognize the whole gamut of human potentialities, and so weave a less arbitrary social fabric, one in which each diverse human gift will find a fitting place." -- Margaret Mead

Discussion: The 20th century was one in which racial and gender prejudice was challenged and diminished, although their institutional impacts still remain. In the 21st century challenges to prejudices of religion and sexual orientation are growing. Claims of exclusive redemption of sin and exclusive access to heaven are made by some religious groups, who are ignorant of the essence and value of other religious practices. Some heterosexuals ignorantly perceive homosexuals as being able to change their sexual orientation just through will power and therefore are prejudiced against them.

Humility and a vigorous commitment to the gathering of accurate information can go a long way to free an individual from prejudice. All the major religions of the world value humility and education. Modern technology now makes it possible for informed educational practices to become universal. What is still lacking is commitment on the part of many insecure and/or uninformed individuals and groups. Injustice around the world still foments violent reprisals.

Local and global educational organizations can all use volunteers. Each one of us can be part of the solution to problems of ignorance and prejudice.

Self-exploratory Question: How can I free myself more thoroughly of prejudice?

Affirmation: I choose to inform myself about others and free myself from prejudices.

November 6   Wise Ways Happiness Step 11: Conscious Contact With A Higher Power

Principle: The Wise Ways Happiness Step Eleven reads, "We seek through prayer and meditation to improve our conscious contact with a Higher Power, praying for guidance and the strength and will to carry the guidance out."

Perennial Wisdom Quote: "Learn to be silent. Let your quiet mind listen and absorb." -- Pythagoras

Discussion: Bill Wilson, a founder of Alcoholics Anonymous, wrote, "There is a direct linkage among self-examination, meditation and prayer. Taken separately, these practices can bring much relief and benefit. But when they are logically related and interwoven, the result is an unshakable foundation for life" (from *The 12 Steps and 12 Traditions of Alcoholics Anonymous*).

Prayer may be seen as talking to a Higher Power of one's own understanding. Meditation may be seen as listening to a Higher Power of one's own understanding. Agnostics and atheists can also medicate and pray, because they can define a Higher Power as any energy or force greater than themselves. Prayer and meditation teach humility and also teach patience and quiet observation of the mind, the heart and the breath. These skills have already been shown in many modern research studies to benefit physical as well as mental health.

New brain studies are showing how meditation practice can actually improve the structure and functioning of the brain. All religions teach some form of meditation to support their ethical guidelines. Without a quiet, self-observing mind, consistent, wise ethical practice is very difficult. Conscious contact with a Higher Power increases emotional awareness and maturity.

Self-exploratory Question: How can I improve my conscious contact with a Higher Power as I understand it?

Affirmation: I commit to meditating and praying on a daily basis.

November 7   Wise Ways Happiness Support Groups' Tradition 11: No Official Fellowship Opinions On Outside Issues

Principle: The Wise Ways Happiness Support Groups' Tradition 11 reads, "The Wise Ways Happiness Support Groups have no opinions on outside issues so that their names are not drawn into public controversy."

Perennial Wisdom Quote: "Concentration is the secret of strength." -- Ralph Waldo Emerson

Discussion: Just as concentration is the secret of personal strength, group concentration can be the secret of group strength. When a group simplifies its purpose, its practices, its organization and its political life, it can become much more effective.

Wise Ways Happiness Support Groups focus primarily on the personal growth of their individual members. They do not take on political or social efforts beyond this purpose. The groups are organized from the bottom up, with the health of group process taking priority. Individual members can have opinions on outside issues, but a group as a whole does not state such opinions. This keeps the purpose of the fellowship concentrated and simple. Everyone benefits.

Self-exploratory Question: When I speak on outside issues, do I speak only for myself?

Affirmation: When I speak on outside issues, I speak for myself, not my group.

Principle: Making unexamined assumptions about others leads to prejudice.

Perennial Wisdom Quote: "Having two ears and one tongue, we should listen twice as much as we speak." -- Turkish saying

Discussion: Fear and emotional insecurity can easily lead to quick judgments based on inadequate information. When we quickly verbalize these judgments, we can get ourselves into even more trouble. They are often false assumptions based on the projections of our own insecure minds. This is why the Chinese developed the proverb: "The sage does not talk; the talented ones talk; the stupid ones argue."

When we make quick assumptions, without checking out real facts, usually we do so because we feel the need to persuade another of our limited point-of-view, because the other's point- of-view feels threatening to us. For example, a person might argue, "Blacks are so different from us that they need separate schools." The fear behind this argument is likely the possibility of having more contact with a race which was enslaved by one's grandparents and is now free to make reprisals. The assumption is "Blacks are so different from us." Actually African-Americans have more in common with Anglo-Americans than differences, especially when it comes to the need for a good education.

The unexamined assumption of great differences leads to prejudice and injustice. In intimate relationships and working place relationships all sorts of inaccurate assumptions can be made which distort communication and promote injustice. It is always important to check out our facts before asserting any point of view.

Self-exploratory Question: How can I be more careful to check out the facts before I present an opinion?

Affirmation: I always check out the facts before I present an opinion.

Principle: Totalitarian government, run by a dictator or oligarchy, is inherently unstable and oppositional to the evolutionary development of human brain functioning.

Perennial Wisdom Quote: "Suffrage is the pivotal right." -- Susan B. Anthony

Discussion: Modern brain research has shown how the evolution of the human brain moves towards increasing complexity. It has also shown how human brains function best when all parts are working well together in an integrated fashion. As the planet's population continues to grow, global warming and virus pandemics threaten everyone, human beings more than ever are in need of democratic governments with leadership which is able to integrate the opinions and needs of all its citizens.

When power resides in the hands of one person or a small oligarchy, which is not responsible to its entire citizenry, evolutionary development is impaired, and wisdom is limited. This is especially true when large parts of the citizenry are impoverished, undernourished, and treated unfairly. Impoverished, undernourished, traumatized people do not have well-developed, integrated brains. This is why the place to start in such countries is with adequate education, nutrition and the rule of just law.

Citizens of modern democracies need to understand the importance of shared global resources and cooperative international organizations such as the United Nations for the safety of the entire world. Nuclear and biological weapons in the hands of dictators and oligarchies are very dangerous. As some corporations become even larger than some nations, it is also important to establish international guidelines for social and economic corporate justice. Through national constitutional amendments and U.N. resolutions, the power of large corporations can also be regulated for the good of the general citizenry.

Self-exploratory Question: How can I be more active in promoting true democracy and responsible international corporate law?

Affirmation: I am advocating for true democracy and fair corporate practices.

November 10   **Freedom From Inappropriate Responses To Fear**

Principle: Fear can lead to dysfunctional "fight," "flight," and "freeze" reactions.

Perennial Wisdom Quote: "The key to change…is to let go of fear." -- Rosanne Cash

Discussion: When adult brains are well-developed and their general functioning is well- integrated, fear is a manageable emotion. Fear primarily is experienced in the amygdala or "low brain" (See Appendix 1.) The amygdala's experience of fear then needs to be regulated by the brain's prefrontal cortex, in order for the mind to determine the best response to the fear. When the "low brain" and the higher parts of the brain, behind the forehead, are not well connected, due to unresolved trauma or inadequate nutrition or education or intense fear, the mind can make poor judgments, and the individual can act out in violence or inappropriate avoidance.

When individuals with this kind of brain functioning achieve unchecked power, the entire citizenry is in danger. When individuals with this kind of brain functioning have the power to do anything they want to their spouses or children, domestic violence and child abuse occur. When individuals with this kind of brain functioning are just temporarily locked up in prisons which are organized as small, totalitarian governments, upon release they can be even more dangerous than when they were first imprisoned.

Medical science now has the ability to diagnose and treat disorganized, unintegrated brain functioning. Compassionate governments need to find ways to provide these services to all needy citizens.

Self-exploratory Question: How can I more responsibly deal with fear?

Affirmation: I use every available resource to make sure that my brain functions well.

November 11   Developing A Coherent Personal Narrative To Improve Parenting

Principle: A parent or teacher's personal narrative matters to the neuropsychological development of his or her children.

Perennial Wisdom Quote: "A big story is a story that teaches that there is something very fine and permanent about you." -- Terry Tafoya, Ph.D., Lecture

Discussion: Terry Tafoya, Ph.D., a Naive American psychologist and storyteller in the Seattle area, teaches that there are three important steps in storytelling: 1) first you create safety and readiness for your listeners; 2) then you tell the story; and 3) then you ask your listeners what the story meant to them.

Dr. Remen, in her *Kitchen Table Wisdom,* tells of a creative storytelling ritual she recommends to all her cancer patients before starting their radiation, chemotherapy or surgery. She asks them to ask their significant friends and family members to select a stone, and then to hold it while sharing a story of some significant crisis which they survived; and the teller then describes the personal quality which most helped them to survive it. After telling the story, each person then says to the cancer patient, "I put__(the quality)__ into this stone for you." She then recommends that the patient holds one of these stones when going into each treatment.

Daniel Siegel, M.D., in his *Parenting From The Inside Out,* helps parents and teachers to understand the importance of healing their own losses and finding meaning in them, so that they can pass on inspirational narratives to their children. Adults who are unable to do this limit the healthy attachment potentials of their children, which further limits the neuropsychological development of the children's brains.

Self-exploratory Question: How can I make my personal narratives more coherent?

Affirmation: My personal narratives are coherent and beneficial to children.

Principle: Young people need accurate neuropsychological information provided by parents and teachers, who can also share their own coherent, personal narratives.

Perennial Wisdom Quote: "Freedom is nothing more than an opportunity to discipline ourselves rather than to be disciplined by others." -- Thomas Murphy

Discussion: Erik Erikson, a famous developmental researcher, asserted that before an individual could adequately deal with the intimacy issues of adulthood, he or she first must, during the ages of 13-25, deal with issues of identity. Modern brain research has also shown that during these ages, young peoples' brains are growing so rapidly that they are more disorganized than during the ages of 8-13 and after 25. Therefore, it is vital that good information about emotional and behavioral social functioning is available to pre-pubescent and pubescent children.

Mental and social health curricula in junior high and middle schools desperately need to be updated with modern brain research information. Children of this age need to see pictures of the holes alcohol and drugs can put into brains. They need to learn about optimal versus dysfunctional brain functioning and how to behaviorally enhance the development of one's brain during the puberty years. This information is available.

Teachers and parents need to be presenting coherent personal narratives (see Nov. 11 reading) to children in middle schools. They need to be encouraging students to share their family stories, as well as their own personal stories, in safe, supportive environments. They can also start after-school Wise Ways Happiness Support Groups for teens or ask a school counselor to start a Wise Ways Happiness Counseling Group.

Self-exploratory Question: How can I give more support to up-dated education?

Affirmation: I support scientifically-based, neuropsychological information in schools.

Principle: Regular exercise is essential to taking care of our hearts and brains.

Perennial Wisdom Quote: "Experts in nutrition, physiology, and medicine all agree that a program of physical exertion on a continuing basis is required to maintain low body fat, a strong and healthy heart, and well-toned muscles." --Danial G. Amen, M.D., *Change Your Brain, Change Your Life*

Discussion: Physical exercise is also essential for maintaining health in the deep limbic system of the brain. This is the part of the brain which, when unhealthy, leads to moodiness, depression and irritability. Exercise increases blood flow through the brain, increases energy, keeps the appetite in check, and promotes good sleep. Exercise allows more of the amino acid L-tryptophan which comes from milk, meat and eggs to enter the brain. L-tryptophan is the precursor of the neurotransmitter serotonin, which, when low, leads to depression.

When choosing an exercise program, choose one which you can enjoy. If walking on an indoor treadmill is a chore, walk outside where you can enjoy Nature, and/or with a friend with whom you enjoy visiting. If you don't like tennis, but enjoy swimming, join a club with a pool. If you like golf, walk and stay off the cart as much as possible. If you enjoy running, do so in a way which protects your legs, knees, and spine. If you like to bicycle, wear a helmet. Have a good time and stay safe.

Self-exploratory Question: How can I improve my exercise routines?

Affirmation: I am committed to regular exercise to take care of my heart and brain.

Principle: Despair thrives in isolation and lack of self-examination.

Perennial Wisdom Quote: "Always continue to climb. It is possible for you to do whatever you choose, if you first get to know who you are and are willing to work with a power that is greater than yourself to do it." -- Oprah Winfrey

Discussion: Oprah Winfrey's TV show has inspired millions of Americans to consider self-improvement. In her above quote she carefully modifies the old American belief that you can do anything you set your mind to do, with the qualifiers that self-examination and connection to a Higher Power are vital, in addition to will power.

Will power alone can lead us down some dysfunctional trails, if we don't know ourselves well, and if we are disconnected from community and spirituality. Bill and Dr. Bob, the founders of the original 12 Step program, Alcoholics Anonymous, knew this well. Bob was a physician and Bill was a financial professional, both very bright men. But both were ruining their lives with addictions to alcohol and were incapable of arresting their addictions by themselves. They realized that despair and addiction thrived in isolation, and they worked with others to build the foundation of a healthy fellowship which facilitates self-examination, connection to a Higher Power (no matter what one's definition of that Power), and service to others in community. They realized that company was much stronger than will power. They created an easy way for alcoholics to find sober, kind company, which offered guidance for those not yet in recovery.

Millions of people around the world have been able to lift themselves out of despair using AA's guidelines. The Wise Ways Happiness Support Groups are founded on similar guidelines, which are available to anyone interested in creating healthy group support. (See Appendix 2 and 4.)

Self-exploration Question: How can I better free myself from despair?

Affirmation: I value self-examination, spirituality and community.

Principle: When a person overly relies on will power for life satisfaction, he or she usually also sinks into dysfunctional power dynamics with others.

Perennial Wisdom Quote: "Do not forget the old adage that a spoonful of honey attracts more bees than a bucket of vinegar. And, finally, lots of friendliness may bring little friendliness in return, but a tiny bit of unfriendliness may result in torrents of hostility." -- Johannes Gaertner, *Worldly Virtues*

Discussion: Exercising healthy will power involves also learning how to negotiate successfully with others without resorting to force or violence. People who rely on force or violence to get their way forget that force always eventually creates an equal and opposite reaction. If we force someone to do something, that person is much more apt to try to force us to do something in return.

Example and modeling are much more influential than verbal instruction. If we want a child to learn non-violence, we need to be non-violent ourselves. If we want a child or another adult to respect us, we have to be respectful ourselves, etc.

Power dynamics also tend to set up what psychologists refer to as the "Drama Triangle," i.e. interpersonal situations in which one or more persons become a "victim," one or more persons become the "persecutors/abusers," and others are drawn into "rescuer" roles (See July 25-28 readings.) These dynamics are very dysfunctional and disempowering to everyone involved. We need to learn these lessons in order to create functional families, communities, nations, and international organizations. The answer is to work towards better communications, respect and understanding, not more force.

Self-exploratory Question: How can I better step out of power dynamics?

Affirmation: I choose not to use force with others and not to allow others to use force with me.

Principle: Real personal power involves creativity, understanding and kindness.

Perennial Wisdom Quote: "When I was young, I used to admire intelligent people; as I grow older, I admire kind people." -- Rabbi Abraham Joshua Heschel

Discussion: Grandiosity involves psychologically needing to be impressive to others. It includes needing the approval and high esteem of others and can create unnecessary dependency. It can include thinking that one is more capable than one really is. It often also involves a need for power and influence.

Many noted teachers have cautioned that real personal power and influence come more from creativity, understanding and kindness than they do from social and political power and influence. The founders of major world religions, including Judaism, Christianity, Buddhism, and Islam, were humble, non-assuming people, who attracted great followings because of their deep understanding, justice and kindness toward others. They did not go out to attract fame and fortune, or to establish new institutions. Rather they were intelligent and creative individuals who listened attentively to their own inner wisdom and the teachings of their elders, and wanted to be of service to others.

It's important to examine our motivations when we take leadership positions. Kindness and understanding are more important than personal influence. Ends don't justify means.

Self-exploratory Question: When I assume leadership, how can I be careful to avoid grandiosity?

Affirmation: I value creativity, understanding and kindness more than influence.

Principle: Reducing wants to needs allows time and energy for satisfying, service-oriented and creative activities.

Perennial Wisdom Quote: "The life that the rich man spends in heaping up gold is in truth like the life of the worms in the grave. It is a sign of fear." -- Kahil Gibran, *The Wisdom of Gibran,* Joseph Sheban, Editor

Discussion: When we feel we must have wealth to have security and influence, we are deluded. Although extreme poverty can interfere with health, and therefore cause unhappiness, still wealth cannot create health and happiness.

Moderation is the key. Reducing our wants to needs, allows us to save energy and resources to give to others, which potentially can create much more happiness than accumulating possessions does. Unfortunately, in modern consumer-oriented cultures, with media dominated by material sales, this principle is very easy to ignore.

Martin Seligman, Ph.D., has researched sources of happiness and has written an excellent book called *Authentic Happiness,* which challenges the consumption road to happiness. He points out that consumption of goods and pleasures can only bring very temporary happiness, and that absorption in creative and meaningful activities, such as service to others by using one's personal strengths is much more satisfying. We have more time and resources for this kind of service when we choose to live simple lives, reducing our wants to needs.

Self-exploratory Question: How can I more effectively reduce my wants to needs?

Affirmation: I buy and consume only what I need, leading a simple life.

Principle: Selling or giving away which we don't need can be very gratifying

Perennial Wisdom Quote: "When people live far from scenes of the Great Spirit's making, it's easy for them to forget his laws." -- Walking Buffalo, American Indian

Discussion: The more we surround ourselves with man-made possessions, the further we usually are from Nature. The further we are from Nature, the further we can drift away from natural laws and become obsessed with the desires of our minds. Having lots of possessions also tends to promote the fear of theft or property damage, as well as excessive work hours to pay for them.

Once a person has made a decision to "downsize" his or her possessions, sometimes it is hard to let them go. One helpful remedy is to begin thoughtful "recycling." This can involve determining who could use a possession more than you and simply giving it to that person. Or this can involve selling a possession and using the proceeds to benefit a needy child in one's local community or through an international charity.

Recycling involves more than the reuse of newspapers and aluminum cans. It involves looking closely at one's possessions and determining who could benefit from them more than yourself, if they are not necessities. It can also involve sharing real estate through hosting foreign exchange students or opening one's swimming pool on certain days to the Boys and Girls Clubs. The idea is to look at possessions, not as status symbols or proofs of worth, but simply as objects which can serve immediate needs and simple pleasures. If an object is just being stored for over a year, it is likely more of a burden than a gift and needs to be recycled.

Self-exploratory Question: What possessions can I productively sell or give away?

Affirmation: I keep only what I use and I give away unnecessary possessions.

November 19   **Freedom from Shopping and Gambling Addictions**

Principle: Shopping and gambling can only bring momentary pleasure, not lasting satisfaction.

Perennial Wisdom Quote: "Rapidly repeated indulgence in the same pleasure does not work. Not only do the pleasures fade quickly, many even have a negative aftermath." -- Martin Seligman, Ph.D., *Authentic Happiness*

Discussion: Dr. Seligman pointed out that even though real income in the U.S. had risen 16% in the previous 30 years, the percentage of people who described themselves as "very happy" had fallen from 36 to 29 percent, and the incidence of depression among young people had risen. Dr. Seligman's research has established that material consumption is simply not an effective route to happiness.

People can become habituated to shopping and gambling, just as they can to using alcohol and drugs, and more and more shopping and gambling leads to less and less satisfaction. The solution is to learn what is truly satisfying and to pursue these behaviors. Research has shown that such behaviors include: 1) sharing with others; 2) building positive memories; 3) self-congratulation; 4) sharpening one's perceptions; and 5) becoming absorbed in creative efforts.

Research has also shown that people who are frequently social and connected to meaningful community activities tend to report more satisfying lives. Shopping and gambling tend to be isolating activities, and include the negative consequence of consuming money which could be used for creative, social and/or service activities. It's helpful to mute TV advertising and to stay out of shopping malls unless you are specifically shopping for a needed item. Energy follows attention, so put your attention on potentially truly satisfying activities.

Self-exploratory Question: How can I put less energy into shopping or gambling and more into truly satisfying activities?

Affirmation: I choose to spend my time on satisfying activities which don't habituate.

Principle: Being able to complete tasks on time is an important element of teamwork.

Perennial Wisdom Quote: "All human power is a compound of time and patience." -- Balzac

Discussion: There is a Korean proverb, "Put off for one day and ten days will pass." Anyone who has a problem with procrastination understands this proverb. Balzac said it well when he talked about human power being a combination of "time" and "patience." Another way to put this is that effective human behavior is a product of timing and patience.

If we rush, usually more errors are made. If we are slow, often we miss the best moments for presentation of our work. If we procrastinate, we may completely miss an opportunity for presentation of our work.

Perfectionism can also lead to procrastination and inaccurate estimates about needed time to meet commitments. This can frustrate team efforts. It is important to learn how to be good estimators of how much time it takes to get our work done. In group projects, as long as the product meets a minimum standard, often the timing of the completion of a product is as important as the excellence of the product.

Balancing one's personal needs for creativity and excellence with meeting the standards and time expectations of others is a skill vital to success in the fast-paced modern world. This requires learning teamwork, time organization, and moderation in self-expectations.

Self-exploratory Question: How can I better avoid procrastination?

Affirmation: I value promptness and follow through with meeting my commitments.

Principle: Rudeness tends to boomerang.

Perennial Wisdom Quote: "To speak ill of anyone is to speak ill of one's self." --
Afghan saying

Discussion: Tecumseh, famous Shawnee American Indian chief, once said, "Show
respect to all men, but grovel to none." Unfortunately, some people feel that others
must be perfect to be deserving of respect, and to be respectful means groveling.
Being respectful does not mean groveling. Being respectful means treating everyone
as a human being, as deserving of human rights. It means treating others as you
would like to be treated yourself.

Rudeness, even to strangers, is unnecessary. People sometimes are
aggressive or thoughtless and in need of assertive confrontation, but this can be
done without rudeness. Rudeness tends to be passive-aggressive. It is behavior
which puts another down in a critical, somewhat passive way.

To be free of this kind of behavior, it can help to remember that someone
else's rudeness does not excuse our own rudeness. Many people say, "Bless you!"
when someone else sneezes. We need to have a similar response to another's
rudeness, because he or she is probably suffering from poor brain functioning. (See
Appendix 1 .) This can be just as threatening to health and quality of life as any virus.
Consider honestly sending "blessings" to anyone who has been rude to you. They
need them.

Self-exploratory Question: How can I better avoid rude behavior?

Affirmation: I practice being respectful to everyone.

Principle: One important way to respect ourselves is to honor our talents.

Perennial Wisdom Quote: "Each man has his own vocation. The talent is the call. There is one direction in which all space is open to him." -- R.W. Emerson, "Spiritual Laws"

Discussion: Have you ever thought of your talents as "calls" to a vocation or avocation or "gifts" from a Higher Power? All of us have some talents which were given to us genetically through our physical and mental make-ups. As Emerson pointed out, when we clearly identify these talents, respect them, and look for ways to use them productively, the universe seems to open doors easily to us.

Sometimes a talent, such as one in music or sports, needs to be developed with diligent practice. Sometimes the talent seems instantaneous, such as the ability to see colors and shapes clearly and to reproduce them accurately on paper or canvas. However easy or difficult it is to develop a talent, it's helpful to remember that opportunities will open to us when we respect and use a talent, especially if we use it in a way which is beneficial to others, as well as invigorating to ourselves.

Dr. Seligman, a leading "positive psychologist", has created a free website (www.authentichappiness.org) which anyone can go to for determining personal "strengths." This is a good place to start. Public high schools and community colleges also offer vocational tests to help identify a person's primary interests and skills and then match them with optimal career options. You will know you are utilizing your talents well when you find employment that you actually enjoy and which energizes you rather than drains you. It's worthwhile to keep looking for such employment. At the very least, it's worthwhile to find a hobby or recreational pursuit which honors your talents.

Self-exploratory Question: How can I better recognize and honor my talents?

Affirmation: I recognize and honor my talents.

Principle: Conflict can only be truly healed through increased empathy, justice, understanding and mutual respect.

Perennial Wisdom Quote: "Nothing in life is to be feared. It is only to be understood." -- Marie Curie

Discussion: Empathy and understanding start "at home." When we have a disagreement or misunderstanding with a family member, it is vital that we don't assign negative intent to the family member, i.e. that we don't assume that he or she is being purposefully hurtful or disrespectful. We can feel hurt or disrespected without someone else's intending that hurt for us. For example, a spouse might unilaterally make plans for a family vacation, thinking it will please his or her partner, not having experience with collaborative vacation planning. His or her spouse might feel disrespected and hurt by not being included in the planning process, and might assign negative intent to the spouse who made the unilateral plans. The spouse who made the plans might feel hurt that his or her efforts to set up a fun vacation weren't appreciated. To undo these hurt feelings, both spouses need to be able to communicate their feelings clearly, carefully listen to the actual intentions and needs of the other, and cooperatively correct the situation as much as possible. This eliminates both of them from an "enemy" role.

When we put someone in an "enemy" role, we are usually fearful and trying to protect ourselves from a repeat of some past injustice, which we are projecting onto the new situation. If we do not take time to respectfully listen and empathize with the feelings and needs of everyone involved, justice is sacrificed.

Self-exploratory Question: How can I empathize more, and think "enemy" less?

Affirmation: When facing conflict, I choose to empathize even with seeming "enemies."

November 24   **Accepting**
Anger

Principle: Violence is unnecessary when we accept anger and are in charge of our own automatic thoughts and behavioral responses.

Perennial Wisdom Quote: "Personality problems result when a person gets stuck in old behavioral patterns which don't work." -- Donald Meichenbaum, Ph.D., Lecture

Discussion: Dr. Meichenbaum has worked with many people recovering from aggressive, behavioral patterns. He teaches how to examine one's past aggressive behavior as if one were looking at four places on a clock:

1) Think of the Stimulus Event as 12 o'clock. It could have been an external or internal stimulus. Ask yourself "What happened?" and reflect on it with the help of another trustworthy person.

2) Reflect on the Primary and Secondary Emotions you experienced in response to the event. Think of this as 3 o'clock. Ask yourself, "Then I felt what?"

3) Next reflect on the Automatic Thoughts you had in response to your emotions Think of this as 6 o'clock. Ask yourself, "Then I thought what?"

4) Finally, reflect on the Behavioral Results of your autonomic thoughts. Think of this as 9 o'clock. Ask yourself, "Then I did what and others responded to my behavior with what?"

        Once you have identified the vicious cycle of aggression, ask yourself, "How can I change what happens at 6 o'clock and 9 o'clock with my automatic thoughts and reactive behaviors, so that the aggression cycle isn't reinforced?" We can accept the emotion of anger without getting stuck in automatic thoughts and aggressive behavior which end up being hurtful to ourselves and others.

Self-exploratory Question: How can I do more to avoid violence?

Affirmation: I can avoid violence by being in charge of my automatic thoughts and choosing non-violent, verbal responses.

Principle: Working through past trauma results in accepted grief and reduced violence.

Perennial Wisdom Quote: "Aggressive kids need to get into pro-social peer groups in which they can work through their losses and grief." -- Donald Meichenbaum, Ph.D., Lecture

Discussion: Recent research has shown that 45% of aggressive boys are suffering from Post-Traumatic Stress Disorder, i.e., they have not recovered from some past trauma. Research has also shown that these aggressive boys have seven times less activity in the left (verbal) sides of their brains than their right sides (non-verbal.) People suffering from the consequences of aggression need to repair their brain functioning by learning how to identify and accept their past losses and grief, and then learning how to respond to their reactive anger with different automatic thought and verbal, behavioral patterns, ones which will remove them from repeated cycles of violence.

Boys, more than girls, often have learned how to suppress and repress feelings of sadness. They can often only identify the secondary feeling of anger. They need to practice looking for the feeling which comes before the anger. It is usually grief and/or fear. When these emotions can be identified and accepted and verbalized, the violence cycle can be interrupted.

The violence cycle can involve violence toward others or violence toward self, which leads to depressed, possibly suicidal, thoughts. In any case those automatic thoughts are dangerous, and the recovering individual needs to learn how to replace those automatic thoughts, so as not to get stuck in destructive automatic behaviors.

Self-exploratory Question: How can I better see the loss and grief under my anger?

Affirmation: I accept my past losses and am responsible for working through my grief, so as to avoid violent behavior.

Principle: Optimal, integrated brain functioning leads to "flow" consciousness.

Perennial Wisdom Quote: "There must be new flowerings, new prophets, new adventures -- always new adventures -- if the heart of man, albeit in fits and starts, is to go on beating." -- Paul Tournier, *The Adventure of Living*

Discussion: Mihaly Csikszentmihalyi in 1990 wrote a book simply called *Flow.* In it he described his research with people who had "optimal experiences" and who creatively lost themselves in activities. These people seemed to have highly specialized individual skills and also a capacity for being socially integrated with others. They had identified their talents, developed them, and found a way to use them beneficially for others, as well as to themselves. They were people who had learned how to focus their attention on present opportunities and respond to them creatively, rather than getting stuck in regrets about the past or anxieties about the future. They had learned how to both avoid boredom and excessive anxiety.

Daniel Siegel, M.D., has shown how "flow" is actually a state of optimal brain functioning in which the entire brain interacts in an integrated, holistic fashion. "Flow" can be learned better in our schools if teachers and parents understand more about its essential qualities and reinforce them in children. The arts, for example, often help teach students concentration and "flow," and if they are cut out of the curriculum due to budget crises, students may learn better math skills but be less successful in life, because they have not learned how to "flow".

Self-exploratory Question: How can I increase "flow" in my life?

Affirmation: I value "flow" in my life and do my best to sustain it.

Principle: Emotions are the body's way of protecting and healing itself.

Perennial Wisdom Quote: "Authentic freedom comes when we refuse to judge any part of our human process…the freedom of feeling every emotion we have, without denial, allows us to access the sacred and empowering gifts of choice." -- Jamie Sams and David Carson, *Earth Medicine*

Discussion: When we repress and avoid certain feelings, we deny ourselves important opportunities to heal and protect ourselves. Some feelings, however, are "secondary" to a "primary" emotion, which needs to be recognized first. For example, rage is almost always secondary to fear of loss or grief. Rage and hatred can also be called "mirroring emotions", because they usually involve certain amounts of reactive projection, comparison, personalization and self-rejection.

To learn to recognize and effectively process all our "primary" emotions, we need to learn to breathe deeply, relax and accept grief, anger, and joy as they arise, carefully watching them and our automatic thoughts, which occur in response to them. Then we can correct our automatic thoughts, if necessary, and make wise behavioral choices.

When we see our emotions as completely tied to other people's behaviors, we lose our independence and our capacity to make thoughtful decisions about our speech and our behaviors. We become reactive and burdened with emotions like jealousy, envy, depression, and hatred. When we can allow our feelings to "flow" smoothly through us without acting out aggressively in anger or any other emotion, we can become truly free.

Self-exploratory Question: Do I deny or react aggressively to certain feelings?

Affirmation: I accept all my feelings, and make thoughtful, non-aggressive choices about how to respond to them.

Principle: When we choose to act out in anger, we choose to enslave ourselves.

Perennial Wisdom Quote: "You have no friends; you have no enemies; you have only teachers." -- Ancient saying

Discussion: Anger signals us that something is not going well. But when we simply "act out our anger," i.e. dump our critical thoughts and angry feelings on others, we are misusing anger. Anger usually follows fear of grief. The grief needs to be experienced before the anger. The primary emotion of grief is the body's way of releasing painful loss, and its accompanying tears have a natural tranquilizer in them, soothing the brain and signaling the brain that a change needs to take place.

   The first change needs to be in our own brain. We need to learn to observe our angry feelings, discover what is not working well for us, examine our automatic thoughts, and respectfully inform those around us of needed changes, ones which would allow everyone to improve the situation.

      Brain research has shown that people who have unintegrated, malfunctioning brains have a disconnect between their amygdala (low brain) and their prefrontal cortex (high brain behind the forehead) (See Appendix 1.) The result is an inability to observe one's feelings and automatic thoughts and the corresponding inability to correct them. Fortunately, many brain malfunctions can be corrected with medication and behavioral education and therapy. People don't have to continue to allow their amygdala's to "hijack" their higher brain functions. They can correct amygdala over-activity and grow new brain cells, which will better connect them to higher brain functioning.

Self-exploratory Question: How can I better integrate my brain functioning?

Affirmation: When angry, I take time to exercise good judgment and not act out.

Principle: When we allow grief to flow through us, taking time to rest and restore our strength, and learning from our loss, we are less apt to become reactively depressed.

Perennial Wisdom Quote: "Affliction comes to us all, not to make us sad, but sober, not to make us sorry, but wise, not to make us despondent, but by the darkness to refresh us." -- Henry W. Beecher

Discussion: Grief has a creative function for all mammals, including humans. Since our human brains are more complex than those of most other mammals, we simply have to learn how to creatively experience grief. When we allow our minds to repress the grief and get stuck in anger or reactive depression, the grief is no longer able to fulfill its healing function.

Grief is an emotion in our body which is designed to slow us down and to cause us to rest and to reach out for emotional soothing and support. This is what Henry Beecher means when he says, "by the darkness to refresh us." When we angrily resist the grief, we imbalance our brains and disallow healing in them. When we repress our tears, we deny ourselves the natural tranquilizer in them which Mother Nature has provided. When we rely on adrenaline to lift us out of reactive depression, we then further increase our hormonal imbalance, caused by our loss in the first place.

Managing grief and loss is a serious business and one which needs to be carefully taught in "grief management" classes for angry, troubled youth and adults. "Anger management" classes alone are insufficient, if they do not sufficiently attend to issues of grief and loss.

Self-exploratory Question: How can I become freer from reactive depression?

Affirmation: I choose to allow my grief to soothe and heal me.

Principle: Learning how to collaboratively problem-solve is an important skill.

Perennial Wisdom Quote: "Don't oppose forces; use them. God is a verb, not a noun." -- Richard B. Fuller

Discussion: A big mistake which is easily made is to oppose force with force. This is like trying to stop a wind by blowing back. It just causes more havoc. Gini Graham Scott, Ph.D., in *Resolving Conflict* explains that collaborative problem-solving seeks to "work out a mutually satisfying solution with others." It is not "competitive" (i.e., seeking only to get one's own way). It is not "avoidant" (i.e., seeking to avoid the conflict situation). It is not "accommodative" (i.e., working cooperatively without asserting one's own concerns). It is not "compromising" (i.e., seeking to work out a solution in which we each give up a little and get some of what we want).

Effective problem solving is "collaborative" and involves these six steps:

1) getting emotions under control;

2) setting ground rules;

3) clarifying positions (including avoiding making judgments about what the other thinks, believes or has done and including looking at the world from the other's point of view);

4) exploring underlying needs and interests;

5) generating alternatives; and

6) agreeing on the best Win/Win option.

These skills need to be practiced in all educational and living situations in order to promote better brain-functioning and emotional health. If you have difficulty with these steps, buy Dr. Scott's book and also secure help in applying its principles.

Self-exploratory Question: How can I improve my collaboration skills?

Affirmation: I am developing my advanced collaboration skills.

Principle: The best way to prevent divorce is for both spouses to take equal responsibility for keeping the marriage current, honest, and joyful.

Perennial Wisdom Quote: "Connecting is *not* magic. Like any other skill it can be learned, practiced, and mastered…. Recent scientific discoveries about the emotional brain, along with the latest observational studies of human interaction, have helped us to form a body of scientifically proven advice for connecting with one another and improving the quality of our lives." -- John Gottman, Ph.D., *The Relationship Cure*

Discussion: According to John Gottman, Ph.D., a noted marriage and couple therapy researcher, the "Four Horsemen of the Apocalypse" which predict likely divorce are chronic 1) criticism, 2) contempt, 3) defensiveness, and 4) stonewalling.

   He reports that in 85% of marriages the "stonewaller" is the husband because men are more easily overwhelmed by marital conflict than are their wives. He believes the reason for this is that the male cardiovascular system remains more reactive than the female's and slower to recover from stress, because evolutionarily men were hunters and women were nurturers.

         In *The Seven Principles For Making Marriage Work,* Dr. Gottman suggests these remedies:

 1) enhancing your "love maps" (i.e., current information about what is going on in your spouse's life, including stresses and aspirations);

 2) nurturing your fondness and admiration for each other;

 3) turning toward each other instead of away, especially when making important choices;

 4) letting your partner influence you;

 5) solving your solvable problems collaboratively together;

 6) continuing to work on your "irresolvable conflicts"; and

 7) creating shared meaning (supporting each other's hopes and aspirations and building a common sense of purpose).

         In order to do all this, couples who thrive devote at least five hours per week to these activities. (See Dec.2 reading & locate Dr. Gottman's books for further help.)

Self-exploratory Question: How can I do more to prevent a divorce?

Affirmation: I do everything I can to keep my marriage current, honest and joyful.

Principle: Thriving marriages take consistent time and attention.

Perennial Wisdom Quote: "Researchers have shown that heart-to-heart rituals have demonstrable positive effects on the heart and immune system. -- Paul Pearsall, Ph.D., *The Heart Code*

Discussion: According to John Gottman, Ph.D., couples who thrive engage in these observable activities:

1) for about ten minutes each morning before leaving for work they find out one thing that each is going to do that day;

2) for about twenty minutes at the end of each workday, they have a low-stress reunion conversation;

3) they take at least five minutes each day to show each other appreciation and affection via touching, holding and kissing, all laced with tenderness and forgiveness; and

4) they take approximately two hours every week to have private "dates" with each other in relaxed atmospheres, updating their love and shared experiences.

       All of these interactions together take only about five hours a week and yet are vital for the maintenance of a healthy marriage. If a marriage looks very different from this, the individuals in it would benefit from reading Dr. Gottman's books and/or seeing a couple therapist. The time to see a couple therapist is before problems and attitudes become intractable, not after.

Self-exploratory Question: What can I do to help my marriage to thrive?

Affirmation: I give time and attention to my marriage, helping it to thrive.

Principle: Successful democracy requires responsible citizens and a constitution which guarantees all citizens the vote and equal representation.

Perennial Wisdom Quote: "To safeguard democracy the people must have a keen sense of independence, self-respect and their oneness." -- Mahatma Gandhi

Discussion: The 21st century is a century of population explosion and also of attempted democratic nation-building. Mahatma Gandhi as early as the middle 20th century wrote about successful democracy requiring:

1) a sense of independence;

2) self-respect; and

3) a people's sense of oneness.

When any of these factors is missing, building and maintaining democracy is difficult. Democracy can also be undermined by big money, special interests, and by apathetic citizens who don't work to keep the political system truly representative. At the community level democracy can also be undermined by disinterest in such vital groups as community councils and boards of education. Self-respecting citizens realize that it takes some time and effort to create and maintain a healthy community. Conflicts of interest need to be collaboratively resolved. Taxes need to be raised to pay for community services.

Government isn't some "they." It is "we." Responsible citizens realize that everyone's safety and security is enhanced when no one is starving or homeless, when everyone is protected by an effective medical system. They work to help their communities to provide economic opportunities for all. They respect themselves and also the basic needs of all their community's citizens. They realize that the common interests of the community need to take precedence over the interests of one person. They do their part for the good of the whole.

Self-exploratory Question: How can I contribute more to the welfare of my community, nation and world?

Affirmation: I take pleasure in being a responsible citizen.

Principle: Absorption in a creative project which benefits the community can make for more satisfaction than self-gratification.

Perennial Wisdom Quote: "Become so wrapped up in something that you forget to be afraid." -- Lady Bird Johnson

Discussion: Martin Seligman, Ph.D., has completed research which has shown that absorption in a beneficial, creative project leads to more happiness and personal satisfaction than does self-gratification through shopping, drinking, eating, or gambling. Unfortunately, many people have not yet learned this, and also are afraid to reach out to contribute to others.

Those who have learned how to do what Dr. Seligman's research suggests are significantly happier than those who have not. Helping to bring joy to another human being brings more joy to one's self than self-absorbed consumption. It is healthier for one's brain, heart and spirit.

It's important to identify your own best talents and then look for ways to use them that will bring joy to others. Don't give in a way which could lead to resentment, if your gift is not acknowledged. Find some way to give with no strings attached, so that the process of giving itself is joyful for you.

Self-exploratory Question: How can I reduce my fear of community participation?

Affirmation: I enjoy service to others more than self-gratification.

December 5   The Wise Ways Happiness Step Twelve: Service & Continued Practice

Principle: The Wise Ways Happiness Step Twelve reads, "Having had a spiritual awakening as a result of these Steps, we commit to practicing these happiness principles in all of our affairs and sharing them with others."

Perennial Wisdom Quote: "When you cease to make a contribution, you begin to die." -- Eleanor Roosevelt

Discussion: Before we can be of the most service to others, we first have to take care of our own spirits, bodies and minds. We need to make sure we are not Hungry, Angry, Lonely and Tired (H.A.L.T.) ourselves. Once we have taken care of our own needs enough to establish a healthy attitude and an honest desire to connect to others, then it is time to find ways to be of service to others.

The Wise Ways Happiness Program, like other 12 Step programs, encourages members to volunteer to be of service to others. However, service needs to be balanced with consistent self-care and attention to one's personal practices of the happiness principles. If an individual is giving too much in service, it is best to relinquish some service commitments in order to pay more attention to personal practices.

Self-exploratory Question: How can I better balance service and personal rejuvenation?

Affirmation: My service work helps me to feel alive and joyful.

December 6   Wise Ways Support Groups' Tradition 12: Public Relations Policy

Principle: Wise Ways Support Groups' Tradition 12 Twelve reads, "The Wise Ways Support Groups may sell this book at their cost. Their principle is always attraction to Happiness Support Groups, not promotion."

Perennial Wisdom Quote: "Attraction is much better than promotion." – a Wise Ways Happiness Slogan

Discussion: It is important to make information about the Wise Ways Happiness Program available to people, giving them an opportunity to be attracted to the Program. However, Wise Ways Happiness Support Group members do not proselytize. They provide information about the program, without using any specific member's name. Members can tell their friends about the Wise Ways Happiness Program and invite them to come to groups, if they are interested. But there is no attempt to push the Program on anyone. If someone is attracted to the Program, fine. If not, that is fine, too.

The size of the membership of Wise Ways Happiness Groups is not important. What is important is the benefit each individual member receives from the Program, and also the availability of the *365 Wise Ways to Happiness* book to any interested individual.

Self-exploratory Question: How can I protect Program members' anonymity and also help make information about the Wise Ways Happiness Program available to others?

Affirmation: Tradition Twelve protects my anonymity and reminds me to attract people to the Wise Ways Happiness Program by example and invitation, not by persuasion.

Principle: It takes courage to be consistently ethical.

Perennial Wisdom Quote: "One isn't necessarily born with courage, but one is born with potential. Without courage, we cannot practice any other virtue with consistency. We can't be kind, true, merciful, generous, or honest." -- Maya Angelou

Discussion: Courage is often recognized on the battlefield. It is less often recognized in one's everyday commitment to be ethical in one's dealings with everyone. A person might have the financial courage to start a big new company, but not have the courage to practice only ethical business practices which are honest and harmful to no one. A person might have the courage to climb a very big mountain, but not be ethical enough to turn around before reaching the summit, in order to help someone who's been hurt.

C.S. Lewis wrote that courage is "not simply one of the virtues, but the form of every virtue at the testing point." Ethics are ultimately more important than physical strength or mental brain power in being courageous and achieving a satisfying life. We have to first be clear about the guidelines of our personal, business and professional ethics. Then we have to have the courage to follow these guidelines even if it means financial or personal loss.

Most ethical mistakes are made out of fear. Most lies are told to avoid the negative consequences from making a mistake. But when we don't admit our mistakes, we can't learn from them. The practice of being ethical is something we need to do for ourselves, not just for others.

Self-exploratory Question: How can I be more courageously ethical?

Affirmation: I am courageously following my ethical principles.

December 8   **Freedom from Ego-centricity and Ethno-centricity**

Principle: Ego-centricity and ethno-centricity in governmental and religious leadership can lead to terrorism and warfare.

Perennial Wisdom Quote: "Christian [or Muslim] leaders who demonize Islam [or Christianity] are contradicting the Bible's [Qu'ran's] spirit of compassion." -- Thich Nhat Hanh, 2004 Public Statement, with editorial additions

Discussion: On December 7, 1941, Pearl Harbor was bombed by the Japanese, and the United States entered a World War against Japan and Germany. This war didn't end until hundreds of thousands of innocent men, women and children were killed. The ego-centricity of powerful national leaders and the ethno-centricity of their citizenry was responsible for these horrors. Ethno-centricity involves believing that one's own nation or tribe is superior than another's so should dominate.

World War II was called "the war to end all wars", and yet warfare has continued, perhaps on a smaller scale, but with ever more lethal weaponry. The world has been at the brink of nuclear disaster several times since 1945, and only with less ego-centric leadership and better communication systems have we been able to prevent disaster.

Ego-centricity involves leaders putting their own egos over the welfare of their citizens. It damages personal lives, family relationships and community-building efforts. Ego-centricity in powerful leaders creates dishonesty, corruption, terrorism, and atrocities being committed on innocent people.

Ego-centricity and ethno-centricity on the part of modern religious leaders, who have lost touch with the fundamental teachings of their group's inspirational teachers, also are very dangerous. Religious practitioners need to carefully examine the fundamental teachings of compassion of their founders and resist ethno-centric teachings which legitimize only one religious group or nation.

Self-exploratory Question: How can I protect myself and my nation better from ego-centric and ethno-centric leadership?

Affirmation: I focus on world-centric rather than ego-centric or ethno-centric thinking.

December 9   **Beyond Ethno-centricity to World-**
centricity

Principle: The world, already linked by the Internet and world news networks, needs to function more and more cooperatively, to promote everyone's national and ecological security and health.

Perennial Wisdom Quote: "Maybe they [the terrorists] have misunderstood us. In that case we can try to correct their perceptions. To correct their perceptions is much better than to drop bombs on them." -- Thich Nhat Hanh, February 2004 Public Statement

Discussion: Thich Nhat Hanh, a Vietnamese Buddhist monk, has brought together groups of Israelis and Palestinians to his Plum Village community in France. At first the two groups were barely able to speak to each other, but after sharing their stories of suffering and engaging in calm, daily meditation together, the two groups were able to listen and empathize with each other. It is this kind of community-building which needs to be supported with national government funds, not just non-profit group funds.

What would you think of a constitutional amendment in the U.S. which would require a certain percentage of the government's "defense" budget to be spent in these peaceful, community-building ways, instead of on spying, weapons and troops? Perhaps its proposal would at least stir up meaningful debate on what efforts really promote homeland security the best. Peaceful volunteers could also visit terrorist prisoners empathizing with their suffering as people and doing their best to correct their distorted beliefs in the morality of killing innocent people.

Self-exploratory Question: What do I think of a constitutional amendment requiring a certain amount of national defense spending to go to world-centric-peace-building?

Affirmation: Understanding our "enemies" is an important part of national defense.

Principle: Effective decision making takes time, practice, humility and retrospective review to see if one's choices reinforce one's priorities, values and principles.

Perennial Wisdom Quote: "Commitment to process can be controlled. Commitment to outcome cannot." -- Gay Hendricks, Ph.D. and Kathlyn Hendricks, Ph.D. *Conscious Loving*

Discussion: Effective decision-making includes at least six elements:

 1) preparing, i.e., collecting as much information as possible about the situation from reliable sources;

 2) clarifying options, i.e., writing down all possible options with as much clarity as possible;

 3) prioritizing the options based on how they relate to one's values and principles;

 4) seeking help, if needed, e.g., consulting with someone to determine if the decision is morally competent and psychologically and physically healthy;

 5) choosing the option which is most consistent with one's priorities, values and principles, taking full responsibility for one's actions and committing to a future review of the consequences of one's choice; and

 6) at a targeted time, reviewing the decision and its consequences and determining if any changes need to be made.

        If a decision involves a partnership, both partners need to be involved in this decision-making process, (see Oct. 17-19 readings), and effective conflict-resolution steps need to be followed, if conflicts arise.

Self-exploratory Question: How can I improve my decision-making skills?

Affirmation: When making a decision, I take time to do it effectively.

Principle: Building trust takes time, commitment, and consistent follow-through.

Perennial Wisdom Quote: "A man who doesn't trust himself can never really trust anyone else." -- Cardinal de Retz

Discussion: Trust is an important part of any important relationship and it must be earned. It can't just be blindly given. How can trust be earned? It can be earned by developing trust in ourselves first, by making behavioral decisions based on consistent priorities, values and principles. When we do this, others gradually come to trust us, if they respect and value our principles and priorities.

      Trustworthy relationships also need to be updated by people's sharing new experiences, feelings and priorities with one another. All people are constantly changing, and these changes vary our priorities from time to time. But if we operate consistently on the basis of such principles as honesty and kindness, then others can continue to trust us, even when our priorities shift to include new options. As we mature and as our family relationships change with birth, death, age and infirmity, our time-commitment priorities may change, but we make these changes within the context of our ongoing ethical principles. Therefore, we can continue to be trustworthy. It is our own responsibility, however, to update those around us about our changing feelings and experiences, so that commitments can continue to be met, within the changing contexts.

Self-exploratory Question: How can I become more trustworthy?

Affirmation: I trust myself and am trustworthy for others.

**December 12   Allow Ourselves to be Influenced by "Soft Start"
Requests**

Principle: Requests for behavioral change, when respectfully presented, need to be respectfully accepted and followed up with by respectful negotiations.

Perennial Wisdom Quote: Women benefit from learning to present requests with "soft starts." Men benefit from learning how to "allow themselves to be influenced." – John Gottman, Ph.D.

Discussion: John Gottman, Ph.D. has recently done extensive studies at the University of Washington on what makes for successful marriages. He found that successful wives begin their problem solving with their husbands with "soft starts," including some appreciations and affection and avoiding criticism. He also found that successful husbands "allowed themselves to be influenced." This means they listened to their wives' feelings, perceptions and requests and respected them, without necessarily agreeing to their wives' proposed solutions. They engaged in cooperative negotiations with their wives, finding solutions which were acceptable to both of them.

When we are secure about our own thoughts and behavioral principles, it is easier to both present our requests respectfully and to also allow ourselves to be influenced. We can accept negative feedback graciously, consider it, and problem solve with others about it without losing self-esteem. We can practice Dr. Gottman's advice both for husbands and wives in all our relationships.

Usually when criticism is harshly given, the intent of the criticizer is to create emotional distance or to prop up a weak sense of self-worth. If we receive such feedback, it is best to allow emotional distance on a temporary basis, and resist the temptation to return the harsh criticism. This eases the situation, reduces dysfunctional interaction and reduces stress.

Self-exploratory Question: How can I deal with criticism more effectively?

Affirmation: I only offer requests for change within a larger context of respect and appreciation. The only criticism which I take to heart is that given in this fashion.

December 13   **Developing Mature**
Strength

Principle: Mature people do not give up easily, and they maintain hope.

Perennial Wisdom Quote: "There are no hopeless situations; there are only people who have grown hopeless." -- Clare Boothe Luce

Discussion: Hope thrives when we are used to being responsible for our own behaviors, and we have experience in taking care of ourselves. When we have held on to childlike dependencies on others and feel abandoned and reliant on outside assistance, hope perishes. Clare Boothe Luce's quote beautifully reminds us that life is so constantly changing that there is always hope. It is only our own minds and attitudes which sometime fail us.

Maturity is about building experience with self-reliance and also about collaborating with others, so that even overwhelming tasks are somehow manageable. Hopeless people are often isolated people who have neither learned how to appropriately ask for help, nor learned how to collaborate with others to make changes in external situations. By learning self-reliance and collaboration, a person can dramatically change his or her life situation and thereby create more hope.

Self-exploratory Question: How can I become more emotionally mature and hopeful?

Affirmation: I am becoming more emotionally mature and hopeful.

Principle: It is more satisfying to work hard and to do one's best than to have success in others' eyes.

Perennial Wisdom Quote: "My mother drew a distinction between achievement and success. She said that achievement is the knowledge that you have studied and worked hard and done the best that is in you. Success is being praised by others. That is nice but not as important or satisfying. Always aim for achievement and forget about success." -- Helen Hayes

Discussion: When we focus on others' opinions of us more than on our own opinion of ourselves, resentment and disappointment result. We live with ourselves day in and day out, and we need to feel good about our own priorities and choices. Others need to feel good about their priorities and choices, not ours. True, if we are in a partnership or functioning in a team, we need to find ways to make our priorities and choices complimentary with those of others. Sometimes this takes effort and good conflict- resolution skills, which need to be a personal priority if we are living within a family or working within a team. Still, it is essential to remember that diligently working hard ourselves to do the best we can is the fundamental route to self-satisfaction, not just pleasing others.

      It also helps to remember Mother Teresa's words, "We can do no great things -- only small things with great love."

Self-exploratory Question: How can I focus more on satisfying achievement rather than on success?

Affirmation: I value working hard and doing my best more than how others perceive my success.

December 15   **Establishing One's Own Emotional**
Boundaries

Principle: Thoughtful, on-going self-awareness and self-care are necessary to keep good emotional boundaries.

Perennial Wisdom Quote: "When one is estranged from oneself, then one is estranged from others, too." -- Ann Morrow Lindbergh

Discussion: Emotional boundaries are needed in order for a person not to lose his or her own personal integrity and peace of mind. Just as we need to balance exhalations with inhalations in order to keep our bodies healthy, we need to balance attention to our inner well-being with attention to others' well-being. We need to have some private time and space in order to be able to connect with others intimately. If we feel emotionally crowded, the natural response is to pull away.

Each person is responsible for affirming his or her own emotional boundaries, because another person cannot keep up with our ever-changing emotional needs. Emotions flow through our bodies so fast that by the time another person guesses what we might be feeling, our feelings have moved on. We are ultimately always responsible for our own feelings, and for protecting ourselves from emotional abuse and neglect. If we don't do this, we start to lose self-respect.

Self-exploratory Question: How can I better maintain my emotional boundaries?

Affirmation: I am aware of my emotional limits and boundaries and protect them.

Principle: Individuals have very different emotional limits and boundary needs. Therefore, we must respect how others set their boundaries.

Perennial Wisdom Quote: "Give to the world the best you have and the best will come back to you." -- Madeline Bridges

Discussion: Most parents learn that different children have different energy and emotional limits and capacities. An effective parent discovers these early on and adjusts expectations, as needed, for each child. One child may get hungry, or angry or tired at a very different time from another. The effective parent accepts this and works with it. He or she does not demand that every child perform in exactly the same way at exactly the same time.

Similarly, as adults we need to recognize that other adults have very different energy and emotional limits and capacities. We cannot demand that every adult protects his or her boundaries in exactly the way we do. If another person calls an "Adult Time Out," we need immediately to give that person time and space to reintegrate himself or herself, so as to be more interpersonally functional at a later time. We need to give such a person time and space to self-soothe, rest or eat.

If someone says he or she is offended by something or feels disrespected by some of our behavior, we need to change our own behavior so that it is no longer offensive or apparently disrespectful. This is true even if we did not intend to be offensive. If we want to maintain a friendly, intimate relationship with the person making such a boundary request, we need to respect the request, even if it may seem foolish. We need to validate the other's feelings and needs, even though we did not intend to be hurtful.

Self-exploratory Question: How can I be more respectful of other peoples' emotional boundaries and limits?

Affirmation: I choose to respect others' boundaries, knowing mine also will be respected.

Principle: Taking periodic Time Out to play is just as important as taking necessary Adult Time Out when one is Hungry, Angry, Lonely, or Tired (H.A.L.T.)

Perennial Wisdom Quote: "'Suzanne will not be at school today,' I once wrote to her teacher. 'She stayed at home to play with her mother.' I don't remember many other days of her elementary years. But, I remember that day." -- Gloria Gaither

Discussion: Play is an important part of adult self-care, not just the self-care of children. Examine your most favorite memories of your own parents. Didn't many of these memories involve play? Mutual play involves shared joy, pleasure, companionship, appreciation, and growth.

Of course, parents need to do more than just play with their children. They need to establish limits for their children and teach their children how to value achievement and self-discipline. But they also need to take time to play. Parents need to take time to recreate with each other within a family context, as well as on a weekly couple "date."

The December 5 reading described five hours of vital couple interaction each week. Similarly, families need to take time to have adult-child interactions which keep awareness, understanding, appreciation and joy current among all family members. Families who have at least three sit-down meals together every week and who have at least one weekly family play time together tend to thrive. Some families set aside a special time each week to plan these occasions together, as well as to problem-solve and express their appreciations toward each other for ongoing shared chores and responsibilities.

Creative play often takes some forethought, although at times it is also spontaneous. It is the vital spice of life. Without it life becomes flat and alienating.

Self-exploratory Question: How can I be sure to take enough time-out-to-play?

Affirmation: I regularly take Time Out from work to play.

Principle: Holidays are meant to rejuvenate, to connect to loved ones and to remind ourselves of important priorities.

Perennial Wisdom Quote: "I learned to love the journey, not the destination. I learned that this is not a dress rehearsal, and that today is the only guarantee you get." -- Anna Quindlen

Discussion: A major challenge when preparing for modern holidays is finding ways to maintain balance, ways to stay focused on creating quality experiences in the present moment, while at the same time not neglecting preparation for the future. Sometimes it is helpful to sit down with one's family several weeks before a holiday and discuss ways the holiday celebration can be simplified and also made more satisfying for the entire family.

Gift-giving at Christmas, for example, can become so all-consuming that the joy and meaning of the celebration can be lost. Resentments and feelings of obligation can accumulate, rather than loving connection being reinforced. Take time to ask yourself: "What is most important about this holiday for me?" "What is most important about this holiday for other members of my family?" "How can I help to make this celebration both simple and deeply satisfying?" Rituals are important (see Dec. 21 reading), but rest and personal and family rejuvenation are also important.

Self-exploratory Question: How can I simplify holiday celebrations to make them more meaningful?

Affirmation: I value and create simple, heart connections during holidays.

Principle: Giving with strings attached never works out.

Perennial Wisdom Quote: Ninety-four-year-old father to his sixty-eight-year-old-son: "One day you wake up and realize that you're not eighty-one anymore. You begin to count the minutes, not the days, and you realize that you're not going to be around. All you have left is the experiences. That's all there is." -- from *Grumpy Old Men*

Discussion: The joy of giving -- of our time, our affection, our admiration, our appreciation, our material gifts, our experience, our wisdom -- is all there really is. We can give of this joy to ourselves, via our moment-to-moment experiences and memories. We can give of this joy to others, via our open-heartedness. We can give of this joy to others, via our examples and our creative efforts, which last beyond our lifetimes. What is most important is that we give with no expectations attached.

      If we give a material gift, we don't measure what we get in return. If we give of our time, we don't measure what time is given in return. If we give of our wisdom and creative efforts, we don't measure how these gifts are received by others. Instead we focus on the joyful experience of the giving itself, one moment at a time. The wisdom of our elders tells us that that's all we really can be sure of. None of us really knows how many of those moments we have.

Self-exploratory Question: How can I give more joyfully, with no expectations?

Affirmation: When I choose to give, it is from my heart with no strings attached.

Principle: Making choices which honor one's priorities takes time and attention.

Perennial Wisdom Quote: "Life does not have to be perfect to be wonderful." -- Annette Funicello

Discussion: Helen Hayes once said, "The story of a love is not important -- what is important is that one is capable of love. It is perhaps the only glimpse we are permitted of eternity."

Have you considered making a top priority of becoming more and more capable of love? Can you drop thoughts about each day's imperfections and instead focus on what was wonderful about each day? Joy exists in the moment, not through perfectly attending to the future.

It's helpful to take special time out at least once or twice a year to reexamine one's priorities. This can be done on a silent retreat or while quietly journaling. Review the last six to twelve months and ask yourself, "Am I making choices which honor my highest priorities? Do I need to make some changes in my life in order to better honor my values and priorities?" Take time later to share your musings with significant others, and ask for their support in helping you to honor your highest priorities.

Clarity and will power is important, and so is company. Perhaps Helen Hayes is right when she reminds us that the capacity to love and the sharing of love is our only real connection to "eternity."

Self-exploratory Question: How can I more effectively establish and honor my priorities?

Affirmation: Today I am honoring my highest priorities and values.

Principle: Sharing meaningful, healthy rituals enhances community.

Perennial Wisdom Quote: "The more you praise and celebrate your life, the more there is in life to celebrate." -- Oprah Winfrey

Discussion: It is natural to create rituals around beginnings, transitions, and endings in one's life. It is even natural to have rituals on a daily basis for these things, such as having a morning cup of tea, reading a newspaper, and brushing one's teeth. What is most important is creating shared, healthy meaning for our rituals and avoiding the creation of unhealthy rituals. For example, we need to avoid the solitary "nightcap" ritual which can create alcohol dependency, the cigarette with every cup of coffee ritual, which can lead to lung cancer, or engaging in addictive shopping around Christmas time.

We need to choose rituals which praise and celebrate life with others in a healthy way, such as attending a religious service once a week and/or attending a 12 Step meeting regularly, celebrating birthdays non-alcoholically with friends and family, and giving creative thought and honor to wedding and birth celebrations.

Malidoma Patrice Some, Ph.D. in *Ritual, Power, Healing and Community,* writes, "Where ritual is absent, the young ones are restless or violent, there are no real elders, and the grown-ups are bewildered." He recommends community support for ritualizing all major life transitions, such as birth, coming into adulthood, marriage, having one's first child, coming into elder-hood at age 50 or 60, and death.

Respecting the religious and cultural rituals of other groups is also important, even if we don't understand them and don't participate in them. As long as they have a praising and non-addictive, celebration function for others, they are valuable.

Self-exploratory Question: How can I create more meaningful ritual in my life?

Affirmation: I respect the place of healthy rituals in my own and others' lives.

Principle: Holidays can become depressing if we focus on past losses or future expectations.

Perennial Wisdom Quote: "The greater part of our happiness or misery depends on our dispositions and not on our circumstances." -- Martha Washington

Discussion: Dorothea Brand once said, "A complete holiday from self-pity is necessary to success." During holiday seasons there is a tendency to become tired and to create too high expectations for ourselves and others. When this happens, disappointment and self-pity is the inevitable result. There is also a tendency to eat too much sugar and create "sugar highs and lows." Food can be tasty without using a lot of sugar. Decorations can be beautiful without being elaborate or expensive.

Many religious people actually abstain from all food for twenty-four hours before a religious celebration as a way of cleansing themselves and heightening their awareness of the celebration. Many rituals focus on making births, transitions or deaths more meaningful. When approaching a holiday, ask yourself, "What is the essence of this celebration? How can I honor it in the most meaningful way?" This will likely bring more satisfaction than engaging in excessive eating or gift-giving behaviors which can lead to the "holiday blues."

Self-exploratory Question: How can I better avoid the "holiday blues?"

Affirmation: I honor holidays in conscious, meaningful, satisfying ways.

Principle: When I clarify my personal intentions and behaviorally follow them, my life becomes more satisfying.

Perennial Wisdom Quote: "You don't get to choose how you're going to die. Or when. You can decide how you're going to live now." -- Joan Baez

Discussion: Having clear intentions and clear priorities makes living a lot easier. Intentions are different from expectations and objectives. Expectations focus on the end results of behavior. Intentions focus on the process and principles of behavior. Objectives focus on external events, which are sometimes unmanageable. Intentions always focus on personal choices, priorities and principles. These are manageable and observable, at least in our own minds.

We can't know for sure about others' intentions, so we need never to assume what they are, especially if we are making negative assumptions about another's intentions. But we can clarify our own personal intentions, and we can share them with others. Then if our behavior leads to an unintended result, we can make amends for it and redirect our current behavior.

Writing down intentions in one's journal can be helpful, because then we can review our journal later and determine whether our behaviors were in line with our chosen intentions. Our intentions usually go along a "high road," but sometimes fear and ego-defenses lead us down behavioral "low roads." When this happens, we need to make amends and correct our behavior, so as to make our "high road" intentions more realizable.

Emily Dickinson once wrote, "If I can stop one heart from breaking, I shall not live in vain." What do you think of that intention? What do you intend to do with your life that will help you to realize, at your death, that you have not lived "in vain"?

Self-exploratory Question: How can I more consistently clarify my intentions?

Affirmation: I work to keep my personal intentions clear, honest, and principled.

Principle: Having close loving relationships is good for one's health.

Perennial Wisdom Quote: "It has been shown that enhancing emotional bonds between people will help heal the limbic system." -- Daniel G. Amen, M.D., *Change Your Brain, Change Your Life*

Discussion: Dr. Daniel Amen is a clinical neuroscientist, child and adolescent psychiatrist and medical director of the Amen Clinic for Behavioral Medicine in Fairfield, CA. In his popular book, *Change Your Brain, Change Your Life,* 1998, he lays out ten relational principles for improving our limbic brain systems and enhancing our emotional bonds:

1) Take responsibility for keeping our relationships strong;

2) Never take a relationship for granted;

3) Protect your primary relationships;

4) Assume the best for them;

5) Keep your primary relationships fresh;

6) Notice the good in them;

7) Communicate clearly;

8) Maintain and protect trust;

9) Deal with difficult issues; and

10) Make time for each other

When we take time to do these things, our brains as well as our relationships benefit.

Self-exploratory Question: How can I take better care of my relationships?

Affirmation: I place great importance on enhancing my primary relationships.

December 25   **Unconditional**
Love

Principle: Unconditional love is free, compassionate, completely in the present.

Perennial Wisdom Quote: "He has no ideas to teach, only presence. He has no doctrines to give, only the gift of his own freedom. Tolerant like the sky, all pervading like sunlight, firm like a mountain, supple like a branch in the wind, he has no destination in view and makes use of anything life happens to bring his way. Nothing is impossible for him. Because he has let go, he can care for the people's welfare as a mother cares for her child." -- Stephen Mitchell's description of Jesus in *The Gospel According to Jesus*

Discussion: Jesus taught his followers how to become like God -- "generous, compassionate, impartial, and serene." (Ibid). Remembering these teachings in the middle of a modern, secular Christmas celebration is not easy. Even the concept of "unconditional love" is difficult for most moderns to understand. To love another "with no strings attached," no expectations, no obligations, no contract, no past, and no future boggles most 21st century minds. It probably has boggled most human minds from the beginning of time. And yet this kind of love, this kind of loving existence is in harmony with the highest teachings of the *Upanishads*, the *Tao Te Ching*, the Buddhist sutras, the Zen, Sufi and Hasidic Masters and *The Bible*. This kind of love is seen as being in harmony with the very essence of the universe.

      This kind of love is most readily present when a person empties herself or himself of desires, doctrines, rules and all that separates a person from precious, present moments. Whatever Christmas has meant to you in the past, consider making it a celebration of this kind of consciousness. Consider doing everything you can to allow this kind of experience for yourself, for one moment, one hour, one day and call it "Christmas."

Self-exploratory Question: How can I deeply experience "Christ consciousness?"

Affirmation: I allow unconditional love to flow through me from a Higher Source.

Principle: Security is something we create inside our minds and our hearts, not our wallets.

Perennial Wisdom Quote: "Do not stop thinking of life as an adventure. You have no security unless you live bravely, excitingly, and imaginatively." -- Eleanor Roosevelt

Discussion: Helen Keller became deaf and blind at age two and yet graduated from Radcliffe. She once said, "Many persons have the wrong idea about what constitutes true happiness. It is not attained through self-gratification but through fidelity to a worthy cause."

When people long for security, they are usually longing for happiness and assuming that happiness will come when economic and political security has been achieved. Economic and political security are important, but they are no guarantee of happiness. The security of a happy heart is mostly created through consistently following one's own values and principles and through lovingly connecting with others. This kind of security may coincide with financial and political security, but it may not.

Financial and political security are sometimes external objectives which we can work toward but have no individual power to attain. This is why it is better to prioritize emotional and spiritual security. When that is established, often economic security follows as a natural outcome.

Self-exploratory Question: How can I prioritize emotional and spiritual security in my life?

Affirmation: I value emotional and spiritual security as the foundation for economic security.

Principle: Healthy brain functioning is necessary for healthy spirituality.

Perennial Wisdom Quote: "Our spirituality is influenced by how the brain functions. It has been my experience that, when the brain is healthy for people with religious beliefs, then God is experienced as loving, compassionate, forgiving, and present. When people struggle with brain problems, God is often perceived as angry, vengeful, controlling, rigid, judgmental, and distant." -- Daniel Amen, M.D., *Healing the Hardware of the Soul*

Discussion: Daniel Amen, M.D., in his popular book, *Change Your Brain, Change Your Life,* discusses how limbic brain functioning is enhanced by exercise and positive physical contact, as well as good nutrition, building positive memories, and spending time with positive people.

Our brains are not static. They are constantly being influenced by how we eat, how we exercise, what medications we take, what thoughts we dwell upon, what behaviors we choose and with whom we hang out. Daniel J. Siegel, M.D., in his book *The Developing Mind, How Relationships And The Brain Interact To Shape Who We Are,* makes similar points. Both psychiatrists are also doing pioneering research on the interactions between brain functioning and behavior. An overview of some of their basic educational material is given in Appendix 1.

All of the readings in this book have been geared toward principles which enhance brain functioning. The 12 Traditions of the Wise Ways Happiness Program are designed to enhance the likelihood that healthy, supportive relationships will form between people who attend Wise Ways Happiness Support Groups. Behavior impacts body. Body impacts behavior. Understanding these interactions is vital for learning how to live wisely.

Self-exploratory Question: How can I improve my brain functioning?

Affirmation: I make daily choices which help to maintain good brain functioning.

Principle: "Inner Guides" teach wisdom. Ego minds teach desire and power. Trust your "Inner Guide."

Perennial Wisdom Quote: "Confusion, anger, depression, violence, and conflict arise when humans forget who they are." – Eckhart Tolle, *Stillness Speaks,* page 46

Discussion: Eleanor Roosevelt said, "Happiness is not a goal. It is a by-product." It is a by-product of being consciously focused on the Now, living fully in each moment, attending to what one truly values. Happiness is a by-product of not giving in to petty desires to have everything we want and to control what happens around us.

Happiness involves trusting our inner guidance and finding security in knowing that we are being true to ourselves and not harmful to others. All the great spiritual teachers of the world have taught the importance of stillness, of listening to one's own inner guidance. Eckhart Tolle, author of *Stillness Speaks* (2003), brilliantly describes the limitations of ego-centric thinking, as well as the importance of dis-identifying from our ego-centric thoughts. He affirms: "I am not my thoughts, emotions, sense perceptions, and experiences. I am not the content of my life. I am Life. I am the space in which all things happen. I am consciousness. I am the Now. I Am (page 47)."

This kind of self-identity frees us from suffering, from attachment to what our egos desire. This kind of self-identity speaks through one's "Inner Guide" and allows a person to embrace Life itself, whatever it brings moment to moment.

Self-exploratory Question: How can I deepen my trust in my own "Inner Guide" and observe my ego-mind, but not give in to its desires and grasping's?

Affirmation: My Inner Guide is loving, kind, and trustworthy. It is part of the Now of Life.

Principle: Periodically reviewing one's priorities helps to maintain a value-based, principled life.

Perennial Wisdom Quote: "There are no shortcuts to any place worth going." -- Beverly Sills

Discussion: Ayn Rand put it this way: "Happiness is that state of consciousness which proceeds from the achievement of one's values." Unfortunately, recently in the United States, "value education" has taken on an exclusive religious tone in many segments of the culture. Other nations even have become fearful of the U.S. as a "superpower," worrying that it will force exclusive Christian or exclusive American political structures onto other nations, all as an umbrella for its desire to maintain hegemony over other nations. Perhaps there are some segments of the U.S. population who are willing, out of fear, to use force in this fashion. In general, however, the U.S. Constitution and the U.S. population are committed to free, democratic choice and not desirous of an international empire.

U.S. leadership and individual U.S. citizens need to convince many parts of the world that they are trustworthy and respectful, not self-centered and greedy. In order for the U.S. to do this, each of us needs to start with reviewing our own values and priorities and targeting ways to make our own efforts more effective. We also need to find ways, as a U.S. culture, to balance individuality with harmonious family life and community. All this will take time and individual effort, one person at a time.

Self-exploratory Question: How can I create time to periodically review my priorities?

Affirmation: I take time to periodically review my priorities and align my behavior with them.

Principle: Rest and renewal allow us to follow our highest priorities.

Perennial Wisdom Quote: "You cannot belong to anyone else until you belong to yourself." -- Pearl Bailey

Discussion: Lao Tze, famous Taoist teacher and author of the *Tao Te Ching*, wrote: "The Tao nourishes by not forcing. By not dominating, the Master leads." When we begin to contemplate New Year's resolutions, we need to keep in mind the principle of leading without forcing. We need to lead ourselves into clearer principles, higher values, and better behaviors. At the same time, we can't force these changes on ourselves or on others. We can clarify our highest intentions and reinforce ourselves when we move closer toward them. We also need to take time to rest and renew ourselves.

As the end of this year approaches, find time to quietly renew your inner resources as well as renew your contacts with loved ones. Rather than celebrating the New Year by getting drunk or getting lost in a crowd, consider celebrating it quietly and soberly, yet joyfully, with those dearest to you. Take some time to contemplate the past year and journal about it, as well as look toward the coming year. Appreciate your loved ones and all the highlights of your last year and share your hopes for the upcoming one. Celebrate with family and/or friends in a way you will remember with gratitude a year from now. Enter the New Year with vigor and joyfulness.

Self-exploratory Question: How can I better balance rest and renewal with celebration?

Affirmation: I take regular time for rest and renewal.

Principle: Stick with "the winners," because company is usually stronger than will power.

Perennial Wisdom Quote: "People are like stained-glass windows. They sparkle and shine when the sun is out, but when the darkness sets in their true beauty is revealed only if there is a light from within." -- Elizabeth Kubler-Ross

Discussion: If we want to have happy, ethical, emotionally and interpersonally satisfying lives, we need to seek people who are practicing these kinds of lives, and we need to hang out with them as much as possible. We need to be ethical, emotionally and interpersonally knowledgeable, and loving persons ourselves. At the end of the year, a possible New Year's resolution might be to "spend as much time as possible with persons I admire, appreciate, and want to emulate." Another resolution might be to "become a person whom I can admire and appreciate." One way to actualize those intentions would be to spend New Year's Eve with these kinds of people and be this kind of person yourself all during New Year's Day.

Self-exploratory Questions: How can I better surround myself with people I like, admire and appreciate? How can I be that kind of person myself?

Affirmation: My friends and associates are ethical, emotionally and interpersonally knowledgeable, loving people.

Principle: True religion is non-competitive, teaching from a compassionate heart, not a competitive mind.

Perennial Wisdom Quote: "Dig as deep as you will, you will never come to a thing called Tao or God. Tao is not a thing…Tao is the law of all things, of all events. Tao is the common ground of all creation." -- John Heider, *The Tao of Leadership,* page 1

Discussion: True religion is easily corrupted by a competitive mind. When a person starts thinking "My God is better than your God" it is a clear sign that that person's religion has become corrupted by a competitive mind. All the great teachers of the world have taught about how God (the Tao, Higher Power, the Great Spirit, the Goddess, etc.) manifests in all of creation and in all that happens in our lives. All the great teachers have taught about how those who would be first will end up last, about how over-determined behavior produces its opposite.

This is why talking about "my God" versus "your God" makes no sense. It is just a frail human mind trying to identify with God and in so doing actually becoming unlike God. As John Heider says, "Tao has no opposites or polarities. Tao is one; Tao is unity" (Ibid, page 7.) When human beings forget this principle of unity which is God and speak competitively and possessively about "their God" or religion, they actually separate themselves from God's principles. They become un-godly.

When we are truly spiritual, we see God in all beings and do not compete for righteousness. We do not judge or put down others' religions. (For a bumper sticker saying "Coexist" showing signs of major world religions go to www.peacemonger.org.)

Self-exploratory Question: Can I see and respect God in all beings, all things, all events?

Affirmation: I see God in everything and do not compete for righteousness.

APPENDIX ONE

BRAIN AND HEART FUNCTIONING RELATED TO HAPPINESS

The Brain: We now know that the brain has a lot of "plasticity". In other words, it is capable of forming new neurons all the time, not just during the early years of childhood.

This is both good and bad news. The good news is that we can change brain functioning even up through our senior years. Learning new tasks, including different ways of managing our emotional and behavioral responses to life, can considerably improve brain functioning at any age.

The bad news is that there is such a thing as "negative plasticity" as well as "positive plasticity". If an individual engages in repetitive behaviors which are damaging to the brain, such as alcohol and drug abuse, irresponsible emotional outbursts and violent behavior, these behaviors create brain patterns which are hard to break. Our thoughts and behavioral choices from day to day impact the way our brain organizes and functions. This is why it is so important to reinforce healthy thoughts and behavioral choices.

What we think, what we do, how we interact with others, all impacts how our brains function. Our brains are growing and changing all the time. The daily choices we make and the people we choose to interact with make a huge difference to that part of our body which guides and directs us every day. There is a "feedback loop" which can be either positive or negative. It's up to us.

Daniel Siegel, M.D., defines the mind as "a process that regulates the flow of energy and information…. It is a verb, not a noun." He adds that "the mind emerges in the transactions of neurobiological processes and interpersonal relationships. The mind develops as the genetically programmed maturation of the nervous system is shaped by ongoing experience." In other words, experience shapes its development. We can "change our minds." As we change our minds, learn Wise Ways Happiness principles and develop more and more "brain fitness," life can become more and more satisfying.

All systems within the brain are intricately interconnected. When one system is affected, usually the others are also affected. Different brain researchers label the systems somewhat differently, but the illustration on the next page generally reflects the understandings of modern neurologists and psychiatrists. If you are interested in learning more about the brain, it is recommended that you read Dr. Daniel Siegel's *The Developing Mind* and Dr. Daniel Amen's *Change Your Brain, Change Your Life.*

New brain research is being advanced every day with the use of new technology such as SPECT tests, functional MRIs and "Referenced EEGs." EEG studies are done in conjunction with a normative database and a clinical database in order to identify abnormal brain activity and to make recommendations for treatment.

A Diagram of the Human Brain

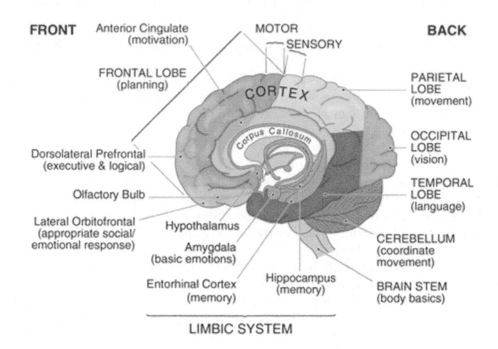

FRONT   Anterior Cingulate (motivation)   MOTOR   SENSORY   BACK

FRONTAL LOBE (planning)

CORTEX

Corpus Callosum

PARIETAL LOBE (movement)

OCCIPITAL LOBE (vision)

Dorsolateral Prefrontal (executive & logical)

Olfactory Bulb

TEMPORAL LOBE (language)

Lateral Orbitofrontal (appropriate social/ emotional response)

Hypothalamus

Amygdala (basic emotions)

Entorhinal Cortex (memory)

Hippocampus (memory)

CEREBELLUM (coordinate movement)

BRAIN STEM (body basics)

LIMBIC SYSTEM

Different Brain Systems, Their Functions and Potential Problems

The **cortex** of the brain plays a very significant role in the brain's ability to change cognitive responses. The **prefrontal cortex** occupies the front third of the brain underneath the forehead and is the most evolved part of the brain. It helps us to watch, supervise, sustain attention, direct and focus our goals and our behaviors. It is involved in such things as time management, judgment, impulse control, planning, organization, critical thinking, and learning from mistakes. It has two hemispheres which are connected by the cingulate gyrus. (The cingulate gyrus is sometimes considered part of the limbic system. See below for more information.)

The prefrontal cortex has many connections to the limbic system (the emotional center of the brain) and is responsible for sending inhibitory messages that help to keep the limbic system under control. Symptoms of prefrontal cortex problems include distractibility, impulse control problems, hyperactivity, Attention Deficit Disorder (ADD), poor time management, disorganization, procrastination, poor judgment, difficulty accessing feelings, trouble learning from experience, short-term memory problems, and social and text anxiety. People with ADD have difficulty achieving sufficient stimulation of their prefrontal cortex and sometimes unconsciously seek conflict as a way to achieve this stimulation. They don't plan to do it, but their prefrontal cortexes crave more activity. Appropriate medications such as Ritalin and cognitive/behavioral therapy to purposefully change thoughts and behaviors can correct many of these problems. Studying and practicing the principles outlined in this book can help to positively change thoughts and behaviors. Brain-wave (EEG) biofeedback training as well as Heartmath biofeedback and stress management computer program training (see www.heartmath.com) are other resources for managing ADD symptoms.

Psychotic disorders occurring in schizophrenia and manic-depressive illness also show up on SPECT brain studies with disturbed prefrontal cortex activity. Appropriate medications and cognitive/behavioral psychotherapy are vital in correcting these problems.

The non-dominant side (hemisphere) of the cortex is usually the right side. It develops first in a child. It processes awareness of facial movements, tones of voice, eye contacts, postures, gestures, rhythms, music, and non-verbal, visual learning in general. Two to three years after birth, the right side of the brain also becomes capable of storing autobiographical information and seeing an integrated map of the body. Problems with the non-dominant side of the cortex result in difficulty recognizing facial expressions, decoding vocal intonation, and developing interpersonal and social skills. Autism is related to problems in this side of the brain.

The **dominant, usually left side of the cortex,** begins developing at about age two years and continues developing at a rapid rate for at least ten years. After that it develops less slowly. It is essential for logical, verbal processes and right/wrong and abstract thinking, intermediate and long-term memory, auditory learning, retrieval of words, complex memories and emotional stability. The left side of the cortex receives information from the limbic system (the lower brain including the amygdala, hippocampus and cingulated gyrus) and sends information back to the limbic system, at least when the brain is working well. This is what allows for the gradual formation of "good judgment" and "impulse control." When the left temporal lobe has problems, people have reading and auditory processing difficulties and are more prone to temper outbursts, irritability, rapid mood shifts, suicidal ideation, memory and learning problems and sometimes even violence and/or paranoia. People with left hemisphere abnormalities can be sensitive to slights and even seem mildly paranoid, appearing to have personality disorders.

Temporal lobe difficulties (both sides of the cortex) can result due to genetics, head injuries and exposure to toxic or infectious materials (either in utero or after birth). Some medications, such as Depakote for aggressive behavior and Ritalin for ADD, as well as cognitive/behavioral and biofeedback therapy can be helpful with these problems. Temporal lobe dysfunction is not an excuse for violence and lawlessness, but it certainly needs to be considered and treated if we want jail populations and suicides to diminish rather than increase. Decreased temporal lobe functioning is also involved in Alzheimer's disease and can be diagnosed early on a SPECT test so that new medications can be used to slow down the progression of this debilitating disease.

It is vital that educators understand temporal lobe functioning and design their **educational curricula** accordingly. Usually a child can't learn until about ages 5-10 that emotions change how you think, that things aren't always how they seem, and different people can have different points of view. These lessons need to be stressed during elementary school years.

At pre-puberty, ages 10-11, a child's learning potential jumps briefly, and this is an important time to educate children about the brain. At puberty (usually starting at age 11-13) the pre-frontal cortex goes "off-line for several years" while it is reorganizing itself for adulthood. (Read *The Primal Teen* for more information about this.) Including brain functioning and drug abuse information in grades 5-8 is vital in order to decrease the likelihood of the puberty years becoming destructive. The use of alcohol and drugs during ages 13-25 is especially destructive because these are the years when the brain is reconstructing itself for adulthood and is temporarily quite disorganized. Even marijuana (frequently seen by teens as less dangerous than alcohol) during these years is toxic to the brain. Students in grades 5-8 need to understand this on a biological level. Dr. Seigel suggests telling middle school children, "If you must drink or use drugs, wait until you are at least 25 years old because by that time your brain will be developed sufficiently to withstand the toxins better. Using alcohol and street drugs before age 25 can seriously derail the healthy development of your brain."

Dr. Seigel also recommends teaching the labeling of emotions and good internal "self-talk" to middle school children. This tends to balance right and left hemisphere functioning. Learning to use language to identify and express emotions calms over-activity in the right hemisphere, which can be a major problem in adolescence. People with under-developed, left hemisphere functioning become flooded by right hemisphere, irrelevant information and can't filter or organize it well. The left hemisphere is the part of the brain which can ask, "What am I feeling right now?" "What do I need right now?" "What do I need to do to get my message across?" "What are my automatic thoughts in response to this feeling?" "Do I need to change my automatic thoughts?" "What behavioral choices will likely have the best results right now?" When this hemisphere is underdeveloped and/or not well connected with the amygdala (lower brain), chaotic thoughts and behaviors occur.

Fortunately, left hemisphere functioning can be improved with good motivation and training and with empathic dialoguing with trained volunteers.

The left brain hemisphere also pulls biographical information out of the right hemisphere and puts it together logically and coherently. Therefore, what Dr. Seigel calls "a coherent personal narrative" requires bi-lateral brain integration. When this integration is still underdeveloped, listening to the personal stories of respected adults and listening to coherent, meaningful stories from high functioning peers can be very helpful. Peer counseling in middle schools and adult volunteers who come in to read inspirational stories, or, better yet, share their own inspirational stories, can be very helpful to children whose brain hemispheres are still not well coordinated. Assigning autobiographical writing, and reinforcing attendance in Wise Ways Happiness Support Groups for teens can also be helpful. By sharing life experiences in such safe groups, a puberty child will have a much better chance of developing a coherent, positive narrative about his or her life.

Recent research has also shown how important having a "coherent, positive narrative" about one's life is to effective parenting. Using *365 Wise Ways to Happiness* with parent support groups in teen treatment centers can help parents to develop such narratives.

Research using this book to help prison inmates to develop coherent, positive life narratives has not yet been done. Likely active participation in Wise Ways Happiness Support Groups while in prison would, not only improve inmates' parenting skills, but also reduce their recidivism rates. There is also a *Wise Ways For Teens* book available through contacting Deborah Stamm, M.S. in Anchorage, Alaska.

Other behavioral approaches to improving temporal lobe functioning include: humming, singing, listening to classical music, dancing, drumming, getting enough sleep, eliminating caffeine and nicotine, improving nutrition, participating in psychological self-examination, learning about ancient wisdom traditions, participating in psychotherapy, facilitating trustworthy and supportive relationships, using EEG biofeedback, and taking up a creative course or hobby.

The **cingulate gyrus** is the part of the brain that runs longitudinally through the central deep aspects of the frontal lobes. It allows a person to shift attention from thought to thought and between behaviors. When this part of the brain is overactive, people have problems getting stuck in certain chains of behaviors or thoughts. Their cognitive flexibility is diminished. They tend to hold onto hurts or grudges, worry, obsess and become emotionally rigid. Some anti-depressant medications such as Zoloft or Prozac or Cymbalta can decrease activity in the cingulate gyrus and help people to shift their attention more freely between topics and become less stuck in depressive thoughts and behaviors. Anafranil, Paxil, Effexor, Serzone, Remeron, Desyrel and Luvox are some medications sometimes effective in healing problems in this part of the brain as well as the basal ganglia. Taking one of these medications for at least a year, while also practicing Wise Ways Happiness principles, can heal over-activity here. Balanced functioning in the cingulate gyrus allows people to set reasonable goals, plan more flexibly and participate in cooperative modes of behavior.

According to Dr. Amen, individuals suffering from hair pulling, nail biting, Tourette's syndrome, kleptomania, body dimorphic disorder (feeling that a part of the body is excessively ugly), hypochondria, autism, compulsive shopping, pathological gambling, chronic pain, addictive disorders, eating disorders, and oppositional defiant disorders usually have problems with this part of their brains. He also reports that he has seen a significant connection, in his practice and research, between a family history of alcoholism and increased activity in the cingulate gyrus. Persons with such a history should abstain from alcohol completely and possibly use one of the above medications to help improve the functioning in the cingulate gyrus parts of their brains.

Having supportive healthy relationships is also important for the healthy functioning of the brain. Naomi Eisenberger and Matthew Lieberman, two UCLA social psychologists, recently found that when 13 UCLA students were intentionally snubbed by their peers as a part of the research project, their anterior cingulate cortexes became more and more active (engorged with blood and redder and redder the longer and stronger they felt snubbed). It was previously known that this part of the brain registers physical pain, and now we know that it also registers emotional distress (*Los Angeles Times* report on Dec. 21, 2003).

Providing safe, supportive learning environments which disallow snubbing and bullying and providing appropriate medication and therapy for some children with cingulate gyrus problems, is a necessity in order to prevent the need for more socially costly remedies for acting-out, future adults.

Higher serotonin levels in the brain can decrease an overactive cingulate gyrus. These levels can be raised naturally with carbohydrate foods such as pastas, bread, potatoes, pastries, pretzels and popcorn. All these foods increase the natural amino acid, l-tryptophan, which is a building block for serotonin. Milk, chicken, turkey, salmon, beef, peanut butter, green peas, potatoes and eggs also are high in l-tryptophan. People with cravings for carbohydrates often have a low serotonin level in their brains and can benefit by taking an anti-depressant medication such as Prozac or Zoloft and by increasing their intake of non-carbohydrate foods high in l-tryptophan, rather than overeating on carbohydrates and causing weight gain. All these dietary issues need to be assertively addressed in public school kitchens as another help to children with cingulate gyrus problems.

Persons who have had traumas to the head and concussions can also develop serious behavioral problems due to brain dysfunctions. Anti-seizure and anti-obsessive, anti-depressant medications can help these problems when they are properly diagnosed.

The **limbic system** of the brain is the emotional powerhouse of the brain. It is the bonding and mood control center of the brain. This part of the brain filters external events through internal states, stores highly charged emotional memories, controls appetite and sleep cycles, directly processes the sense of smell, tags events as internally important, and modulates motivation and libido. When this part of the brain is over-active, people struggle with moodiness and negativity. When the limbic system is less active, a person's state of mind is generally positive and hopeful. Sexual orgasm is a "mini-seizure of the limbic system and tends to release or lessen deep limbic activity." (Amen, page 41) This is one reason why humans have an increased sense of wellbeing after sexual orgasm. This is also why sexuality can become addictive if a person does not know other ways of lessening deep limbic activity. Moderate, healthy, sexual activity can help to reduce limbic system over-activity when practiced in line with healthy relationship choices.

When the limbic system is over-active, emotions tend to take over and depression can ensue, shutting down access to the prefrontal cortex. People with overactive limbic systems tend to lose their appetites and have trouble sleeping even when they are chronically tired. Anti-depressant medications increase certain neurotransmitters in the brain (norepinephrine and serotonin) and this, in turn, decreases the metabolism or inflammation of the deep limbic system. Using behavioral approaches (through psychotherapy and/or group support) for decreasing automatic negative thoughts also decreases over-activity in the deep limbic system. Mark George, M.D. from the National Institute of Mental Health did excellent research showing how thinking happy thoughts lowers the metabolism in the deep limbic system and having sad thoughts increases its activity. When the limbic system has lower metabolism, more activation is possible in the cortex, and sleep, mood and appetite generally all improve.

The limbic system is near the center of the brain, resting in a ring above the brain stem and between the brain stem and the cortex. It is made up of the following parts:

1) The **amygdala**: The amygdala is the main processing area for memories which have emotional impacts. It plays an integral role in shaping the perceptions of interactions between people. The amygdala also is responsible for storing implicit (unconscious) information about trauma and loss. It forms earlier than the hippocampus and is involved in infant attachment. The amygdala implicitly encodes experiences and emotionally biases perception. It is involved in fear responses. The cortex is designed to regulate the amygdala, but emotional trauma and loss and alcohol abuse can result in a disconnect between the amygdala and the cortex, which results in emotionally unaware, behavioral reactions. Anxiety comes about when the fear system in the amygdala breaks loose from its cortical controls.

The good news is that, with attention, direction and sometimes medication, the negative effects on the brain of past traumas and losses can be considerably healed. When children can heal emotional damage to their brains, they can have more satisfying adult lives. When adults can heal damage to their brains, they can stop passing on their damage to their children and others.

2) The **hippocampus**: The hippocampus is involved (along with the cortex) in the control and regulation of learning. It is the brain's primary explicit (conscious) memory center. It is not fully developed until an infant is about 18-24 months old. It integrates external and internal sensations. When the body is not traumatized, the hippocampus sends memories to the cortex. During a traumatic situation or an alcohol binge the hippocampus does not do this, and a memory "blackout" happens. Also, if the hippocampus is storing unresolved trauma information, it will bias the perceptual

information it passes on to the cortex. This will make it more difficult for the cortex to have wise perceptions and direct wise decisions.

    3) The **corpus collasum** links the right and left hemispheres of the cortex. The biggest growth in this part of the brain is between the ages of 3 and 7. Educational instruction needs to keep in mind individual brain development, as well as general stages of brain development. The task of learning to read can only effectively begin after the corpus collasum has sufficiently developed. This can happen for healthy children any time between the ages of 3 and 7. Trying to teach a child to read before this part of the brain has developed is not wise.

Other parts of the brain

The **thalamus** is the gland which picks up incoming sensory messages (except smell) and relays them to the appropriate centers in the brain. Its job is to make sense of the body's constant sensory bombardment.

The **hypothalamus** receives messages from the thalamus and sends them to bodily muscles, organs and the cortex. It controls the sleep and appetite cycles of the body.

The **pituitary** is a pea-sized gland that directs the entire endocrine system. It receives messages from the hypothalamus and helps the body to produce the hormones it needs to respond to different situations.

The **cerebellum** is behind the brain stem and controls movement and "muscle memory."

The **brain stem** regulates basic body function such as heartbeat and breathing.

The **basal ganglia** are large structures deep within the brain which control the body's idling speed. When this part of the brain works too hard, anxiety, panic, fearfulness and conflict avoidance can result. People can become overwhelmed by stressful situations and have a tendency to freeze or become immobile in thoughts or actions. People who are chronically irritable or angry often have left-sided basal ganglia problems. Mood stabilizers such as Lithium, Tegretol, or Depakote can be helpful in calming down the over-functioning of the basal ganglia. The benzodiazepine anti-anxiety medications such as Valium, Xanax, Ativan, Serax and Tranxene are addictive and should be avoided for everything but occasional, severe panic attacks. BuSpar is not addictive and can be effective in treating long-term anxiety. It also can have calming effects on aggressive behavior. Workaholism can also be created by over-functioning basal ganglia. These people have their internal idling speed set too high, and their energy levels don't allow them to rest.

Behavioral techniques such as guided imagery, diaphragmatic breathing, combating automatic negative thoughts, mindfulness meditation, self-hypnosis, and learning how to deal with conflict all can have a positive effect on the functioning of the basal ganglia. Spreading one's nutritious food intake out throughout the day to prevent hypoglycemic episodes can also improve basal ganglia over-activity. Eliminating caffeine and alcohol, both of which can aggravate anxiety, is also helpful. (Alcohol in small doses decreases anxiety, but in large doses it increases anxiety, especially during withdrawal. Its chronic use also leads to insomnia, which upsets entire brain functioning. Caffeine in large doses is addictive and increases irritability and hyperactivity.)

When the basal ganglia are under-active, people struggle with concentration and fine motor control problems and sometimes develop Attention Deficit Disorder (ADD). People with ADD often have poor handwriting due to difficulty with fine motor coordination. Psycho-stimulant medications such as Ritalin, Dexedrine or Adderall increase the production of the neurotransmitter dopamine in the basal ganglia and increase their activity. (These medications taken by people who already have well-functioning or over-functioning basal ganglia can lead to increased panic and anxiety.)

The basal ganglia also integrate feeling and movement, enhance motivation, suppress unwanted motor behaviors, and mediate pleasure. People with Parkinson's disease and Tourette's syndrome have a deficiency of dopamine in the basal ganglia.

Gender Differences

Recent research has shown that females in general have larger deep limbic systems than males. This explains why it is generally easier for them to get in touch with and express their feelings, as well as bond with and be emotionally connected with others. It also explains why, for females, it is more difficult for them to experience sex as just recreational, rather than bonding. This also explains why men and women and teens need to learn why it is best not to be sexual, unless they want to be emotionally bonded with and committed to a partner.

Dr. Amen has found that over-activity in the deep limbic system, especially on the left side, can correlate with cyclical tendencies toward depression and irritability. This part of the brain has a higher density of estrogen receptors than other parts of the brain, so it is vulnerable in some women, causing serious "PMS" symptoms of irritability. Anti-depressant medication can sometimes be helpful with this irritability, as can some herbal remedies.

The amygdala, according to Louann Brizendine, M.D., author of *The Female Brain,* is larger in men. She calls it the "instinctual core" which can only be tamed by the pre-frontal cortex. Perhaps this, along with social and cultural influences, helps to explain why men tend to be more violent than women.

Dr. Brizendine also points out that the hypothalamus, which she calls "the conductor of the hormonal symphony," starts pumping earlier for girls than for boys, helping to explain why girls tend to reach puberty before boys.

The hippocampus, involved with memory, is larger and more active in women than in men, again according to Dr. Brizendine. She suggests this may be why women tend to remember "a fight, a romantic encounter or a tender moment" better than men.

The prefrontal cortex, which is responsible for putting the brakes on the amygdala and keeping one's emotions from running wild, is somewhat larger in women than in men. It also matures faster in women by one to two years. This does not mean that women are necessarily smarter than men. It does possibly explain why many women are less violent than men.

The anterior cingulated cortex, which weighs options and makes decisions, is also larger in women than in men. Dr. Brizendine hypothesizes that this may be responsible for the fact that women tend to "worry" more than men.

The pituitary gland in women produces hormones of fertility, milk production and nurturing behavior. This production is stimulated by holding an infant and nursing an infant. When a man holds an infant, his pituitary gland can also be stimulated to produce hormones which promote nurturing behavior.

Some Common Causes of Brain Damage

Alcohol use by a pregnant woman can have a devastating effect on the developing brain of a fetus, even in such small amounts as one to two drinks a week. Drinking in

the first trimester can lead to malformations of the face. Drinking in the second trimester can interrupt new nerve formations in the brain. During the third trimester alcohol consumption can kill existing neurons and interfere with nervous system development.

Recent brain research has shown that alcohol actually causes more extensive damage on a fetus than even cocaine or crack heroin. MRI research has shown that alcohol use damages the corpus callosum, the band of nerve fibers that connects the left and right hemispheres of the brains of fetuses. The frontal lobes of **fetal alcohol effect and fetal alcohol syndrome children** are also often smaller than other children. Some children are more affected by the alcohol consumption of their mothers than others. Researchers still do not know why. According to the National Institute on Alcohol Abuse and Alcoholism, alcohol "is the leading cause of birth defects due to an ingested environmental substance in this country."

Chronic, heavy alcohol use in adults over many years can lead to what is called adult **"wet brain."** Every time a drinker has a "blackout" (i.e. loses memory while drinking, but does not necessarily lose consciousness) brain cells are destroyed. Enough of this destruction can eventually cause "wet brain." Symptoms of "wet brain" are similar to other forms of dementia among elders, so the syndrome is sometimes not properly diagnosed.

Every year hundreds of college students die of **alcohol poisoning** from binge drinking. Every year thousands of people die of alcoholism and resulting impaired judgment. Most of the hundreds of thousands of people in U.S. prisons are there because of alcohol and drug related impairments. All of society pays for these incarcerations and yet alcohol taxes are still resisted to help pay for all these alcohol-related societal problems.

Various forms of accidents, some, of course non-alcohol related, also can injure the brain. Much brain damage is also caused by warfare which is socially sanctioned.

Anyone suffering from any form of brain trauma or toxicity should always have a complete medical exam to determine the extent of the damage and possible treatment options. The good news is that the brain, if treated soon enough, can often repair itself. The bad news is that extensive damage to the brain often cannot be repaired.

The Heart: Less research has been done on the impact of heart functioning on human happiness levels than on the impact of brain functioning on human happiness levels. We do know, however, that emotional stress negatively impacts the heart by causing its beating rhythms to become more irregular and faster. There are new biofeedback devices now available (from www.heartmath.com in California) which can help individuals to learn how to manage stress more effectively. We know that the heart is not just a pump necessary to oxygenate the brain's blood flow. It also secretes hormones which interact with hormones secreted in the brain and in other organs of the body. The HeartMath Institute of California is doing some exciting new research and publishing some good books both for adult and teen consumption. Their emphasis at this time is on teaching people how to maintain more "coherent," rhythmic, heart beats which are associated with optimal brain functioning. More research clearly needs to be done on the interactions between heart and brain functioning.

APPENDIX TWO
WISE WAYS HAPPINESS SUPPORT GROUP
MEETING FORMAT GUIDELINES

Instructions for Chairperson: Chairperson roles are voluntary and rotate so that this service is shared. Usually the chairperson selects the sharing topic and the relevant readings from our book.

It is recommended that a new group start with Step Study, using Appendix 4 for an overview of the Steps. Afterwards the group can proceed to broader topics.

The Chairperson is responsible for doing her or his best to provide time for everyone to share for at least five minutes. If the group is too large for this, the Chairperson can begin the sharing and then call on people who raise their hands to share.

The Chairperson can optionally also call on the next person to share, and then ask each new sharer to call on the next person. Another option is for the chairperson to declare the topic completely "Open" to whatever is uppermost on each person's heart and mind, using our book's Subject index to find a relevant reading.

Generally, the sharing period lasts about 45-60 minutes. The chairperson is always responsible to make sure there are no interruptions or "cross talk" and that the meeting begins and ends on time.

Meeting Preamble (Read by the Chairperson)

"Hello, Welcome to the __(location of the group)_____ Wise Ways Happiness Support Group meeting. My name is (first name only)____and I am volunteering to be your chairperson today. We will now begin the group with a minute of silence.

"Now we will go around our circle and introduce ourselves by our first names only. If this is your first group meeting, please let us know so we can welcome you and get to know you better. My name is _____.

"Wise Ways Happiness Support Groups are a fellowship of persons gathered together to study perennial wisdom and positive psychology principles. We believe that happiness is an inside job and that changed attitudes and perceptions can lead to greater life satisfaction. Wise Ways Happiness Support Groups are not allied with any sect, or denomination, political cause or organization. We do not engage in any controversy. We gather together for the sole purpose of personal growth and interpersonal fellowship, support, and service. There are no dues for membership. Our groups are self-supporting through voluntary contributions.

"At our group meetings we keep the focus on ourselves -- our own attitudes, perceptions and behaviors. We do not gossip, question each other or cross talk in meetings. We take turns sharing, and we stay focused on studying Wise Ways Happiness principles as they apply to our lives. We start and end our meetings on time. We introduce ourselves by our first names only before we speak, and we conclude our sharing with "I pass." We listen in silence. We are free to "pass" and not speak."

Reading the Steps and Traditions

"We will now go around the circle, each of us reading one of the 12 Wise Ways Happiness Steps and 12 Happiness Support Groups' Traditions" as follows:

THE 12 STEPS OF WISE WAYS HAPPINESS SUPPORT GROUPS

1. Humility

We humbly give up our fearful escapes from awareness and our reactive attempts to control others.

2. Love

We become willing to accept reality and to connect our low brains to our high brains, surrendering to love, not to fear.

3. Trust

We learn to trust a Higher Power or energy of our own understanding, One which supports life, love, beauty, harmony, freedom and diversity.

4. Honest Self-Assessment

We make honest assessments of our assets and our shortcomings.

5. Self- Disclosure

We share our self-inventories with our Higher Powers, and confidentially with a loving, accepting other, without self-recrimination or shame.

6. Letting Go

We continue strengthening our assets and letting go of our shortcomings.

7. Emotional Connection

We humbly let go of our pride and reach out of our emotional isolation to lovingly connect to others.

8. Self - Forgiveness

We learn self-forgiveness and how to make amends to others and to ourselves for our past mistakes.

9. Making Amends

We make direct amends, whenever possible, to those we have harmed, except when to do so would harm others.

10. Continual Honesty

We continue honest, daily self-examination, and when mistakes are found, we promptly admit them.

11. Prayer and Meditation

We seek, through prayer and meditation, to improve our conscious contact with a Higher Power, praying for guidance and the will and strength to carry it out.

12. Service and Continued Practice

Having had a spiritual awakening as the result of these steps, wo commit to practicing these happiness principles in all our affairs and sharing them with others.

THE 12 TRADITIONS OF WISE WAYS HAPPINESS SUPPORT GROUPS

1. Unity and Respect for the Common Welfare: Unity and respect for the common welfare of the group promotes individual progress for the greatest number of members.

2. Maintaining Anonymity, Confidentiality and Trust: Personal anonymity and confidentiality (use of first names and last initials only at meetings, and respect for confidential sharing) are the foundations of trust within the Happiness Program.

3. Clear Purpose and Mutual Support: The primary purpose of Wise Ways Happiness Support Group meetings is to study the happiness principles in this book and to support each other in the practice of these principles.

4. Autonomous Support Groups: Each Wise Ways Happiness Support Group

is autonomous.

5. <u>Group Leaders are Trusted Servants:</u> Group leaders are but trusted, elected servants. They do not govern, nor have more status than any other group member.

6. <u>Group Membership:</u> Group membership is based on attendance at meetings and on commitment to practicing the Wise Ways Happiness Steps and Traditions.

7. <u>Self-supporting Groups:</u> Wise Ways Happiness Support Groups are always self-supporting.

8. <u>Principles, Not Personalities:</u> In Wise Ways Happiness Support Groups principles are always more important than personalities.

9. <u>Group Decisions:</u> Wise Ways Happiness Support Group

decisions are made by a "group conscious" meeting, ideally by a

consensus of the group at the meeting.

10. <u>No Other Group Affiliations:</u> Wise Ways Happiness Support Groups have

no other affiliation and neither endorse, finance, nor lend their

names to any other enterprise, lest problems of money or prestige

divert them from their primary purpose. Professionally facilitated

Wise Ways Happiness Counseling Groups have permission to use

the Wise Ways Happiness name as long as they are using this book

for their meetings.

11. <u>No Official Fellowship Opinions on Outside Issues:</u> The Wise Ways

Happiness Support Groups have no opinion on outside issues so

their names aren't drawn into public controversy.

12. <u>Public Relations Policy:</u> The Wise Ways Happiness Support Groups

may sell this book at their cost. Their principle is always attraction

to Happiness Support Groups, not promotion.

<u>Sharing and Listening</u>

"The topic I have selected for this meeting is _____. I will begin by reading a brief selection from our literature and then sharing from my own experience with this topic. Then we will go around the circle sharing one at a time either on this topic, or on anything you need to talk about."

<u>Closing</u>

"Let us close by forming a circle, holding hands and saying the Serenity Prayer"

THE SERENITY PRAYER

(Adapted from Reinhold Niebuhr's prayer)

Higher Power/Great Spirit/God, grant me the serenity

To accept the things I cannot change,

The courage to change the things I can,

And the wisdom to know the difference.

(*The term "Higher Power" may be adapted to read, "God," "Great Spirit" or some other universal name for Higher Power, as long as a group conscience decision supports this choice.

Business Meetings & Group Inventory Discussions

If business issues or announcements come up for a Happiness Support Group, we use the last 15 minutes of a group for that, after announcing the issue at the previous meeting. Decisions are made by a democratic vote with a simple majority vote needed to pass a decision, although a group consensus is ideal.

Below is a suggested Group Inventory list of questions. It is suggested that after a group has been meeting for 12 sessions or more, the group set aside one business meeting a month to address one or more of these questions.

Some Wise Ways Happiness Support Group Inventory Questions

1. Does our group meet on time, end on time, and respectfully share time to talk at meetings? If not, how can this be improved?

2. Does our group keep names of participants and what is shared at meetings strictly confidential? If not, how can this be improved?

3. Does our group welcome newcomers by speaking to them personally before and after the meetings and by giving them a time to ask questions or share their

comments for at least ten minutes at the end of each meeting? If not, how can this be improved?

4. Does our group keep some extra copies of this book available at each meeting for newcomers? If not, how can this be improved?

5. Does our group allow "cross talk" (i.e. interruptions, direct and personal questioning, advice giving and feedback, etc) during sharing time? If so, how can this be changed?

6. Does our group focus on self-improvement and sharing about personal experiences, strengths and hopes, rather than focusing on other people, places or things? If not, how can this be improved?

7. Does our group focus on talking about solutions to problems rather than the problems themselves? If not, how can this be improved?

APPENDIX 3: INVENTORYING AND BUILDING ON OUR STRENGTHS

Martin Seligman, Ph.D., has developed an excellent strength-self-assessment tool which he has generously posted on a website for free public access. Go to the website

www.authentichappiness.org to take this inventory. It will identify your strengths from this list of what he calls the "Really Big 24 Strengths:"

1. Wisdom and Knowledge

   curiosity/interest

   love of learning

   judgment/critical thinking

   originality/ingenuity/creativity

   perspective

2. Courage

   valor

   industry/perseverance

   integrity/honesty

   Zest/enthusiasm

3. Love/humanity

   intimacy

   kindness/generosity/nurturance

   social intelligence

4. Justice

   citizenship/duty/loyalty/teamwork

   equity/fairness

   leadership

5. Temperance/moderation

   forgiveness/mercy

   modesty/humility

   self-control/self-regulation

   prudence/caution

6. Transcendence

   appreciation of beauty/awe

   gratitude

   hope/optimism

   humor/playfulness

   spirituality/sense of purpose

To build on one or more areas of your strengths, you can use the following "Strengths Index" to find *Wise Ways Happiness* readings which relate to each area.

STRENGTHS INDEX

Wise Ways **Happiness Readings Relating to Wisdom and Knowledge:**

Jan. 2,5,6,10,16,21,23,27,28,30,31; Feb. 7,8,11,12,13,23,27; March 10,17,21,22; April 2,13,17,18,19; May 4,9,14,22,29; June 2,6,8,9,15,28; July 6,12,25,28; Aug. 10,11,12,15-17, 20, 25, 26; Sept. 2,10,11,12,15-17,19, 22,23,25,27,28; Oct 2,3,9,13,21,22,26,27, 30,31; Nov. 5,8,12,13,24,25-29; Dec. 6,10,14-16,20,26,27,31; Appendix 1,2,3.

Wise Ways Happiness Readings Relating to **Courage, Industry, Integrity, Honesty, Zest:June14June14**

Jan. 1,4; Feb. 2,4,5,9,10,11,20,21,27; March 7,9,24,26-29; April1,5,6,9,10,11,12,21,26-30; May 1,6,12,15,17,18,28,31; June 10,11,19,21,22; July 5,11,13,18,26,30; Aug. 5,17; Sept. 6,20,25; Oct.1,3,17-19,28; Nov.10,15,16,23,5,27-29; Dec.11,13,23,29

Wise Ways Happiness Readings Relating to Love, Humanity, Kindness, Generosity:

Jan. 3,8,15,18,24; Feb. 3,4,9,22,25,26,28; March 1,23,31; April 20,24,25,28; May 2,5,8,10,11,20-21,23,25,27,30; June 1,7,12,14,16-18,20,23-24,27,29; July 1,3,4,8,19-24; Aug. 1-4,24; Sept. 6,8,9,17,18,20,21,24; Oct. 6-16,25,30,31; Nov. 1,3,23,27; Dec. 1,2,12,15-16,18-19,21,24-25,31; Appendix 2.

Wise Ways Happiness **Readings Relating to Justice, Citizenship, Fairness, Leadership:**

Jan. 3,7,10,14,17,20,29; Feb. 1,6,27; March 2,3,5,10,11,30; April 3,8; May 7; June 3,25,30; July 10,14,16-17,22-23,29,31; Aug. 8,21,23,27-28; Sept. 1,4,5,7,10,18,29; Oct. 2-3; Nov. 9,17,18,20,21,30; Dec. 3,4-6,8-9,19,21; Appendix 1.

Wise Ways Happiness **Readings Relating to Temperance, Moderation, Forgiveness, Caution:**

Jan. 11,19,25-26; Feb. 8,12,14,23; March 12-16,18-20; April 14-16,22; May 3,13,16,19; June 4; July 9; Aug. 9,15,24-25,28-29; Sept. 3,13-14,30; Oct. 4,20-23,25; Nov. 4,6,7,13,17,19; Dec. 5,17,30.

Wise Ways Happiness **Readings Relating to Transcendence, Beauty, Gratitude, Hope, Humor:**

After taking time to identify and build on your areas of strength, it is time to identify your shortcomings and the correlated strengths which you need to work on. You can use the following Wise Ways Happiness Comprehensive Self-Inventory to locate what you think are some of your shortcomings. Then use the inventory to identify the correlated strength for each of your shortcomings. Use the General Index to select readings related to these potential, auxiliary strengths. Work on owning and developing your primary as well as auxiliary strengths, possibly with the help of a Wise Ways Happiness Support Group.

You might want to mark the continuum lines only in pencil, so that you can review your self-inventory every 6-12 months to see how you have been able to strengthen your assets. Focus on strengthening your assets will gradually also help you to reduce your correlated shortcomings.

MY HAPPINESS SKILLS SELF-INVETORY - Date: _____

Assets	**Shortcomings**
Life Enhancing Qualities	**Life Depleting Qualities**

_____

Accepting, tolerant - ___/___/___/___/___ - Intolerant, resentful, rejecting
Able to concentrate - ___/___/___/___/___ - Distractible, hyperactive
Able to validate feelings - ___/___/___/___/___ - Unable to validate feelings
Active - ___/___/___/___/___ - Passive, lethargic
Appreciative of others - ___/___/___/___/___ - Envious, critical
Assertive, proactive - ___/___/___/___/___ - Submissive
Attentive, good listener - ___/___/___/___/___ - Inattentive, scattered
Aware of others - ___/___/___/___/___ - Self-centered
Aware of dreams - ___/___/___/___/___ - Lack of dream awareness
Balanced, moderate - ___/___/___/___/___ - Unbalanced, excessive
Boundaries, emotional - ___/___/___/___/___ - Enmeshment
Calm, present focused - ___/___/___/___/___ - Worrisome, dramatic, living in past/future
Clean, orderly - ___/___/___/___/___ - Unhygienic, disorderly
Cheerful, contented - ___/___/___/___/___ - Sad, malcontented
Clarifying preferences - ___/___/___/___/___ - Forcing solutions
Comfortable with solitude - ___/___/___/___/___ - Afraid of aloneness
Community minded - ___/___/___/___/___ - Isolated
Committed - ___/___/___/___/___ - Uncommitted

Confident - ___/___/___/___/___ - Unconfident, fearful
Consistent - ___/___/___/___/___ - Inconsistent
Constructively critical - ___/___/___/___/___ - Judgmental
Cooperative, agreeable - ___/___/___/___/___ - Uncooperative, disagreeable
Even-tempered - ___/___/___/___/___ - Irritable
Courageous - ___/___/___/___/___ - Cowardly, fearful
Courteous - ___/___/___/___/___ - Discourteous, rude
Creative - ___/___/___/___/___ - Uncreative
Curious - ___/___/___/___/___ - Bored
Enthusiastic - ___/___/___/___/___ - Anxious
Emotionally Intelligent - ___/___/___/___/___ - Emotionally immature
Mature - ___/___/___/___/___ - Immature
Empathic - ___/___/___/___/___ - Insensitive, critical
Feelings aware - ___/___/___/___/___ - Unaware of feelings
Faithfulness - ___/___/___/___/___ - Cynical
Faithful - ___/___/___/___/___ - Disloyal
Flexible - ___/___/___/___/___ - Rigid, stubborn, caught in black and white thinking
Focused, have clear intentions - ___/___/___/___/___ - Ambivalent, confused
Forgiving - ___/___/___/___/___ - Judgmental, resentful
Free - ___/___/___/___/___ - Constrained, imprisoned
Friendly - ___/___/___/___/___ - Unfriendly
Generous, helpful - ___/___/___/___/___ - Self-indulgent, selfish
Grateful, thankful - ___/___/___/___/___ - Ungrateful, self-pitying,
appreciative   victim attitude, complaining
Happy - ___/___/___/___/___ - Unhappy, depressed
Healthy parenting - ___/___/___/___/___ - Unhealthy parenting
Healthy exercise - ___/___/___/___/___ - Sedentary lifestyle
Healthy sexuality - ___/___/___/___/___ - Unhealthy sexuality
Honest - ___/___/___/___/___ - Dishonest
Hopeful - ___/___/___/___/___ - Despairing, despondent
Humor, with a sense of - ___/___/___/___/___ - Overly serious
Humble - ___/___/___/___/___ - Arrogant, prideful
Independent - ___/___/___/___/___ - Dependent
Industrious - ___/___/___/___/___ - Lazy
Integrity, with - ___/___/___/___/___ - Divided, duplicitous
Intuitive - ___/___/___/___/___ - Concrete, disinterested
Involved, outgoing - ___/___/___/___/___ - Withdrawn, disconnected
Joyful - ___/___/___/___/___ - Joyless
Kind, compassionate - ___/___/___/___/___ - Unkind, cruel, hostile, evil
Knowledgeable - ___/___/___/___/___ - Ignorant
Learning from mistakes - ___/___/___/___/___ - Denying or hiding mistakes
Loving, caring - ___/___/___/___/___ - Indifferent, hating, uncaring

Neat, clean, organized - ___/___/___/___/___ - Messy, dirty, disorganized
Non-addicted - ___/___/___/___/___ - Addicted
Non-personalizing - ___/___/___/___/___ - Personalizing
Non-possessive, simple - ___/___/___/___/___ - Possessive, greedy
Non-stealing - ___/___/___/___/___ - Stealing, coveting
Non-violent - ___/___/___/___/___ - Violent
Nutritious eating habits - ___/___/___/___/___ - Unhealthy eating habits
Open, genuine - ___/___/___/___/___ - Manipulative
Patient - ___/___/___/___/___ - Impatient
Peaceful - ___/___/___/___/___ - Agitated, irritated, angry
Persistent - ___/___/___/___/___ - Easily discouraged
Positive thinking, optimistic - ___/___/___/___/___ - Pessimistic
Prompt - ___/___/___/___/___ - Procrastinating, tardy
Purposeful, decisive - ___/___/___/___/___ - Aimless
Questioning - ___/___/___/___/___ - Assuming
Realistic - ___/___/___/___/___ - Perfectionistic, grandiose
Reasonable - ___/___/___/___/___ - Unreasonable
Recycling, conserving - ___/___/___/___/___ - Wasteful
Relaxed - ___/___/___/___/___ - Tense
Renewing - ___/___/___/___/___ - Depleting
Respectful - ___/___/___/___/___ - Discourteous, neglectful
Responsible - ___/___/___/___/___ - Irresponsible, over-responsible -
Self-accepting - ___/___/___/___/___ - Self-shaming
Self-respecting, self-caring - ___/___/___/___/___ - Self-neglecting
Self-aware - ___/___/___/___/___ - Avoidant, projective
Self-contained - ___/___/___/___/___ - Prone to gossip
Self-disciplined - ___/___/___/___/___ - Undisciplined
Serene - ___/___/___/___/___ - Anxious, agitated, fearful
Sober, moderate - ___/___/___/___/___ - Chemically dependent
Silent, quiet - ___/___/___/___/___ - Noisy, loud
Spiritual - ___/___/___/___/___ - Non-spiritual
Stable - ___/___/___/___/___ - Unstable
Strong - ___/___/___/___/___ - Weak
Supporting diversity - ___/___/___/___/___ - Prejudiced
Thoughtful, contemplative - ___/___/___/___/___ - Thoughtless
Thrifty - ___/___/___/___/___ - Extravagant
Trusting - ___/___/___/___/___ - Suspicious
Trustworthy - ___/___/___/___/___ - Untrustworthy
Using talents/abilities - ___/___/___/___/___ - Disinterested in self/wasteful of talents
Willing to seek help - ___/___/___/___/___ - Smug, complacent
Wise - ___/___/___/___/___ - Unwise

Appendix 4: How to Start a Happiness Support Group

There are many ways to start a Wise Ways Happiness Support Group. If you have been in a Book Club, you might ask yourself, "How did my Book Club start?" Maybe you could start a Wise Ways Happiness Support Group the same way. Maybe you are a member of a church, fellowship, synagogue, mosque, temple, or non-profit organization which might be interested in starting a Happiness Support Group.

Ideally the membership should be about 5-9 members. Seven members is ideal. Maybe you could just share this book with some of your friends and ask if some of them are interested in joining you in such a support group.

If you are a counselor or therapist, perhaps you are interested in using this book to start a support group in your agency or private practice. The first edition of this book has been used in community mental health centers and in correctional facilities to structure and facilitate effective support groups. Clients select their own topics to be considered in each gathering (using any part of this book.).

The fundamentals of an effective Happiness Support Group include members making the following basic commitments:

1) A commitment to confidentiality,

2) A commitment to attendance (weekly, or monthly at a specified time and place.)

3) A commitment to openness and honesty, and not interrupting others,

4) A commitment to not giving direct advice or feedback to another person during a meeting,

5) A Commitment to focus on sharing about one's own personal experiences, strengths and hopes, and not on the behaviors of others,

6) A commitment to NOT gossiping about a group member outside of the meeting,

7) A commitment to taking turns "chairing" the meetings, by opening and closing the meeting on time, and selecting a topic for that meetings sharing, by using one of the 365 readings and self-discovery questions in the 365 meditations or in one of the Appendices. (The Subject Index in the back of this book can help.) And

8) A commitment to Not allow discussions about specific religions or any one member's stories to dominate the group.

9) If a member decides to leave the group, a commitment to tell the group in person. The group opening can then be filled by the group.

If a Wise Ways Happiness Support Group is started in a mental health agency, the group might be larger than 7 members and with more drop-in attendance, if the facilitating therapist decides that best meets the needs of the agency's population.

It is recommended that the Happiness Steps and Traditions (simplified in bold print in the following pages) be read at the beginning of each meeting. It is also recommended that each meeting close with a moment of silence, or an affirmation from that day's reading or with the Serenity Prayer:

God, grant me the Serenity to Accept the things I cannot change,

The Courage to change the things I can,

And the Wisdom to know the difference.

DISCUSSION OF THE 12 HAPPINESS STEPS AND SUPPORT GROUP TRADITIONS

We can choose to learn through fear and resistance and suffering, or we can choose to learn through wisdom and the experience of those who have come before us. Wise Ways Happiness Support Group members commit to learn through wisdom. When fear and resistance and suffering do appear in our lives, we choose to consciously look for how we ourselves have contributed to the creation of that reality. We do not blame others. We do not judge or reject others. We learn to compassionately relate to others, as we learn to compassionately relate to ourselves. Wise Ways Happiness Support Groups study spiritual principles and positive psychology.

The Wise Ways Happiness Program can be summarized in the following 12 Steps. These Steps are organized into the "3 A's" of the Wise Ways Happiness Program. Steps 1-4 focus on the first "A," Awareness. These Steps involve studying humility, love, trust, and self-assessment. Steps 5-8 focus on the 2nd "A," Acceptance. These Steps involve studying self-disclosure, letting go, emotional connection, and self-forgiveness. Steps 9-12 focus on the 3rd "A," Action. These Steps involve studying how to make amends, how to be continually honest, how to practice daily prayer, meditation and self-evaluation, how to practice "principles in all our affairs" and how to involve oneself in service to others. Below is a brief discussion of each of these steps. We recommend a new group reviews the Steps and Traditions first and then goes on to study chosen topics from the daily meditations.

Step One, HUMILITY: We humbly give up our fearful escapes from awareness and our reactive attempts to control others.

In Step One we humbly accept the futility of pursuits of external power over others. We become aware that accepting this kind of powerlessness over other people, places and things actually empowers us to establish internal happiness and peace.

In Step One we learn that authentic power is always internal. It is based on our ability to not react unconsciously to fear. By not reacting unconsciously to fear we don't generate anger, jealousy, loneliness, greed, self-pity, resentments, and feelings of inferiority or superiority. Instead we learn to feel connection to and love for our true selves and the true selves of others. We grow in this form of authentic power, by giving up useless attempts for external power.

Gary Zukav in *The Seat of the Soul* (page 221) defines authentic power as energy formed by the intentions "of love and compassion, guided by wisdom." When we are fearful or distrustful, energy leaves us through our solar plexus areas. We experience anxiety or anger. If we fear our ability to love or be loved, we literally experience heartache. We lose power whenever we are afraid. An authentically empowered person "does not release energy except in love and trust" (Ibid, page 224). He or she is humble, reverencing life in all forms, feeling free to love and be his or her self, not competing for external power. Such a person gives with purpose and joy and consciousness, forgiving, not holding others responsible for his or her own experience.

In Wise Ways Happiness Support Groups, we strive together to become this kind of authentically empowered person. We strive to learn through wisdom rather than through fear and doubt and all their consequences. With acceptance, we listen to each other's personal experiences, feelings, and perceptions. We trust in the gifts present in every shared experience. We learn from each other by focusing on solutions to problems and avoiding complaining or blaming. We grow together in authentic, internal power. We grow in our capacity to love, accepting that love is an active force, yet one incapable of harm or domination. We seek to nurture ourselves and each other in a fellowship of love.

Unhealthy pride blocks awareness and seeks to dominate others. It masks our faults and separates us from others. Humility expands awareness and connects us to others. Humility helps us to see common human vulnerabilities and needs. It also helps us to see creative human diversity.

To be fully aware we need to be aware of ourselves, aware of others and aware of life's interaction patterns. We also need to be fearless. To be fearless we need to have well-functioning brains. Wise Ways Happiness Support Group members learn about human brain anatomy and development. (See Appendix 1.) Group members learn to take responsibility for healing unhealthy brains and maintaining healthy ones.

To be fearless involves calmness in the amygdala, part of the low brain's limbic system. When this center of the brain becomes over-stimulated by fear or anger, energy does not flow sufficiently to the prefrontal cortex, the higher part of the brain which helps us to understand and make good judgments about what we are seeing, hearing, experiencing and saying. An excited amygdala shuts down our awareness and judgment capacities and causes us to exclusively focus on a perceived threat.

Fear assumes external danger, pulls blood away from our extremities (feet, hands and high brain) and pumps it in to our hearts and chests and pelvic areas so we can fight or flee. Unfortunately, often the real source of danger is ourselves. We are often being "triggered" by a threat of our own making, for example, our unhappiness over a perceived weakness or misbehavior of a loved one. Often our perceptions are skewed by past grief and loss, which we have repressed out of awareness. At the same time, we are unconsciously afraid of new losses, so we act out to attempt to prevent them. But this very acting out can often alienate the very people who might be most capable of helping us to heal our past emotional wounds.

In Step One of the Wise Ways Happiness Program we learn to humbly witness our fearfulness when it appears and stay calm, rather than acting it out. We witness our physiological reactivity -- such as our racing heartbeat, sweaty arm pits, or tense neck muscles. We also witness our automatic thoughts which may be judgmental, shaming or blaming. We don't verbalize these defensive, automatic thoughts, but instead witness them in our minds and look for our own feelings underneath these thoughts. We look for the fear underneath the anger, the grief underneath the fear, and the exhaustion underneath the grief. We take no verbal or physical action unless it promotes our safety and is not harmful to others. We do not use our fear to try to angrily control others. We give our "low brains" time and energy to connect to our "high brains." We humbly accept the limitations of our will powers and respect others' rights to make their own choices. We let go of pride and humbly permit ourselves to honestly see ourselves in relationship to others.

Step Two, LOVE: We become willing to accept reality and to connect our low brains to our high brains, surrendering to love, not to fear.

Step One (Humility) makes room for Step Two (Love). A fearful body and mind have no room for love. Fear constricts the body's energy into the torso, to provide for fleet-footed escape or strong-fisted fight. It protects physical survival, so contains a fundamental gift. But, if it is triggered when our physical survival is not threatened, it prevents loving contact with others.

When human brains are the healthiest and functioning optimally, all of their cells have good blood flow and are moderately stimulated by nerve impulses. There are no "hot spots" (over-stimulated brain centers) and no "cold spots" (under-stimulated brain centers). The low brain centers and the high brain centers are both working well together. The low brain centers, where emotions such as anger, fear and grief form, are not so over-stimulated that there is no energy left to send messages to the high brain centers, the prefrontal cortexes where understanding, self-responsibility and good judgment forms. Instead healthy low brains have energy to send to their high brain centers. They stay calm (only moderately stimulated) enough to allow the high brain centers to help them to move beyond the primary emotions of anger, fear and grief into awareness of self-responsibility, and understanding of connection with others. This high brain experience can then finally develop into what we call "love."

When we are Hungary, Angry, Lonely, or Tired (H.A.L.T.) we cannot move into love energy. We must first have something to eat, calm our low brains, find human supportive connection or sleep. Only after we have taken care of these primary needs can we then move into love energy.

Appendix One includes an illustration of a human brain. It shows a person's high brain (prefrontal cortex) and low brain (amygdala and entire limbic system). When optimal high brain functioning does not happen, we remain stuck in denial, anger and fear.

To experience more love in our lives we need to allow the energy from the lower parts of our brains to flow freely up into our high brains. We need to practice silence until what we say and do reflects optimal functioning in our high brains, as well as our low brains. As our brain energy moves up and peripherally out, grasping, attachment and revenge impulses in the low brain move up and out. Questions such as "How can I change or punish this person?" are replaced by questions such as "How can I heal this grief and loss?" We then are empowered to take effective action on the higher-level questions rather than on the lower level questions. The lower level questions create resistance and self-defense in others. The higher-level questions stimulate self-responsibility, creative action and attract support.

Our brains are designed to dissolve fear into love, unless we are physically threatened. Human culture has only recently evolved to a level at which we are not always threatening each other with physical extinction. Our brains, if we use their higher levels well, are now capable of creating peaceful human community. But, we have to take careful responsibility for our reactive, fearful, angry low brains, or such peaceful community becomes impossible.

In Step 2 we allow our minds to follow the leadership of our hearts because healthy hearts are designed to pump blood effectively throughout our whole bodies. When our low brains dominate our lives with fear and anger, we cannot feel the underlying emotions of grief and loss. We are then not aware of how much of ourselves we lose by denying our feelings and denying and avoiding the feelings of others.

We all need support in learning how to better love one another. In Wise Ways Happiness Support Groups, we learn how to offer each other this kind of support, even though we may not even like each other, nor approve of each other's behaviors.

Step Three, TRUST: We decide to trust a Higher Power or energy of our own understanding, One which supports life, love, nature, beauty, harmony, freedom and diversity.

Step 3 is about looking for a wisdom higher than that in our ego-minds. It is about learning to say to the Universe, "Thy will be done." It is about letting go of what mind says is right and trusting the Universe to give what is authentically needed, moment by moment. It is about looking for guidance from non-physical teachers, Divine Intelligence, God, Mother Nature -- whatever name is given to the Source of life and wisdom beyond our individual brains and minds.

Relaxing into this level of receptivity may not be easy at first. We may at first just trust
in the larger wisdom of the Wise Ways Program or of our Wise Ways Happiness Support Group but, over time, we see that the Source of Wisdom is beyond even that. We learn to see the wisdom radiating through the eyes of persons of many different cultures, nations, races and religions. We come to see good radiating through all of life and experience.

Step 3 involves allowing ourselves to pray for more wisdom and awareness, for connection to a divine partnership with an intelligence beyond our own. Anthony de Mello in *Walking on Water* wrote "That is the great benefit of prayer: concentration. You start doing one thing at a time, and you are completely present to each act you undertake." (page 29) This kind of concentration is not often reinforced in our modern multi-tasking world. Yet this kind of concentration is what is involved with optimal, integrated, brain functioning.

Take for example the simple Serenity Prayer: "Higher Power, give me the serenity to accept the things I can not change, the courage to change the things I can, and the wisdom to know the difference." This prayer helps us to distinguish between things we can change and external people, places, and events which we can't change. It helps us to slow down and concentrate on this difference. It reminds us that it takes patience and courage to determine non-reactive, effective actions. This prayer-full concentration is very self-empowering. It also helps to align our authentic personal power with Higher Power energy. When we don't take time to prayer-fully slow down, observe all of our thoughts and feelings, check our perceptions out with others and take action only where we can make an effective difference, we are usually just reacting out of our low brains and we end up taking a "low road," not a "high road." Usually the consequences are negative. When we take the time to trust all of our perceptions and feelings, and to check these out with trusted others before we take action, usually aggression, violence, and pain and suffering can be avoided.

When our brains are the healthiest and most integrated, we humans are the most loving. There is a universal energy (Higher Power) which keeps creating life so that it grows towards light and love. When human minds focus on fear and hatred this same Higher Power energy furthers their early destruction, through illness, accident or aggression. Of course, every early death is not the result of that individual's own choices. Sometimes innocents die because of the fear and hatred of others. Fear and hatred is very contagious. It can spread through whole communities, causing them to turn on other communities and to start or continue escalating spirals of violence.

In Step Three we learn to trust our bodies and our minds and to experience how they can connect to a Higher Power energy beyond ourselves. We begin to experience the supportive energy of other Wise Ways Happiness Group members. We begin to experience moments of balanced, integrated brain energy in which we feel connected to other people and the natural world, with love and appreciation. We may not like everyone in our group and our life, but we learn how to love and accept them anyway.

In the Wise Ways Happiness Program, we can define a Higher Power of our own understanding. No one forces a creed or a doctrine on us. We can be members of an organized religion or not. We can be atheists and agnostics or deists or goddess worshippers. We are free to keep discovering deeper and deeper aspects of our Higher Powers. We can experience Higher Power energy with others, or we can be very private with our Higher Power experiences. We can experience Higher Power inside, outside or everywhere.

In the Wise Ways Happiness Program, we learn the difference between healthy and unhealthy spirituality. We practice a spirituality which is joyful, accepting, grateful, trusting, egalitarian and democratic. We advocate the separation of church and state. Our groups do not acquire property or engage directly in political activities. We do not make negative judgments of others or isolate ourselves from people of differing beliefs. All are welcome in our Groups. We support the free expression of feelings, as long as it is done safely and respectfully, within the guidelines of our 12 Traditions.

The deeper we look into the natural world the more we see how interconnected everything is. We literally breathe in and swallow new cells which have formerly been part of other persons, plants and animals. Our largest organ, our skin, replaces its cells approximately every four weeks. The rest of our body is renewed (through breathing, eating and eliminating) approximately every five months. Nothing alive is static. We are forever changing and the energy supporting all this change is beyond personal power. This energy, this Higher Power, promotes life, balance, harmony and freedom. When we make choices in line with this Power we thrive. When we make choices not in line with this Power, we wither and die early.

How we behave affects not only ourselves, but others as well as the plants, animals, minerals and space around us. Trusting in these interconnections and the principles which sustain them is trusting in a Higher Power. When we don't have this trust, we tend to fall into the illusions of separateness and become self-centered, angry and controlling. When we have this trust, we are generous toward all which is in and around us. We feel part of a wisdom and energy greater than our own.

With time and the help of Step Three, we learn clearer intentions, deeper trust and more appropriate action and timing. We trust that, as our negativities manifest in our lives, they are coming up to be healed. The more we can see our lives with clear awareness, the more we can experience authentic power, power linked to trusting the Universe.

Step 4: HONEST SELF-ASSESSMENT: We make an honest assessment of our assets and our shortcomings.

The journey to authentic power involves becoming conscious of all our feelings, thoughts and actions. Unearthing and healing our negativities happens gradually, but consistently, as we learn to daily examine our attitudes, behaviors and their consequences. When we do this with compass ion towards ourselves, we also see our growing strengths, and we offer these strengths to others, as well as ourselves. We challenge our fears. We become more mindful of our thoughts and our choices, as well as their impact on others. We take regular 4th Step Self-Inventories, using the outline in Appendix 3. We start out focusing on our assets, checking four or five of them every time we do an inventory. We note what shortcomings may arise when we grow lax in these assets, and we celebrate our successes. We focus on four or five shortcomings which we want to guide into their correlated assets. We look up helpful readings in this book focusing on one needed asset at a time. When we are ready, we move on to Step 5 sharing our inventory with a trusted other.

If we are members of another 12 Step program due to our past abuses of drugs or other substances or processes, we abstain, one day at a time, from that abuse while we are members of Wise Ways Happiness Support Groups. If we have not developed substance abuse problems, we still are alert to how substance abuse can hinder our emotional and spiritual progress, and we use alcohol and prescription drugs only in moderation and as prescribed.

We do our self-inventories without self-recrimination or shame, knowing that this is the beginning of change and the beginning of making amends to ourselves for past mistakes. We keep writing our self-inventories, until we are able to accept all our assets and limitations. We humbly remind ourselves that our human imperfections are not reasons to feel shame and reject or isolate ourselves. We also remind ourselves that we are capable of change. We are aware that, as we strengthen our characters and virtues, so we also heal and integrate our brains. We take seriously the need to keep our brains healthy and developing so as to enhance, not only our own happiness but the happiness of those around us. (Also see the website www.authentichappiness.org for more help in doing self-inventories which identify our strengths.)

Step Five: SELF-DISCLOSURE: We share our self-inventories with our Higher Powers, and confidentially, with a loving, accepting other, without self-recrimination or shame.

Step 5 reminds us that in Wise Ways Happiness Support Groups we do not attempt to solve our problems in isolation. We trust our Higher Powers and other group members or dialogue partners, confidentially and honestly sharing our experiences in our meetings.

In Step Five we learn to be honest about our behaviors and our mistakes. We also learn to identify our fears, own them, identify the other feelings they generate and communicate these feelings with acceptance and emotional connection with others. We focus on ourselves, not others. We focus on substituting assets for our shortcomings and on supporting others in attempting to do the same.

Patricia and Ronald Potter-Efron in *The Secret Message Of Shame* define shame as "self-conscious judgment," and "a painful belief in one's defectiveness as a human being." They define the asset which replaces shame as healthy pride, i.e. "a positive belief in one's basic worthiness as a human being." A person can have this healthy pride and still practice the humility of Step One. Healthy pride is earned and real. It is the result of doing something well, of showing caring and love to others and feeling quietly good about it. It is the result of taking regular self-inventories and noticing progress in building assets and diminishing short-comings.

Healthy pride does not make comparisons between self and others. Healthy pride only makes comparisons between past levels of personal development and present ones. Healthy pride does not heat up the low brain. It is a calm, quiet, internal experience which builds confidence and energy to keep on making self-improvements.

The Potter-Efrons in *The Secret Message Of Shame* describe how this kind of healthy pride builds strength, vigor, purpose, competence, honor, respect, dignity, humility, acceptance, wholeness, integrity and independence. Regularly doing self-inventories and regularly sharing them, including noted progress, with trusted others builds this kind of healthy pride. Sharing parts of our self-inventories in Happiness Support Group meetings and in private conversations with other Group members helps us to let go of unhealthy shame and self-recrimination and accept our daily progress, even if it seems slow.

Step Five is the first of four steps which focus on acceptance. Step Six goes on to focus on ways of strengthening our assets and letting go of our shortcomings.

Step Six: LETTING GO: We continue strengthening our assets and letting go of our shortcomings.

Happiness Support Groups are not for perfect people. They are for perfectly imperfect people. We ALL really are perfectly imperfect. Some of us just avoid awareness of this more than others, out of our fear of shame, judgment, or punishment.

In Happiness Support Groups we learn to accept the natural consequences of our mistakes and to humbly learn from them. We realize that is how each of us learns. Through experiencing our pain, and accepting it, and not running away from it, our pain becomes manageable, not endless suffering. We gradually even learn to humbly laugh about our "slips" and mistakes. Through this deep level of acceptance, we learn to love ourselves and others more completely.

One way to strengthen our assets is to quietly note and share our successes. This we learn to do in our group meetings and in our one-to-one get-togethers and "dialoguing partnerships." (See Appendix 5.) We learn to help each other to celebrate increasing ability to put Wise Ways Happiness principles into practice. When we have "slips" in this application, we don't shame ourselves or others. We realize that backward steps are sometimes necessary in order for us to be reminded of the pain which results from not practicing wise principles.

We realize that one way of letting go of our shortcomings is to simply share our "slips" with humor and honesty with other Happiness Support Group practitioners. We know we will not be judged or rejected by other members for this kind of self-disclosure. Rather, other members will simply likely share in more detail how they have been working on overcoming similar shortcomings.

Another way to help ourselves to let go of shortcomings is to keep a private journal. There are many ways to keep journals but one way includes noting the following experiences: negative emotional experiences, correlated reactive automatic thoughts, corrective Wise Ways Happiness principles or thoughts, corrective Wise Ways Happiness actions. Just the very process of keeping a journal itself can be helpful in noting needed changes and successful progress. Dreams can also be recorded in these journals and used to develop more self-understanding. Reference to dream work principles in Appendix 6 can help to keep a more meaningful journal and also to share these dreams with others in a more meaningful way.

Eventually modern brain research will likely show how taking our night dreams seriously, and working on making them less anxiety-provoking, can actually help to heal our physical brains. As we know, healing our physical brains can also gradually improve our minds and our abilities to create authentic happiness in our lives.

Another way to help ourselves to let go of our shortcomings is to spend more time meditating and studying spiritual literature. This can be done alone or with the help of a spiritual advisor or a spiritually aware psychotherapist. Whatever ways we choose to strengthen our assets and let go of our shortcomings, what is most important is patience and ongoing clear intention. Attending regular Happiness Support Group meetings and helping group newcomers is very important in doing Step Six work.

Step Seven: EMOTIONAL CONNECTION: We humbly let go of our pride and reach out of our emotional isolation to lovingly connect to others.

In Step Seven we focus on strengthening and broadening our connections to other people, especially fellow group members and "dialogue partners." We let go of our old "know it all" pride, our old fears and shyness and we build stronger, deeper, more honest relationships with others.

Through studying the 12 Steps, attending meetings and reading the *365* Wise Ways Happiness meditations, we gradually develop better self-care and interpersonal skills and wider trust in the ability of support group meetings and to help us mature emotionally. We recognize the dangers of isolation and self-pity.

Modern brain research has shown how connecting with other people in a loving and appreciative way actually helps to heal imbalanced brains. When we are afraid, meeting with others who have overcome similar fears is very calming. When we are angry, it is very valuable to have a safe place to express our anger without any negative repercussions. When we are grieving, having others there to quietly listen to our grief, accept our tears, and perhaps even give us warm hugs, is very therapeutic. All of these experiences are very soothing and healing to brain activity which may be imbalanced due to stress and/or illness.

Offering this kind of support to others in Wise Ways Happiness Support Group meetings and in on-on-one get-togethers is very therapeutic. Discussing our experiences applying Wise Way Happiness principles is also very therapeutic. When we give support to others, we also support our own understanding of the principles and our own progress in the program.

Step Eight: SELF-FORGIVENESS: We learn self-forgiveness and how to make amends to ourselves for our past mistakes.

Step Eight reminds us that we can not begin to authentically forgive others if we have not first taken the time to forgive ourselves. In any given situation in which we feel we have been harmed, there is always some part of it which is our own responsibility. Perhaps we were not cautious enough. Perhaps we were critical of another and therefore were verbally attacked in retaliation. Even if our own error was very small in comparison to the reactive error of another, it is important to first see our own part in a negative interaction, and forgive ourselves for it.

We cannot always remain perfectly rested, aware and able to practice Wise Ways Happiness principles in all our affairs. This is our intention, but not the full reality of any of our actual experiences. None of us are perfect. Therefore, self-acceptance and self-forgiveness is vital. Self-rejection and unhealthy pride can block us from making amends both to ourselves and others, keeping us stuck in our old mistakes so that we repeat them over and over.

An honest willingness to "give away" our shortcomings is the foundation of self-forgiveness. When we honestly regret having made a mistake, when we are completely aware of the pain we have exposed ourselves to because of our mistake, it is easier to release our mistaken attitudes, choices and behaviors.

Trusting in a Higher Power, a loving Universe (as we learned in Step 3) to accept us despite our mistakes is an important part of self-forgiveness. If we see our ego-wills as ultimate powers we can become easily discouraged. When we step back from our ego-wills and remind ourselves of the awesome power of the rains, the winds, the sun and the entire natural Universe it is easier to humbly forgive ourselves, align ourselves with our Higher Powers and go on to do better the next time.

A wise teacher once taught that the only real mistake one can ever make is not to admit a mistake. Once the mistake is admitted it can be released, and we can learn from it sufficiently not to repeat it. We can see how we bring suffering upon ourselves and set ourselves up to be treated badly by others, by not acting on loving Wise Ways principles. When we can take full and complete responsibility for all our suffering, seeing it within a larger context of our relationships and our community's and nation's decisions and yet also taking deep, personal responsibility for our own part in the cause of the suffering, self-forgiveness is necessary. We are all only human.

The Wise Ways Happiness Program, along with many other 12 Step programs, uses the slogan, "Principles, not personalities." This slogan reminds us that what's really important is doing our very bests to follow our highest principles. What others think of our personalities is not as important as our own evaluations of how we did or didn't live up to our Wise Ways principles. Self-condemnation is a waste of time. Instead we need to just get busy understanding what allowed us to undermine our own principles and what is necessary to get back on a "high road."

Learning the Wise Ways Happiness principles of self-care of the brain can go a very long way to keep us on a "high road." Even when others go down a "low road," short-circuiting their high brains, with over-activity in their low brains, we don't have to follow right along with them. When we do mistakenly go down the "low road," we can quickly admit it and redirect ourselves to the "high road." We don't have to wait for anyone else to do the same.

Step Nine: MAKING AMENDS: We make direct, whenever possible, to those we have harmed, except when to do so would harm others.

In Step Nine we actually begin making direct amends to others we have harmed, unless by doing so we would harm them more. We put others' needs ahead of our own selfishness, and we make restitution for our past mistakes by changed new behavior, by paying back debts, by making direct verbal or written amends, or by engaging in any process which will help ourselves and others to let go of the painful past, with respect.

Step Nine is the first of four "action" Steps which naturally progress from the earlier "awareness" and "acceptance" Steps. In this Step we carefully engage in new behaviors, ones which may help to correct past mistakes. Sometimes there is not anything concrete we can do to make amends to another we have harmed, other than to acknowledge our mistake and express our regret over it. Other times we can redo something in a corrective way, for example returning something or giving someone voluntary labor or financial payment. Often the best we can do is make a big effort to change our attitude toward a person or a situation so that we no longer contribute to feelings of separation and anger.

When there is nothing we can do to make direct amends to someone we have harmed, we can do our best to help out others who might be in need of help. For example, if we have financially cheated someone who is already dead, we can give financially to a worthy charity. Or if we have treated an ex-spouse badly, we can treat a second spouse lovingly. If we have been dishonest with someone with whom it is no longer safe to have contact, we can be absolutely honest in all our new relationships. All these measures are ways of making amends to the larger universe of beings. Since we all are spiritually connected in unfathomable ways, making amends even to strangers can also be very healing. The important thing is that we take effective new action.

Step Ten: CONTINUAL HONESTY: We continue honest, daily self-examination and when mistakes are found we promptly admit them.

In Step Ten we remind ourselves to do daily, honest self-evaluations and to promptly note and make amends for any new mistakes or "slips" we have made in practicing our 12 Step Program. We don't procrastinate. We don't go to bed at night having treated someone else badly without admitting it to them and making amends. We stay current with our moral inventories.

In Step Ten we humbly come to realize new aspects of ourselves which need examination and loving attention. We continually turn to new aspects of our self-inventories to look for ways we can make improvements.

By watching how others respond to us, by taking responsibility for all our actions and feelings, we keep discovering new places in our lives to apply the Wise Ways Happiness principles. We do this cheerfully and without shame. We do not make ourselves into martyrs. We do make ourselves into responsible, growing, spiritual beings. If we are members of an organized religion, we work on harmonizing and integrating our Wise Ways Happiness principles with the teachings of our religion. If we are agnostics or atheists, we integrate the Wise Ways Happiness principles with our secular knowledge.

Attendance at a weekly Wise Ways Happiness Support Group, and/or getting together with another Wise Ways practitioners on a one-to-one basis to dialogue, (see Appendix 5.) helps to keep our daily inventories current. We use these times of fellowship, not only to listen to and emotionally support others, but also to share our own progress reports and insights from our daily inventories.

Company is much stronger than will power. We do our best, not only to be completely honest in all our own affairs, but also to surround ourselves with honest, self-examining and self-responsible people. When we discover unconscious dishonesties, we immediately correct them and go on to privately examine what led us to become so unconscious. The Wise Ways Happiness Program is a daily program both of self-care and self-responsibility. We take it seriously, and also observe ourselves with humor and self-forgiveness.

Step Eleven: PRAYER AND MEDITATION: We seek through prayer and meditation to improve our conscious contact with a Higher Power, praying for guidance and the will and strength to carry it out.

Prayer and meditation are processes which Wise Ways Happiness Group members can learn to do as practitioners of any religion or even as agnostics or atheists. Prayer does not have to be addressed to an organizationally-defined concept of God. Prayer in its essence is offering gratitude and petition to any power greater than self. Praying with one's family can help a person, not only to define areas of gratitude and need for help, but also to interpersonally communicate these things. Some people find it very difficult to communicate gratitude and to make requests for help in respectful, non-demanding ways. Prayer and quiet, thoughtful meditation are processes which teach us how to do these things and can be shared with others.

As an anonymous person once said, "Prayer doesn't change God. Prayer changes me." The same can be said for quiet periods of meditation when we sit alone and watch our thoughts, read meditative literature or express our gratitude and requests for spiritual support from sources beyond our ego-minds.

In our modern, multi-tasking world, finding time for thoughtful, calm contemplation and meditation is not easy but, it is necessary. Otherwise we begin to feel out of balance and anxious and reactive, and suffering soon arrives. When we have a daily mediation practice, even for just a few minutes a day, our experiences go more smoothly, and we can learn to soothe our own brains and spirits. We also learn to be more soothing and supportive of the brains and spirits of our loved ones.

Step Twelve, SERVICE AND CONTINUED PRACTICE: Having had a spiritual awakening as the result of these steps, we commit to practicing these happiness principles in all our affairs and sharing them with others.

Step Twelve is about selfless service and sharing the Wise Ways Happiness principles, book and practices with others. Step Twelve is not about forming a bigger fellowship or convincing others of the rightness of the Wise Ways Happiness principles. Step Twelve is about the benefits of service to the server, not to the person served. When we share our experience, strength and hope with others, our own spirits are strengthened. When we discuss Wise Ways Happiness principles with others, our own understanding of them grows. When we start a Happiness Support Group in our community, we grow in personal confidence and in compassion for others. When we offer to network with Wise Ways Happiness Support Group members in other communities, we expand our friendship and support circles.

Selfless service is service done without expectation of reward or acknowledgement. It is service done for the purpose of the joy of giving and the joy of lovingly connecting to others. There are few places in our modern, highly competitive, highly individualistic and speedy culture for us to easily engage in this kind of connection to others. As a result, we have to individually take responsibility for creating these kinds of connections.

Selfless service creates loving connection to others more readily than any other behavior. Parenting inspires selfless service. Romantic love inspires selfless service. Violent attacks on the homeland and pandemics inspire self-less service. The relationships we form with our spouses, our partners, our children, our comrades in self-defense, all inspire great loyalty and love.

In Wise Ways Happiness Support Groups, we learn how to offer this kind of service to other group members, to family members and to friends. We also learn how to ask for this kind of help and receive it graciously. By doing this we learn to practice healthy principles in all our affairs on an ongoing basis, and by so doing to carry the Wise Ways Happiness Program message to others.

THE HAPPINESS GROUP 12 TRADITIONS

Happiness Group Tradition One: <u>Unity and respect for the common welfare</u>. Unity and respect for the common welfare of the group promotes individual progress for the greatest number of members.

Happiness in any group requires respect for the common welfare over and above respect for any one individual's opinions or needs. If an individual is out-voted by the majority "consciousness vote" of any group, then that individual needs to either respect the needs of the majority of the group, or leave the group to form another Happiness Support Group.

Happiness Group Tradition Two: <u>Maintaining Anonymity & Confidentiality, and Trust:</u>

Personal anonymity and confidentiality (use of first names only at meetings, and respect for confidential sharing) are the foundation of trust in the Wise Ways Happiness Program.

Happiness Group Tradition Three: <u>Clear Purpose and Mutual Support:</u> The primary purpose of Wise Ways Happiness Support Group meetings is to study the happiness principles in this book and to support each other in the practice of these principles.

The primary purpose of Happiness Support Group meetings is to study this *365 Wise Ways to Happiness* book and to support each other in our practice of the Wise Ways Happiness Program.

Happiness Group Tradition Four: <u>Autonomous Support Groups:</u> Each Wise Ways Happiness Support Group is autonomous.

Happiness Support Groups may network with one another, but their group decisions need to always be autonomous.

Happiness Group Tradition Five: <u>Group Leaders Are Trusted Servants:</u> Group leaders are but trusted, elected servants. They do not govern, nor have more status than any other group member.

Group meeting chairpersons rotate and are volunteer. If the group decides it needs a leader to open up and close a space for a meeting that can be rotated too, or someone can be elected by the group to do that service for 6-12 months at a time.

Happiness Group Tradition Six: <u>Group Membership:</u> Group Membership is based on attendance at meetings and on commitment to practicing the Wise Ways Happiness Steps and Traditions.

Groups can pass around a signup sheet for members to volunteer to sign their first names and last initials, and their email and/or phone numbers. This is also so members can be supportive of each other on the phone, if they wish to be. It is vital, however, that individual members do not talk about other members who are not present in a phone conversation. Two person conversations are meant to be for personal support, not for talking about others. That is gossiping and tends to break down group cohesiveness.

Happiness Group Tradition Seven: <u>Self-supporting Groups:</u> Wise Ways Happiness Support Groups are always self-supporting.

There are no dues for Wise Ways Happiness Support Groups. If they are meeting within a mental health agency, there may be fees for attendance, but that is up to the agency. If rent is needed for a gathering place, then a basket is passed at meetings to pay for the rent. Different Wise Ways Happiness Support Groups can network with each other, but there is no larger organization with dues.

Happiness Group Tradition Eight: <u>Principles, Not Personalities:</u> In Wise Ways Happiness Support Groups' principles are always more important than personalities.

If personality conflicts develop between group members, it is best that they be worked out by each person individually working the 12 Steps on the issue to see if amends can be made and the conflict resolved. If that isn't possible, it is best for one of the individuals to leave the group and start a new one, so that the conflict does not undermine the group.

Happiness Group Tradition Nine: <u>Group Decisions:</u> Wise Ways Happiness Support Group decisions are made by a "group conscious" meeting, ideally by a consensus of the group at the meeting.

If a consensus can't be reached on a group decision then a majority of those present should make the decision on the question being raised.

It's a privilege to be a leader. Leadership should always be rotated and shared. No one has higher status than others in a Happiness Support Group.

Happiness Group Tradition Ten: <u>No Other Group Affiliations:</u> Wise Ways Happiness Support Groups have no other affiliation and neither endorse, finance, nor lend their names to any other enterprise, lest problems of money or prestige divert them from their primary purpose. Professionally facilitated

Wise Ways Happiness Counseling Groups have permission to use the Wise Ways Happiness name as long as they are using this book for their meetings.

The focus of meetings needs to stay on learning about and applying the Wise Ways Happiness Principles. Agencies and correctional institutions may use this book and the Wise Ways Happiness Support Group Traditions, but they need to follow the suggested format suggestions and limit discussions to studying this book,.

Happiness Group Tradition Eleven: <u>No Official Fellowship Opinions on Outside Issues:</u> The Wise Ways Happiness Support Groups have no opinion on outside issues so their names aren't drawn into public controversy.

It is important to keep the focus on studying Wise Ways Happiness Principles. Debating and stating opinions on outside issues can dilute the focus and effectiveness of the groups.

Happiness Group Tradition Twelve: <u>Public Relations Policy:</u> The Wise Ways Happiness Support Groups may sell this book at their cost. Their principle is always attraction to Happiness Support Groups, not promotion.

Groups may purchase this book from various book sellers, but they should always resell books at their own cost. Members can attract others to attending the groups, but it is important that the policy always be attraction, not promotion.

APPENDIX 5: WORKING WITH OUR DREAMS

First take a few moments to review the Jan. 5th meditation on why it is important to start remembering your dreams. Then review the Sept. 19th meditation with some dream recall aids.

There are at least two levels of dream exploration: Interpersonal and Intrapersonal. At the Intrapersonal level the "I" in the dream represents your most conscious self. Other people, animals and objects in your dream represent less conscious aspects of yourself. If there is conflict in your dream, at the intrapersonal level, this conflict represents conflicts between different parts of yourself. This is very important to consider because often our inner conflicts are unconscious, so we can have a hard time healing them.

Here are two questions you can ask yourself which can help to heal these inner conflicts:

- What inner conflict does this dream suggest?

- How would I like this dream conflict to be resolved?

Now write down how you would like the dream conflict to be resolved. You can use any imaginary characters or forces you want. It is your dream.

At the Interpersonal level of dream exploration, the "I" in the dream represents yourself and other people, animals or images in the dream represent real people, animals and situations with them. Therefore, it is helpful to ask yourself, "What does this pattern of conflict remind me of from my past or my life right now?"

Then it can help to journal about those memories or present situations which seem like your dream conflicts. You can even go on and write down an imagined conversation between yourself and these people or pets or strangers which might clarify the conflict, as well as how you would like the conflict to be resolved.

Then imagine the dream actually ending the way you want it to end. Conclude with the self-statement, "Next time I will dream it this way." This is especially helpful to do with nightmares. It makes them less scary and more manageable.

Dream work can also be used for problem solving

You can write down a problem as a brief phrase or sentence and place the note next to the bed. Then review the problem for a few minutes before going to bed, and once in bed, visualize the problem as a concrete image, if possible. As you drift off to sleep, 1) tell yourself you want to dream about the problem and 2) keep a pen and paper, and perhaps a flashlight or a pen with a lit tip, on the night table. No matter what time you wake up, lie quietly before getting out of bed, note whether there is "any trace of a recalled dream and invite more of the dream to return if possible." Then write down everything you remember. Later you can use some of the ideas above for exploring answers which your dream may have given you for your question.

APPENDIX 6

HAPPINESS SLOGANS

AND RELATED HAPPINESS READINGS

Listen and Learn.................. .April 17-18; Sept. 2; Oct.17 & 23

Principles first...................... Dec 20, 23, 29-30

Keep life simple.................. March 14-16; April 13; Nov. 17-18; Dec. 18

Be honest.........................Jan.10; March 27-29; April 7; May 6 & 15; Oct.3

One day at a time............... Jan. 20; Feb. 1-2; June 9

Hope and be grateful............ Feb. 17; Dec. 13

Live and let live................... Feb. 7, 11, 19, 22, 25; May 13-17; July 28

Stop expecting. Start accepting. Feb. 12; May 27-28; Nov. 25; Dec. 19 & 23

Let go, with love................... Jan. 16; Feb. 7 & 23; June 7; Nov. 25 & 29

Appreciation, not judgment....... June 27; May 20-21

Principles, not personalities....... March 9; Aug. 10; Dec. 29-30

Mind my own business............. May 13-17, 22-23, 27-28; June 1; July 8

Stick with the winners............... April 8; July 30-31; Oct. 6; Dec. 31

Win/Win, not Win/Lose............. June 13; July 12-14 & 22; Nov. 30

Make plans, don't plan outcomes. Feb 12; April 17; May 13-17; Dec. 18 & 23

Progress, not perfection.............. March 19-21

Attraction is better than promotion.... Dec. 1

Appendix 7: Partnership Dialoguing Guidelines

If you aren't a member of a group you might want to form a Dialoging Partnership and study the Wise Ways Happiness principles with a family member or friend. Or you might already be a member of a Happiness Support Group but want to also have a Dialoging Partner at home. Following these dialoguing guidelines and the happiness principles can improve any relationship, as well as the individuals in it.

1) Have an agreed upon beginning and ending time for your dialoguing session. (This is usually a minimum of 30 minutes.)

2) Do not attempt to dialogue when under any influence from alcohol or any other mind altering drug.

3) Listen carefully. Focus your attention on what the other is saying. Do not let your mind wander or rehearse your reply. Do not interrupt.

4) Agree on the question or topic about which you want to dialogue. (Choosing a topic from the Subject Index or a Self-discovery Question in this book can be a helpful option.) Clarify out loud a commitment to keep confidential any material shared in the dialoguing session.

5) Remember that the purpose of the dialogue is to deepen understanding of yourself and another, not to come into agreement. Each person is entitled to his or her own feelings, thoughts, attitudes and opinions and some time to express them.

6) Make it a point neither to respond defensively nor to engage in argument.

7) Do not look for flaws in what others say. This is not a debate. Focus on being a good listener when you listen, and when you speak, focus on expressing yourself clearly and ending with "I pass."

8) Don't criticize your dialoguing partner, defend yourself or apologize for your point of view.

9) When responding to your dialoguing partner, as much as possible, simply be silent or limit your responses to:

A) "I understand," or some other understanding statements" or

B) "I don't understand. Please say more."

10) It is important to end each dialoguing session at the agreed upon time and with appreciation for the time taken and the commitment to learn to understand one's self and one's dialogue partner better, along with a commitment to better practice happiness principles.

12) At the end of each dialoguing session, clarify when another dialoguing session will be available in the future.

AUTHORS AND SOURCES

Abrams, Jeremiah -- Aug. 29

Acharya, Sri Ananda -- May 14

Adams, Dennis D., M.A. -- May 18

Aeschylus -- Aug. 6

Afghan saying -- May 5; Nov. 21

African proverbs and sayings -- Jan. 28; March 12; May 7; May 17; July 26

Akbar, Na'im -- April 22

Alcott, Louisa May -- Feb. 15; April 21

Amen, Daniel G., M.D. -- Sept. 8, 9, 17,18 & 21; Oct. 5, 20, 21-24; Nov. 4 & 13; Dec. 24 & 27, Appendix 2

Anderson, Margaret -- Oct. 12

Andrews, Lewis, Ph.D. -- Feb. 8

Angelou, Maya -- Dec. 7

Anthony, Susan B. -- Nov. 9

Aristotle -- January 18,

Asante, Molefi -- May 4

Ash, Mary Kay -- Sept. 2

Astor, Brooke -- June 10

Atlantic Monthly Magazine -- Sept. 16

Avery, Bylle -- March 1

Bacon, W.T. -- June 30

Baez, Joan -- Dec. 23

Bailey, Pearl -- Dec. 12 & 30

Bakole wa Ilunga -- Feb. 14

Baldwin, James -- May 11

Balzac -- Nov. 20

Bateson, Gregory -- March 13

Beattie, Melody -- Nov. 3

Beal, Louse -- Oct. 31

Beecher, Henry Ward -- June 25; Nov. 29

Bibee, Bruce – March 11; April 26; May 30

Bible, The -- Jan. 8 & 15; Feb. 26; March 2; April 13; May 10; June 23 & 28; Sept. 30; Oct. 14

Bierce, Ambrose -- Oct. 27

Blake, William -- Aug. 23 & 31

Bob, Dr. -- Nov. 14

Boorstein, Sylvia, Ph.D. -- July 17; Aug. 17; Sept. 5 & 12

Booth, Father Leo -- Aug. 29

Bovee, Christian -- Oct. 3

Boyle, Thomas, M.D. -- Aug. 14

Brand, Dorothea -- Dec. 22

Branden, Nathaniel -- July 6
Bridges, Madeline -- Dec. 16
Briggs, John -- March 21
Briggs, John and Peat, David -- July 2
Buchman, Frank -- June 2
Buddha -- Jan. 13; March 14; April 14 & 28; May 10; Aug. 27; Sept. 12; Oct. 1
Buddhist teachings & references -- Jan. 13, March 1 & 14; May 10, June 5, 8, 23 & 28; July 22; Aug. 23, 27-28, 31; Sept. 5 & 12; Nov. 16; Dec. 8, 9 & 25
Bulgarian saying -- May 9
Burnett, Carol -- Dec. 12
Bush, Barbara -- July 30
Byron, George G.N. -- Oct. 26
Caddy, Eileen -- June 29
Campbell, Bebe Moore -- Aug. 7
Campbell, Susan, Ph.D. -- Oct. 12-17
Camus, Albert -- February 18, Aug. 2
Capra, Fritjof -- June 10-11
Carnes, Patrick, Ph.D. -- July 9
Carson, David -- July 27; Aug. 22; Nov. 27
Cary, Phoebe -- Oct. 16
Casarjian, Robin -- Sept. 27- 30; Aug. 9 & 24
Cash, Rosanne -- Nov. 10
Character Strengths and Virtues, A Handbook and Classification -- March 30
Chief Luther Standing Bear -- Aug. 16
Child, Lydia M. -- July 31
Chinese proverbs -- Jan. 26; March 20, 25 & 30; April 30; May 26, Nov. 8
Chittister, John -- June 24
Christian teachings & references-- Feb. 26; March 14 & 22; April 13; May 10; June 23 & 28; Aug. 23, 27, 28 & 31; Sept. 30; Oct. 14; Nov. 16; Dec. 8, 9, & 25
Cicero -- March 28; April 17; Aug. 25
Clark, Glenn -- May 15
Collins, Frederick L. -- May 30
Cohen, Sheldon -- Feb. 20
Confucius -- Jan. 21; March 27; April 28; May 19; July 3; Oct. 19
Course in Miracles -- Feb. 20; May 10
Cousins, Norman -- March 4
Covey, Stephen, Ph.D. -- April 4, July 12
Cowper, William -- Feb. 5
Creole saying -- June 27
Csikszentmihalyi, Mihaly -- Nov. 26
Curie, Marie -- Nov. 23
Dag Hammarskjold -- June 20
Dalai Lama, The -- March 1
Danish saying -- Jan. 10; March 12; June 23; July 28

419

King, Martin Luther, Jr. -- March 31
Kipling, Rudyard -- Feb. 20
Kohlberg, Lawrence, Ph.D. -- Sept. 10 & 12-13
Korean proverb -- Nov. 20
Krishnamurti, Jiddu -- Jan. 25; July 13
Kronenberger, Louis -- March 5
Kubler-Ross, Elizabeth, M.D. -- July 4; Sept. 13; Dec. 31
Lamm, Maurice -- Feb. 17
Landor, Letitia Elizabeth -- July 14
La Rochefoucauld, Francois -- May 27; July 23
Larson, Noel, Ph.D. -- May 28
Laotian saying -- April 7
Lao-tze -- Feb. 12 & 28; Aug. 10; Dec. 30
Lebanese saying -- Jan. 7; March 10; June 21
Le Guin, Ursula K. -- June 17
Lessing, Doris -- Aug. 20
Levine, Michael -- Sept. 14; Oct. 9
Lewis, C.S. -- December 7
Lewis, Hunter -- Sept. 20
Lindbergh, Anne Morrow -- Dec. 15
Lincoln, Abraham -- Feb. 4 & 19; April 12
Lippman, Walter -- April 28
Liszka, James Jakob, Ph.D. -- April 29; May 23; Aug. 5
Levine, Michael -- Sept. 14
Long, Vonda Olson, Ph.D. -- May 28
Longfellow, Henry Wadsworth -- July 29
Lord, Nogah -- Sept. 6
Lovett, Sidney -- April 23
Luce, Clare Boothe -- Dec. 13
Luecke, David L. -- July 19
Lyubomirsky, Sonja, (with C. Tkach & K.M. Sheldon) -- March 1
McKibben, Bill -- Sept. 16
Mahabharata, The -- April 28; Oct. 23
Mahaiyaddeen, Bawa -- Jan. 14
Malcolm X -- Jan. 23
Mandela, Nelson -- May 10
Mansfield, Katherine -- Aug. 1
Maori saying -- Feb. 27
Maslow, Abraham, Ph.D. -- Sept. 11-12
Ma-tzu-lau -- Feb. 11
May, Rollo -- Sept. 7
Mayfield, Curtis -- April 8
Mead, Margaret -- Nov. 5
Meichenbaum, Donald, Ph.D. -- Nov. 24 & 25

Yakima Indian Nation Museum publication -- <u>March 19</u>
Yogananda, Paramahansa -- <u>April 4</u>

SUBJECT INDEX

Made in United States
North Haven, CT
20 February 2022

16297022R00239